Gait Disorders

Evaluation and Management

Gait Disorders

Evaluation and Management

edited by

Jeffrey M. Hausdorff, MSME, PhD

Tel Aviv Sourasky Medical Center
Sackler School of Medicine, Tel Aviv University
Tel Aviv, Israel
Harvard Medical School
Boston, Massachusetts, U.S.A.

Neil B. Alexander, MD

University of Michigan
Ann Arbor VA Health Care System GRECC
Ann Arbor, Michigan, U.S.A.

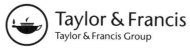

Taylor & Francis
Taylor & Francis Group

Boca Raton London New York Singapore

Published in 2005 by
Taylor & Francis Group
6000 Broken Sound Parkway NW, Suite 300
Boca Raton, FL 33487-2742

International Standard Book Number-10: 0-8247-2393-7 (Hardcover)
International Standard Book Number-13: 978-0-8247-2393-4 (Hardcover)

Library of Congress Cataloging-in-Publication Data

Catalog record is available from the Library of Congress

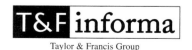

Taylor & Francis Group
is the Academic Division of T&F Informa plc.

**Visit the Taylor & Francis Web site at
http://www.taylorandfrancis.com**

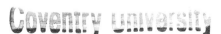

Preface

The ability to walk safely, easily, and in an aesthetically pleasing manner is a skill learned early and highly prized. Although it is typically taken for granted, gait is key to mobility and functional independence and at the core of our ability to carry out many activities of daily living. In older adults and patients with neurological deficits, ease and safety in walking may become compromised, and gait is often viewed as abnormal, i.e., as a disorder. While not an inevitable part of aging, gait disorders are common among older adults and in patients with neurological disease. By some estimates, as much as 20% of non-institutionalized older adults admit to walking difficulties or require the assistance of another person or special equipment to walk. Left untreated, gait disorders may contribute to reduced physical activity, impaired mental health, falls, fear of falling, frailty, nursing home admission, and loss of independence.

Fortunately, when a gait disorder appears, a diagnostic and management strategy can be developed that may limit the extent of the disorder and its functional impact. When properly managed, the risk of falling, for example, can often be reduced. A major goal of this book is to provide clinicians, therapists and others treating gait disorders with an understanding of the mechanisms underlying gait disorders and how to best manage these disorders. To a large extent, the content in this book is self-contained and assumes minimal pre-requisite understanding of motor control and gait. As such, it should also prove helpful to patients and their caregivers who want to better understand and manage their own gait disorders as well as to students and investigators in a variety of disciplines who would like to learn more about this field.

The book is divided into three major sections. Section I serves as the foundation. Here, experts in the field summarize the motor control, physiology and biomechanics of walking; review the current understanding of how and why gait and balance often change with aging and neurological disease; and describe gait disorders that are common in older adults and in patients with neurological disease. Section II examines clinical tools available for the evaluation of gait disorders and falls and provides a detailed, practical plan for the evaluation and assessment of gait disorders and fall risk. In Section III, experts describe the current state-of-the-art of management of gait disorders in general and offer a guide to the management of certain specific problems that commonly affect gait in older adults, in patients with foot and ankle disorders, hip fracture and replacement, and neurological disease.

Describing a wide range of assessment tools, diagnostic evaluation strategies, and clinical approaches to gait, this reference:

- introduces as new classification scheme to encompass the full range of mobility capacity in all older adults
- reviews the physiology and biomechanics of gait and common gait disorders
- covers cognitive and behavioral influences on gait and falling
- details clinical and evidence-based methods for gait disorder and fall analysis, as well as techniques for gait optimization in patients with neurological disorders, foot and ankle disorders, and post-hip surgery,
- presents a state-of-the-art strategy for multidimensional fall risk assessment and fall reduction
- features a detailed review of exercise strategies including Tai Chi to improve balance and gait

People of all ages may have gait disorders. While there is much overlap in the evaluation and management of gait disorders in the young and the old, there are also unique differences. In many young adults, a single cause of a gait disturbance can often be pinpointed. Older adults often have multiple deficits that may contribute to or exacerbate the gait disorder. Many older adults often have multiple conditions that affect their gait, further complicating evaluation and management. In this book, we place a special focus on the gait disorders of older adults and in patients with common neurological diseases, but note of course, that much of the presentation may be applicable to other populations as well.

Gait is influenced by many factors and can be studied from multiple perspectives. One key to successful evaluation and management of gait disorders is appreciation of this diversity and the interaction among a variety of apparently disparate factors. Neurologists, geriatricians, neuropsychologists, biomechanists, physiatrists, neuroscientists, and physical therapists are actively involved in the study and treatment of gait disorders among older adults. Reflecting this wide spectrum, we note that experts from numerous and varied disciplines have contributed to this book. We hope that this product will produce a synergistic effect and prove useful to students, clinicians, patients and investigators, who may be interested in improving their understanding and treatment of a multi-factorial problem common to many older adults and patients with neurological disease.

Jeffrey M. Hausdorff
Neil B. Alexander

Acknowledgments

Dr. Hausdorff acknowledges the support of the National Institute on Aging (NIA) Grant AG08812 (Harvard Medical School Claude D. Pepper Older Americans Independence Center) and Grant AG14100, the National Center for Research Resources Grant RR13622, the National Institute of Child Health and Human Development Grant HD39838 as well as support from the US-Israel Bi-National Foundation.

Dr. Alexander acknowledges the support of the National Institute on Aging (NIA) Grant AG08808 (University of Michigan Claude D. Pepper Older Americans Independence Center) as well as the Office of Research and Development, Medical Service and Rehabilitation Research and Development Service of the Department of Veterans Affairs. Dr. Alexander is a recipient of a K24 Mid-Career Investigator Award in Patient-Oriented Research AG109675 from NIA.

Contents

Contributors

Neil B. Alexander Mobility Research Center, Division of Geriatric Medicine, Department of Internal Medicine, Institute of Gerontology, University of Michigan and Ann Arbor VA Health Care System, Geriatric Research Education and Clinical Center, Ann Arbor, Michigan, U.S.A.

James A. Ashton-Miller Biomechanics Research Laboratory, Department of Mechanical Engineering, University of Michigan, Ann Arbor, Michigan, U.S.A.

Richard Baker School of Physiotherapy, La Trobe University and Hugh Williamson Gait Laboratory, Royal Children's Hospital, Victoria, Australia

Yacov Balash Movement Disorders Unit, Department of Neurology, Tel Aviv Sourasky Medical Center and Sackler School of Medicine, Tel Aviv University, Tel Aviv, Israel

Belinda Bilney BPT, School of Physiotherapy, La Trobe University, Victoria, Australia

Bastiaan R. Bloem Department of Neurology, Radboud University Nijmegen Medical Center, Nijmegen, The Netherlands

Frank-Erik De Leeuw Department of Neurology, Radboud University Nijmegen Medical Center, Nijmegen, The Netherlands

Sonia Denisenko BPT, School of Physiotherapy, La Trobe University, Victoria, Australia

Fiona Dobson   School of Physiotherapy, La Trobe University and Hugh Williamson Gait Laboratory, Royal Children's Hospital, Victoria, Australia

Karen Dodd   BPT, School of Physiotherapy, La Trobe University, Victoria, Australia

Joyce Fung   School of Physical and Occupational Therapy, McGill University, Montreal, Jewish Rehabilitation Hospital Research Centre, Laval, Quebec, Canada

Nir Giladi   Movement Disorders Unit, Department of Neurology, Tel Aviv Sourasky Medical Center and Sackler School of Medicine, Tel Aviv University, Tel Aviv, Israel

Bruno Giordani   Neuropsychology Section, Department of Psychiatry, University of Michigan, Ann Arbor, Michigan, U.S.A.

Allon Goldberg   Ann Arbor VA Health Care System, Geriatric Research Education and Clinical Center, Ann Arbor, Michigan, U.S.A.

Mark D. Grabiner   Department of Movement Sciences, University of Illinois at Chicago, Chicago, Illinois, U.S.A.

Jeffrey M. Hausdorff   Movement Disorders Unit, Tel Aviv Sourasky Medical Center, Sackler School of Medicine, Tel Aviv University, Tel Aviv, Israel and Division on Aging, Harvard Medical School, Boston, Massachusetts, U.S.A.

Jennifer Healey   Cambridge Research Laboratory, Hewlett–Packard, Cambridge, Massachusetts, U.S.A.

Jeremy A. Idjadi   NYU—The Hospital for Joint Diseases Orthopedic Institute, New York, New York, U.S.A.

Karen R. Josephson   Geriatric Research Education and Clinical Center (GRECC), VA Greater Los Angeles Healthcare System, Sepulveda, California, U.S.A.

D. Casey Kerrigan   Department of Physical Medicine and Rehabilitation, School of Medicine, University of Virginia, Charlottesville, Virginia, U.S.A.

Kenneth Koval   Dartmouth-Hitchcock Medical Center, Orthopedic Surgery, Lebanon, New Hampshire, U.S.A.

Anouk Lamontagne   School of Physical and Occupational Therapy, McGill University, Montreal, Jewish Rehabilitation Hospital Research Centre, Laval, Quebec, Canada

Stephen R. Lord   Prince of Wales Medical Research Institute, Randwick, North South Wales, Sydney, Australia

Jane Mahoney   Section of Geriatrics and Gerontology, University of Wisconsin Medical School, Elder Care of Dane County, Madison, Wisconsin, U.S.A.

Jennifer McGinley   School of Physiotherapy, La Trobe University and Hugh Williamson Gait Laboratory, Royal Children's Hospital, Victoria, Australia

Hylton B. Menz   Musculoskeletal Research Centre, School of Physiotherapy, La Trobe University, Bundoora, Victoria, Australia

Tanya A. Miszko   Department of Physical Education and Sports Studies, The University of Georgia, Prescriptive Health, Inc., Snellville, Georgia, and Veterans Affairs Medical Center, Decatur, Georgia, U.S.A.

Meg Morris   BPT, School of Physiotherapy, La Trobe University, Victoria, Australia

Elif K. Orhan   Department of Neurology, Medical School, University of Istanbul, Istanbul, Turkey

Carol C. Persad   Neuropsychology Section, Department of Psychiatry, University of Michigan, Ann Arbor, Michigan, U.S.A.

Robert J. Przybelski   Section of Geriatrics and Gerontology, University of Wisconsin Medical School, Falls Prevention Clinic, Madison, Wisconsin, U.S.A.

Karen L. Reed-Troy   Department of Movement Sciences, University of Illinois at Chicago, Chicago, Illinois, U.S.A.

James K. Richardson   Department of Physical Medicine and Rehabilitation, University of Michigan, Ann Arbor, Michigan, U.S.A.

Patrick O. Riley   Department of Physical Medicine and Rehabilitation, School of Medicine, University of Virginia, Charlottesville, Virginia, U.S.A.

Laurence Z. Rubenstein UCLA School of Medicine, Geriatric Research Education and Clinical Center (GRECC), VA Greater Los Angeles Healthcare System, Sepulveda, California, U.S.A.

Stephanie Studenski Schools of Medicine, Nursing and Allied Health, University of Pittsburgh, and Staff Physician, GRECC, VA, Pittsburgh Healthcare System, Pittsburgh, Pennsylvania, U.S.A.

Sharon L. Tennstedt New England Research Institutes, Watertown, Massachusetts, U.S.A.

Steven L. Wolf Departments of Rehabilitation Medicine, Medicine (Division of Geriatrics), and Cell Biology, Emory University School of Medicine, and Nell Hodgson Woodruff School of Nursing, Emory University, Atlanta, Georgia, U.S.A.

Joseph D. Zuckerman NYU—The Hospital for Joint Diseases Orthopedic Institute, New York, New York, U.S.A.

1

Gait, Mobility, and Function: A Review and Proposed Classification Scheme

Stephanie Studenski

Schools of Medicine, Nursing and Allied Health, University of Pittsburgh, and Staff Physician, GRECC, VA, Pittsburgh Healthcare System, Pittsburgh, Pennsylvania, U.S.A.

I. INTRODUCTION

Mobility limitations are so endemic among older adults that they are used as a common lay idiom for aging itself. The image of a hobbling man with a cane to represent aging speaks to this universal phenomenon. Mobility limitations are a major contributor to loss of independent functioning. The causes of mobility limitations involve the complex interactions of multiple systems. Since so many biopsychosocial processes influence mobility, dysmobility (defined here as abnormal mobility that interferes with function) can be considered a final common pathway. Dysmobility may represent one important way to summarize the integrated effects of aging and multiple comorbidities on health and functioning. Treatment strategies for mobility disorders are diverse (for more details see Chapters 13–19) and only partially based on evidence. New opportunities for prevention and treatment are evolving rapidly. A more organized approach to the underlying causative mechanisms and consequences of dysmobility is needed to integrate what we are learning and apply it to clinical care.

In this chapter, we briefly review the epidemiology and significance of dysmobility. We then describe current assessment tools, diagnostic evaluation

strategies, and approaches to intervention. We propose a broad simple classification schema that encompasses the full range of mobility capacity in older adults.

II. EPIDEMIOLOGY

A. Prevalence and Incidence

Mobility limitations are usually reported at either basic or higher levels of
mobility. Basic mobility problems include getting around inside the home
and transfers from bed or chair. Higher-level mobility problems include
getting around outside the home, ability to walk one-quarter to one-half
mile and ability to climb stairs. Basic mobility problems are rare among
community dwelling persons over age 65. According to the Supplement
on Aging of the National Health Interview Survey, in 1994, 2.0% of persons
over age 70 need help from another person to get in and out of a chair or
bed and 5.0% need help in walking inside the home (1). In contrast, among
institutionalized Americans over age 65 (data from the National Nursing
Home Survey, 1999), 80.4% need help getting around (2). Mobility disability
increases with age in the community; dependence in walking increases from
7.4% of persons aged 70 to 74 to 15.93% of persons aged 85+ years (1).
Women tend to have higher rates of mobility disability than men and non-
whites than whites (1). Higher-level mobility problems are more common
than basic mobility problems among older adults. About 7.5% of community-living Americans aged over 70 years have difficulty going outside the
home alone (1). Difficulty walking modest distances increases with age;
30.4% of people aged 65 to 74 vs. 67.3% of people over age 85 report difficulty walking one-quarter mile (3). The annual incidence of new higher-level
mobility disability increases with age and remains higher in women than in
men (at age 70, 11% for women and 7% for men; at age 85, 33% for women
and 25% for men) (4,5). Education influences mobility disability; older persons with low educational levels have both increased prevalence and incidence compared to persons with higher levels of education (6). The
prevalence of mobility disability appears to be decreasing; in 1997, 41.5%
of those aged 65 and older reported difficulty walking one-quarter mile,
compared to 39.3% in 2002 (3).

B. Natural History

Mobility status predicts future disability. Poor mobility performance as
measured by the Short Physical Performance Battery is an independent
predictor of nursing home placement and new basic or mobility disability
(7). Poor mobility as measured by timed chair stands is one of four factors
proposed to be common risk factors for geriatric syndromes including
incontinence, falls and functional decline (8). Conversely, good mobility,
along with good cognition and nutritional status, is an independent predictor of recovery of independence after a period of disability (9).

Mobility status predicts more than disability. Older people who report difficulty walking 2 km (a little over a mile) or climbing one flight of stairs are twice as likely to die over the next 8 years compared to those with no difficulty, even after controlling for age, chronic conditions, smoking, marital status, and education (10). Poor mobility performance predicts hospitalization independent of baseline health status, with increased risk primarily associated with hospitalization for geriatric conditions, such as dementia, pressure ulcer, hip fractures, other fracture, pneumonia, and dehydration (11). In addition to discriminating differences in risk between persons in a population based on status at one time, change in mobility over time is also a predictor of future events. In a sample of 439 community dwelling older adults, persons who declined in gait speed over 1 year were over twice as likely to die in the ensuing 5 years, even after accounting for baseline gait speed, age, gender, comorbidity, utilization, functional status and change in function (12). Mobility may be one of a constellation of domains that link multiple outcomes associated with aging and has been proposed as a core indicator of frailty (8,13).

The impact of physical mobility limitations on mobility disability may be modified by other important factors, including cognition, upper extremity limitations, vision and hearing loss, affect, self-efficacy, social support, and the environment (14–18). It is possible for older adults to be mobility disabled without physical mobility limitations, especially in the face of cognitive deficits. For example, a person with dementia may be able to walk but be unable to navigate in order to find the bathroom inside the home or the neighbor's house outside the home. Conversely, persons with physical mobility limitations who do not have limitations in other areas may be better able to cope and solve problems to reduce the impact of physical mobility limitations on function, compared to those who lack these resources for compensation. Thus, an older adult with intact cognition and good coping skills may be able to live independently despite severe mobility limitations.

III. THE LANGUAGE OF MOBILITY ASSESSMENT

Mobility is the ability to move one's body through space. While walking may be considered the most common manifestation of mobility, mobility capacity can be considered to range from rolling over in bed to running a marathon or walking a tightrope. In this sense, much of mobility capacity is hierarchical or ordered. Some tasks are easier than others. Ability to do harder tasks generally implies ability to do easier ones, and inability to perform easier tasks predicts inability with more difficult ones.

The language of mobility often focuses on capacity to perform common activities. Mobility can also be described quantitatively by timing or counting elements of common tasks or by performing more complex assessments of body part motions. While detailed assessments of aspects of mobility can be used to gain insights into mechanisms, more general assessments are useful for classification and for assessing clinical impact. Clinical impact can be defined generically in terms of overall health and function, or can be disease-specific. Indicators of mobility capacity can be obtained from self-report, professional assessment or observed performance. Each source of information has strengths and weaknesses, almost none assesses the full range of mobility capacity.

A. Self-Report

Self-report measures of mobility are common and often include items related to transfers, walking ability and stair climbing. They may focus on specific limitations or on more general mobility functions. Self-report measures are valuable because they represent the perspective of the person with the most at stake and can sometimes summarize effects that vary over a period of time. Self-report measures are limited in that responses depend on wording; for example, whether the inquiry is about inability versus difficulty. Difficulty, frequency of performance, or altered strategy (for example, going up stairs one step at a time instead of step over step) may be much more sensitive to change but require longer and more detailed surveys to assess. When multiple items about mobility are combined in a scale that is based on degree of difficulty for each item, it can be difficult to interpret a summary score. Is mild difficulty on two items worth the same as much difficulty on one item? Self-report measures must also resolve conflicts about potential capacity versus recent experience with performance (19). A person who hasn't walked a mile in years may have no idea if they actually could do it, or if it would be difficult. Mobility self-report is probably most reliable when targeted toward activities that are attempted by the respondent reasonably frequently. Self-report also depends on the insight and accuracy of the respondent, sometimes a problem in the presence of cognitive or affective disorders. Because mobility is often considered a central part of functional status, self-report mobility items are rarely isolated into separate items or mobility-specific scales and more commonly form parts of more global approaches to functional disability, as in commonly used scales such as the Katz Activities of Daily Living, Lawton–Brody Instrumental Activities of Daily Living, Nagi items, or the Short Form-36 Physical Function (20–23). All of these scales use mobility status as an inherent powerful indicator of function but are not mobility-specific. Self-report of mobility items are also important indicators in disease specific scales for many conditions including arthritis (24), angina (25), and stroke (26). Self-report also depends on the reference time frame. Many commonly used self-report forms of mobility assessment assume stability over short periods of time or else require the ability to integrate function over time, whereas short-term variability within chronic states and wide swings with acute illness are common. "Time in state" or queries about frequency address this issue. Since physical activity is based largely on mobility, information about number of days spent in bed, number of restricted activity days, or frequency of physical activities offer another perspective on mobility (27). Other perspectives best obtained from self-reports of mobility include confidence in mobility (28) and extent of mobility in terms of life space (how far one can get independently— bedroom, home, neighborhood, community, large distances) (29). A major advantage of self-report items is that they do not require the physical presence of the older adult; information may be collected by self-completed question- naires or by telephone. The information might be reported by the older adult or a significant other, although there are likely to be some differences between self- and proxy reports.

B. Professional Rating

Professional assessment of mobility capacity is widely used in rehabilitation for clinical and reimbursement purposes as a major, but not exclusive, component of disability assessment. These assessments tend to focus on limitations in tasks like transfers, walking, and stair climbing rather than disabilities like carrying groceries or bathing, which are heavily mobility dependent. Common measures such as the Functional Independence Mea- sure, require trained assessors to assign one of seven levels of performance to activities such as transfers, walking, and stair climbing, based on need for assistance (30). The simpler Barthel score includes common mobility tasks based on need for help from another (31). Professional assessment of mobility is an important element of disease-specific scales for conditions such as stroke (32) and Parkinson's disease (33). These types of measures can provide an integrated professional assessment and have strong psychometric properties. Many of them are focused on major clinical limitations, are limited to simpler mobility tasks and are insensitive to difficulties at higher levels of mobility. They are more costly because they require professional training and time. They also require the physical presence of the older adult and the professional rater.

C. Performance Measures

Performance measures of mobility can be simple timed or counted scales of a single task such as gait speed, 6 minute walk time, or one foot standing, or can combine tasks as in the short physical performance battery or the "get up and go" test (7,34–37) (see also Chapter 2). Performance measures are increasingly used in specific disease assessments. The 6 minute walk has become incorporated into assessments in CHF and COPD (38). More com- plex performance tests of mobility and balance such as the gait abnormality rating scale (GARS) or the Berg balance scale cover more details of body part motion or specific postural control-related tasks (39,40). They require more judgment than the timed and counted tasks and may be useful for finer discrimination, diagnosis, or outcome assessment. Performance measures can be brief and simple to perform and have strong psychometric properties. They tend to represent performance at one moment in time, and thus are vulnerable to error when there is high day-to-day variability. In some performance measures, small differences in technique can have large effects on results. For example, gait speed measured over a short distance (3 or 4 m) will have radically different results depending on whether the protocol calls for a standing start or a steady walking speed. The difference between the two gait speed measures gets worse at faster walking speeds (see Table 1 for an illustration of this effect). Simple timed and counted measures may require less professional expertise and time, and thus can be less costly to collect. They do still require the presence of the older adult and the rater.

D. Capturing the Range of Mobility

Virtually no single measure captures the range of mobility from rolling over in bed to highly trained activities such as running. In long-term care, many people are not ambulatory. The ability to transfer independently and move around in bed discriminates groups with different care needs. In this setting, it is therefore important to discriminate levels of mobility capacity within a nonambulatory population. Mobility-independent older adults may have similar levels of daily function but are also not a homogeneous group. Non-disabled older persons may be classified as "usual" and "successful" based on fitness and ability to perform challenging tasks and their prognosis for survival and risk of disability is different (41). Among typical ambulatory elders, mobility characteristics such as speed, amount of difficulty, and ability to perform mildly challenging activities are powerful indicators of higher levels of function and future events. Since it is important to both (1) place mobility in context within the full range of performance and (2) to examine mobility in finer detail, a two-level assessment may make the most sense, with a simple classification within the full range followed by a more detailed assessment based on goals and needs. For the initial classification, consider the seven-level descriptive scale described in Table 2. These levels are derived from the author's clinical experience and are linked to the metabolic demands of movement described in Table 2. All older adults should be classifiable on such a scale. More detailed assessments could follow and be linked to the initial level. For lower levels of mobility, detailed assessments of the degree of assistance with bed mobility and transfers may be important for care planning, prevention of complications of immobility or fall risk. For persons at higher levels, performance of difficult balance tasks like one foot standing or tandem walking would be appropriate. Such a classification scale could potentially be linked to activity capacity as measured by METs, physical

Table 1 Walking Indicators, Energy Capacity, and Function: An Example of How Mobility Is Related to Function

Functional status	Mph	m/sec: 4 m walk		6 min walk distance		400 m walk time	METs	Typical history of fatigue with activity
		Stand	Roll	Meter	Feet			
Overt disability	1.0	0.41	0.46	165	541	14 min 24 sec	<2	Self care, walking very short distances
Subclinical disability	1.5	0.57	0.69	248	813	9 min 36 sec	<2	
	2.0	0.75	0.93	335	1,098	7 min 12 sec	2.5	Household activities, walking one-quarter mile
Usual healthy elders	2.5	0.88	1.15	414	1,358	5 min 45 sec	3.0	Carrying groceries or light yard work
	3.0	1.0	1.38	497	1,630	4 min 48 sec	3.5	Moderate housework, several flights of stairs
	3.5	1.1	1.60	576	1,889	4 min 7 sec	4.0	Carrying loads up stairs or up hills, heavy household or yard work
Fit elders	4.0	1.25	1.84	662	2,171	3 min 36 sec	>4	Heavy work or sports

Walking speed calculations performed by the author. The relationship between standing and rolling start was calculated based on the author's prior work. The relationship between 4 m walk speed and miles per hour, 6 minutes walk and 400 m walk time are standard conversions of velocity, distance and time calculated by the author. The relationship between MPH, METs and activity is derived from Appendix A: American College of Sports Medicine ACSM Resource Manual. 3rd ed. Baltimore: Williams and Wilkins, 1998: 657–665.

Abbreviations: MPH, walking speed in miles per hour; m/sec, walking speed as velocity in meters per second; stand, timing from a standing start; roll, timing begins after walking has started; METs, metabolic equivalents.

Source: From Studenski S. Exercise. In: Landefeld, ed. Clinical Geriatrics. Lange, 2004.

Table 2 Example of a Seven-Level Classification of Mobility

Level 1	Able to perform sustained physical activity for at least 30 min at a vigorous pace like running, jogging, tennis. Greater than 4 METs, sustained activity
Level 2	Able to perform sustained physical activity for at least 60 min at a usual pace like walking one or more miles. 3.5–4 METs, sustained activity
Level 3	Able to perform physical activity at a usual pace for at least 15 min like walking one-half mile. 2.5–3.5 METs, limited duration of activity
Level 4	Physical activity limited. Able to walk one block. May have slowed gait speed. May use an assistive device like a cane to walk. 2.0–2.5 METs
Level 5	Physical activity limited. May have difficulty walking one block but able to walk across a room. May use assistive device like a cane or walker. <2 METs
Level 6	Mobility severely limited. Requires wheelchair for indoor mobility. Transfers independently. 1.5 METs
Level 7	Mobility profoundly limited, requires assistance with transfers from chair or bed. 1 MET

Levels are initial estimates based on relationships to energy demand, ability to sustain activity and functional limitations. This preliminary classification schema is derived by the author and is currently undergoing further field testing.

performance, and mobility-dependent activities (Table 1). Existing scales might be characterized in terms of where they distribute along the full range of mobility capacity (Table 3). Scale scores might then be interpreted based on likely placement within the overall mobility range. Modern scaling techniques based on ordered categories such as Rasch analysis, item response theory, and item banks could be used to carry out a two-step mobility assessment. The first step would be a "range finding" assessment, in order to initially place the individual on a part of the full range scale (Fig. 1). A person could be classified initially as ambulatory or nonambulatory. If ambulatory, further classification could be based on a short walking test as "fit" or "not fit" based on some threshold such as walking speed or SPPB score at a ceiling level. For persons who are at ceiling on the short test (the "fit"), testing for discrimination at a higher level would assess "mobility reserve" with more difficult balance or endurance tests. The nonambulatory could have detailed testing of bed mobility and transfers. A two-step classification and assessment strategy would allow for better discrimination without increasing the burden of testing, since testing would be targeted. This paradigm requires further validation. It might be further refined for use in various settings as a way to target rehabilitation interventions or types of injury prevention. Change in classification level over time might be an indicator of decline or improvement.

Table 3 A Theoretical Plot of Mobility Measures Against the Range of Mobility Capacity Using the Seven Level Classification Scheme

1	2	3	4	5	6	7
Vigorous	Active/fit	Usual Aging	Subclinical mobility disability	Overt mobility disability	Not ambulatory Able to transfer	Not ambulatory, Unable to transfer
	Gait speed, SPPB, get up and go test, 6 minute walk					
	FIM, Barthel					
tandem walking and 1 foot standing?						
	Berg Balance Scale					
	SF-36 Physical Function					
METs >4	METs 3.5–4	METS 2.5–3.5	METs 2–2.5	METs 1.5–2	METS <2	
			Difficulty with IADL	Difficulty with PADL		

E. Interpreting Measures of Mobility

There is no common language for mobility in health care practice or research. While health professionals who are involved in rehabilitation tend to be familiar with measures of mobility, very few other health professionals and almost no consumers or health system decision makers have any exposure to these measures. Since mobility is so central to the health and function of older adults, we need to promote some structured forms of mobility measurement for common use in practice, research, and health care systems. We should all be able to describe the mobility of our populations using a common set of terms. While many options are available, brief measures like the seven-level classification schema proposed here and brief

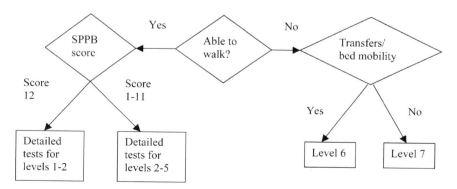

Figure 1 Two-level screen for mobility level.

tests like the short physical performance battery or gait speed might be useful as initial indicators. Such simple terms and classifications might help make dysmobility a recognizable condition for use by patients, families, primary care providers, health care systems, and insurers.

This lack of common language affects our ability to communicate our research findings as well. In current research studies on mobility and balance of older adults, the populations are diverse and hard to characterize. Study samples may be very healthy volunteers or may have varying amounts of clinical and subclinical mobility disability. Since it is hard to understand or compare the severity of dysmobility between study populations, it can be difficult to compare studies or apply research findings from mobility and balance research to practice. A classification strategy like the one proposed here would allow research studies to describe each sample population in common terms that are more universally interpretable. This kind of classification strategy would be amenable to evaluation as a clinical measurement test. It could be directly assessed for reliability, validity, feasibility, and clinical acceptance. We have implemented a field study of such an instrument and expect to have results in the next few years.

IV. AN OVERVIEW OF APPROACHES TO THE CAUSES OF MOBILITY DISABILITY

While there are many potential causes of mobility disability, the practical value of evaluation for the causes of dysmobility is not known. Like many areas in health care today, the potential for testing is much greater than the proven utility of testing. The justification for pursuing the root causes of a problem is often that the treatment or prognosis will differ based on which of several causes is detected. Disease-specific prognosis is clearly affected by severity of mobility problems for conditions like stroke and Parkinson's disease. We do not yet have a clear idea about when causation is important for treatment of dysmobility and when it is not (19). While it is valuable to develop and test models of causation for many reasons, it is important to consider when they are helpful in clinical management. As we gain new knowledge about the causes of mobility disability, we should continue to evaluate how evaluation further informs treatment and prognosis.

There are numerous research studies about the causes of mobility and balance problems. Some studies focus on older persons without clear medical diagnoses that would explain the mobility disorder. Others target a specific condition like arthritis or stroke, with or without consideration of coexisting conditions. In all such studies, the characterization of the population, the types of contributing factors examined and the types of mobility deficits assessed vary widely. Findings from such studies are often provocative and insightful but can be conflicting and often are difficult to incorporate into a common understanding. Since common understanding depends on common terms and approaches, the field would benefit from some consensus on frameworks. In general, frameworks tend to be biomechanical or pathophysiologic and to focus on physical health causes. Since psychological, cognitive, social, and environmental factors also contribute to mobility problems, they should also be incorporated into an assessment framework. Several frameworks exist (34,42,43, Alexander in this book, Chapter 8) for dissecting the causes of mobility deficits. Whatever the framework used, it is important to keep several confounding issues in mind. First, some common causes of mobility deficits, like weakness and reduced endurance, might be primary causes or might be secondary to any underlying cause that reduces activity and precipitates deconditioning. Thus, there is an intimate feedback relationship between physical activity, conditioning, and mobility. Almost anyone who has a mobility problem will become less active and have resulting deconditioning, weakness, and decreased endurance. Most anyone who has a low activity level, even without any other cause, is likely to become deconditioned, weak and have low endurance. For this reason, strength and endurance deficits are almost always found in persons with dysmobility, may or may not be causal and interventions on these deficits are almost always part of the treatment plan.

Evaluation of the causes of mobility disorders is likely to be broader than the causes of gait disorders, since gait itself can be normal in persons who have mobility limitations due to conditions such as visual loss or cardiopulmonary disease with loss of endurance.

Great strides are being made in our understanding of some causes of mobility disorders. Recent studies have focused on the influence of peripheral neuropathy and vestibular dysfunction on mobility and balance in older adults (44,45). There are major developments in our understanding of previously poorly characterized central nervous system contributors to dysmobility such as nonmemory cognitive functions like attention and motor planning, and subtle extrapyramidal abnormalities (46–48). There is an increasing awareness of potential mediating effect on dysmobility of white matter disease in the brain as a consequence of diffuse cerebrovascular disease (49,50). We are more aware of psychological, emotional, and environmental factors that affect mobility (16–18).

V. TREATMENT OF DYSMOBILITY TO IMPROVE FUNCTION OR PREVENT DISABILITY

Treatment for dysmobility includes many types of exercise, adaptive equipment, medical management, and environmental modifications. We do not yet know when treatment of dysmobility requires a differential diagnosis prior to specific interventions based on unique causes or when dysmobility could be treated directly through a generic mobility exercise program. Perhaps management of dysmobility could resemble current strategies

applied to management of hypertension. In modern hypertension management, most hypertension is treated without extensive initial diagnostic testing.
Further evaluation is limited to cases with special features or poor response to
intervention. In dysmobility, it might sometimes be appropriate to initiate
interventions like generic therapeutic exercise as a first step, and reserve thorough evaluations for those who do not respond or have special barriers to
exercise (Fig. 2).

A strategy is needed to determine the presence of a "rate limiting
barrier" to starting exercise. Such a barrier would be expected to require
separate prior management and such persons might need a more in-depth
assessment of causes and an individualized treatment plan first. Clinical
examples of scenarios requiring initial further diagnosis and management
might include poorly controlled congestive heart failure or low vision due
to macular degeneration. A strategy to help decide on treatment might be
to examine the current evidence on the causes of mobility and balance
disorders for insights into potential cause specific barriers and strategies
for evaluation and management. Future research could compare the effects
of various combinations of initial assessments, generic interventions, and
cause-specific interventions.

Since almost everyone with dysmobility has reduced physical activity
and deconditioning, interventions on strength and endurance are almost
always indicated. While the weight of the evidence convincingly supports

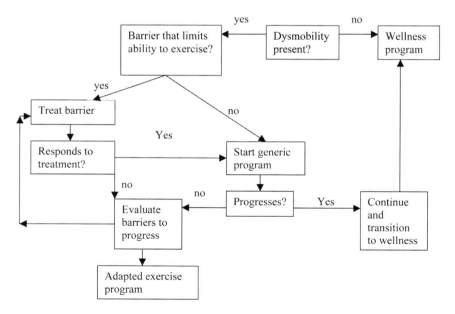

Figure 2   Decision making about exercise for mobility limitation.

benefits to strength and endurance from targeted exercise, the impact of these gains on function are more limited (51). Gains in strength or endurance might be constrained by coexisting physical impairments like pain or nonphysical factors like motivation. Gains in mobility function from gains in strength or endurance might be limited by impairments in central nervous system motor control, affect, cognition, self-efficacy, or the environment.

There are numerous unresolved issues within the field of exercise for mobility. What kind of strength training is most effective for improving mobility? Are we interested in improving ability to move a maximum load or are we interested in improving the rate of force development or perhaps the maximum total force and speed (often measured as muscle power)? What are the optimal strategies for improving balance? For global balance skills, what combinations of skills should we target among options like control of weight shifting, size of the base of support, speed of response, ability to modify response to conditions, and ability to perform dual tasks while moving? Are there deficits in components of postural control such as among sensory inputs, sensory integration or motor control that require specific adaptations to the exercise program? How much practice of complex motor responses is needed to induce automaticity and neuroplasticity?

Once gains are achieved, we know little about how to sustain them. Adherence with most programs that improve endurance, strength, balance, and mobility can be achieved with aggressive and expensive personal attention and support for participants, but rates of long-term sustained activity have been almost uniformly disappointing (52). We need to understand more about keys to long-term motivation and reward. It is this author's opinion that important factors include convenience and personal gratification. Interventions to improve and maintain mobility should be designed to be recreational and fun.

VI. SUMMARY

Mobility problems are endemic, increase with age, cause serious disability and signal risk for multiple serious negative outcomes such as institutionalization and death. Many measures of mobility have been developed for diverse purposes. There are no standards for communicating about mobility between providers, specialists and investigators. To move forward, we need simple and widely accessible common terms, classifications, and measures. There are no clear standards and no evidence base for preferring one strategy versus another for the evaluation of mobility disorders. We need to test and compare explicit evaluation strategies based on explicit conceptual frameworks of causation and consequences. Similarly, there are no clear standards or evidence for one intervention strategy versus another. We need to develop, test, and compare treatment approaches that accommodate both common manifestations and unique contributors to dysmobility. We need to better incorporate behavioral and medical interventions to overcome barriers to progress or maintain gains. There are numerous emerging opportunities to improve the mobility of older adults.

REFERENCES

1. Activities of Daily Living (ADLs) by Sex, Race, and Age. SOA, SOA II National Center for Health Statistics, Data Warehouse on Trends in Health and Aging, http://www.cdc.gov/nchs/agingact.htm (September 2004).
2. Health, United States. Chartbook on Trends in the Health of Americans from the National Nursing Home survey 1999. 2003:287. http:www.cdc.govnchsdata-hus-tables-2003–03hus097.pdf (September 2004).
3. Difficulty in Physical Functioning by Age, Sex, Race, and Hispanic Origin: United States, 1997–2002. NHIS National Center for Health Statistics, Data Warehouse on Trends in Health and Aging, http://www.cdc.gov/nchs/agingact.htm (September 2004).
4. Guralnik JM, LaCroix AZ, Abott RD, et al. Maintaining mobility in late life I: demographic characteristics and chronic conditions. Am J Epidemiol 1993; 136:845–857.
5. Leveille SG, Penninx BWJH, Melzer D, Izmirlian G, Guralnik JM. Sex difference in the prevalence of mobility disability in older age; the dynamics of incidence, recovery and mortality. J Gerontol Soc Sci 2000; 55B:S41–S50.
6. Melzer D, Izmirlian G, Leveille SG, Guralnik JM. Educational differences in the prevalence of mobility disability in old age: the dynamics of incidence, mortality, and recovery. J Gerontol B Psychol Sci Soc Sci 2001; 56(5):S294–S301.
7. Freedman VA, Martin LG. Understanding trends in functional limitations among older Americans. Am J Public Health 1998; 88(10):1457–1462.
8. Guralnik JM, Ferrucci L, Simonsick EM, Salive ME, Wallace RB. Lower-extremity function in persons over the age of 70 years as a predictor of subsequent disability. N Engl J Med 1995; 332:556–561.
9. Tinetti ME, Inouye SK, Gill TM, Doucette JT. Shared risk factors for falls, incontinence and functional dependence. JAMA 1995; 273:1348–1353.
10. Gill TM, Robison JT, Tinetti ME. Predictors of recovery in activities of daily living among disabled older persons living in the community. J Gen Intern Med 1997; 12(12):757–762.
11. Hirvensalo M, Rantanene T, Heikkinen E. Mobility difficulties and physical activity as predictors of mortality and loss of independence in the community-living older population. J Am Geriatr Soc 2000; 48:493–498.
12. Penninx BWJH, Ferrucci L, Leveille SG, Rantanen T, Pahor M, Guralnik JM. Lower extremity performance in nondisabled older persons as a predictor of subsequent hospitalization. J Gerontol Med Sci 2000; 55:M691–M697.
13. Perera S, Studenski S, Chandler JM, Guralnik JM. Magnitude and patterns of decline in health and function over one year affect subsequent survival over five years. J Gerontol. In press.
14. Fried LP, Tangen CM, Walston J, et al. Frailty in older adults: evidence for a phenotype. J Gerontol A Biol Sci Med Sci 2001; 56:M146–M156.
15. Lundin-Olsson L, Nyberg L, Gusafson Y. Attention, frailty, and falls: the effect of a manual task on basic mobility. J Am Geriatr Soc 1998; 46:758–761.

16. Maino JH. Visual deficits and mobility. Clin Ger Med 1996; 12:803–823.
17. Penninx BWJH, Guralnik JM, Bandeen-Roche K, et al. The protective effect of emotional vitality on adverse health outcomes in disabled older women. J Am Geriatr Soc 2000; 48:1359–1366.
18. Hausdorff JM, Levy BR, Wei LY. The power of ageism on physical function of older persons; reversibility of age-related gait changes. J Am Geriatr Soc 1999; 47:1346–1349.
19. Ostir GV, Markides KS, Black SA, Goodwin JS. Emotional well-being predicts subsequent functional independence and survival. J Am Geriatr Soc 2000; 48(5):473–478.
20. Studenski S. Mobility. In: Hazzard W, ed. Principles of Geriatric Medicine and Gerontology. 5th ed. New York: McGraw-Hill, 2003:947–960.
21. Ware JF, Sherbourne CD. The MOS 36-Item Short-Form Health Survey (SF-36): 1. Conceptual framework and item selection. Med Care 1992; 30:473–483.
22. Katz S, Ford AB, Moskowitz RW, et al. Studies of illness in the ages. The index of ADL: a standardized measure of biological and psychosocial function. JAMA 1963; 185:94.
23. Lawton MP, Brody E. Assessment of older people: self-maintaining and instrumental activities of daily living. Gerontologist 1969; 9:179–186.
24. Nagi SZ. An epidemiology of disability among adults in the United States. Milbank Mem Fund Q 1976; 54:439–467.
25. Meenan RF, Gertman PM, Mason JH. Measuring health status in arthritis. The arthritis impact measurement scales. Arthritis Rheum 1980; 23(2):146–152.
26. Spertus JA, Winder JA, Dewhurst TA, Deyo RA, Prodzinski J, McDonell M, Fihn SD. Development and evaluation of the Seattle Angina questionnaire: a new functional status measure for coronary artery disease. J Am Coll Cardiol 1995; 25(2):333–341.
27. Duncan PW, Wallace D, Lai SM, Johnson D, Embretson S, Laster LJ. The stroke impact scale version 2.0. Evaluation of reliability, validity, and sensitivity to change. Stroke 1999; 30(10):2131–2140.
28. Kosorok MR, Omenn GS, Diehr P, Koepsell TD, Patrick DL. Restricted activity days among older adults. Am J Publ Health. 1992; 82(9):1263–1267.
29. Lachman ME, Howland J, Tennstedt S, Jette A, Assmann S, Peterson EW. Fear of falling and activity restriction: the survey of activities and fear of falling in the elderly (SAFE). J Gerontol B Psychol Sci Soc Sci 1998; 53(1):P43–P50.
30. Baker PS, Bodner EV, Allman RM. Measuring life-space mobility in community-dwelling older adults. J Am Geriatr Soc 2003; 51(11):1610–1614.
31. Keith RA, Granger CV, Hamilton BB, Sherwin FS. The functional independence measure: a new tool for rehabilitation. Adv Clin Rehabil 1987; 1:6–18.
32. Mahoney FI, Barthel DW. Functional evaluation: the Barthel index. Md State Med J 1965; 14:61–65.
33. Kalra L, Crome P. The role of prognostic scores in targeting stroke rehabilitation in elderly patients. J Am Geriatr Soc 1993; 41(4):396–400.
34. Henderson L, Kennard C, Crawford TJ, Day S, Everitt BS, Goodrich S, Jones F, Park. Scales for rating motor impairment in Parkinson's disease: studies of reliability and convergent validity. J Neurol Neurosurg Psychiatry 1991; 54(1):18–24.

35. Studenski S, Perera S, Wallace D, Chandler J, Duncan PW, Rooney E, Fox M, Guralnik JM. Physical performance measures in the clinical setting. J Am Geriatr Soc 2003; 51:1–10.

36. Podsiadlo D, Richardson S. The timed "Up & Go": a test of basic functional mobility for frail elderly persons. J Am Geriatr Soc 1991; 39(2):142–148.

37. Guyatt GH, Sullivan MJ, Thompson PJ, Fallen EL, Pugsley SO, Taylor DW, Berman LB. The 6-minute walk: a new measure of exercise capacity in patients with chronic heart failure. Can Med Assoc J 1985; 132(8):919–923.

38. Simonsick EM, Newman AB, Nevitt MC, Kritchevsky SB, Ferucci L, Guralnik JM, et al. Measuring higher level physical function in well-functioning older adults: expanding familiar approaches in the health ABC study. J Gerontol Med Sci 2001; 56A:M644–M649.

39. Celli BR, Cote CG, Marin JM, Casanova C, Montes de Oca M, Mendez RA, Pinto Plata V, Cabral HJ. The body-mass index, airflow obstruction, dyspnea, and exercise capacity index in chronic obstructive pulmonary disease. N Engl J Med 2004; 350(10):1005–1012.

40. Berg KO, Wood-Dauphinee SL, Williams JI, Maki B. Measuring balance in the elderly: validation of an instrument. Can J Publ Health 1992; 83(suppl 2):S7–S11.

41. DiPietro L. Physical activity in aging: changes in patterns and their relationship to health and function. J Gerontol A Biol Sci Med Sci 2001; 56(Spec No 2): 13–22.

42. Wolfson L, Whipple R, Amerman P, Tobin JN. Gait assessment in the elderly: a gait abnormality rating scale and its relation to falls. J Gerontol 1990; 45(1):M12–M19.

43. Ferrucci L, Bandinelli S, Benvenuti E, di Iorio A, Macchi C, Harris T, et al. Subsystems contributing to the decline in ability to walk: bridging the gap between epidemiology and geriatric practice in the In CHIANTI study. J Am Geriatr Soc 2000; 48:1618–1625.

44. Richardson JK, Thies SB, DeMott TK, Ashton-Miller JA. Interventions improve gait regularity in patients with peripheral neuropathy while walking on an irregular surface under low light. J Am Geriatr Soc 2004; 52(4):510–515.

45. Herdman SJ. Role of vestibular adaptation in vestibular rehabilitation. Otolaryngol Head Neck Surg 1998; 119(1):49–54.

46. Hausdorff JM, Nelson ME, Kaliton D, Layne JE, Bernstein MJ, Nuernberger A, Singh MA. Etiology and modification of gait instability in older adults: a randomized controlled trial of exercise. J Appl Physiol 2001; 90(6):2117–2129.

47. Shumway-Cook A, Woollacott M. Attentional demands and postural control: the effect of sensory context. J Gerontol A Biol Sci Med Sci 2000; 55(1): M10–M16.

48. Wilson RS, Schneider JA, Beckett LA, Evans DA, Bennett DA. Progression of gait disorder and rigidity and risk of death in older persons. Neurology 2002; 58(12):1815–1819.

49. Wolfson L. Gait and balance dysfunction: a model of the interaction of age and disease. Neuroscientist 2001; 7(2):178–183.

50. Onen F, Feugeas MC, Baron G, De Marco G, Godon-Hardy S, Peretti II, Ravaud P, Legrain S, Moretti JL, Claeys ES. Leukoaraiosis and mobility

decline: a high resolution magnetic resonance imaging study in older people with mild cognitive impairment. Neurosci Lett 2004; 355(3):185–188.
51. Keysore JJ, Jette AM. Have we oversold the benefits of late-life exercise? J Gerontol 2001; 56A:M412.
52. Van der Bij AK, Laurant MGH, Wensgin M. Effectiveness of physical activity interventions for older adults. Am J Prev Med 2002; 22:120.

2

Clinical Evaluation of Gait Disorders: No-Tech and Low-Tech

Neil B. Alexander

Mobility Research Center, Division of Geriatric Medicine, Department of Internal Medicine, Institute of Gerontology, University of Michigan and Ann Arbor VA Health Care System, Geriatric Research Education and Clinical Center, Ann Arbor, Michigan, U.S.A.

Assessments and interventions to improve gait are commonly used in older adults. In a recent survey, clinical physiotherapists noted that they had no systematic standardized gait assessment tool, and that less than one-quarter utilized a gait laboratory for assessment (1). The vast majority of these therapists requested a gait assessment tool, a "low-tech" measure that could be used easily and quickly within a busy schedule without compromising reliability and validity. This chapter reviews the various "no-tech" and "low-tech" gait assessments, from self-report measures to performance-based set of multiple tasks. Outcomes are simple and at most require measures of distance and/or timing.

I. SELF-REPORT MEASURES

In self-report measures, respondents rank the presence of absence of a problem with walking or a walking-related task, with rankings ranging from no difficulty in task performance (independent), to unable to perform the task either with or without human assistance (dependent). Difficulty and disability in walking an increased distance and stair climbing are commonly

19

assessed as part of this assessment, as is the use of a cane or other assistive device. One of the few batteries with multiple measures of walking difficulty and disability is the EPESE self-report battery, assessing the ability to walk across a room with or without help (Katz ADL item) and the ability to use stairs and walk one-half mile (two Rosow–Brelau items) (2). These self-report measures of walking difficulty and disability may not only be good indicators of walking function but of overall functional mobility (3). Modifications to walking performance, such as reporting "having slowed down," may provide another means to ask about difficulty in walking (4). Certain factors, such as advanced age (> 85), three or more chronic conditions at baseline and the occurrence of stroke, hip fracture, or cancer predict a less progressive but "catastrophic" loss of walking ability (5). In community-dwelling older adults, self-reported difficulty in walking, in this case walking a quarter-mile (2–3 blocks), increases with age and poorer self-rated health, and the effect is independent of measured gait speed (6). Test–retest reliability of these self-report measures depends on the interval noted and the functional level of the sample tested. For example, kappa values for two-day test–retest were good (0.69–0.75) for walking on stairs and three or more city blocks in relatively functionally able old (7), while small consistent changes occur weekly in those with already documented ADL and mobility disability (8). Note that in older adults in a primary care setting, gait speed or measures of lower extremity performance (i.e., short physical performance battery, SPPB, see below) were better than self-report functional measures in predicting outcomes such as hospitalization and functional decline (9).

II. PERFORMANCE-BASED MEASURES

High-tech assessments that involve formal kinematic and kinetic analyses (see Chapters 3 and 4) have not been applied widely in clinical assessments of older adult balance and gait disorders. Instead, a set of functional gait and balance tasks (which includes gait-related tasks such as turning while standing) has been proposed as a means to detect and quantify abnormalities and direct interventions. These tasks are either timed or scored semi-quantitatively, usually based upon whether a subject is able to perform the task and if able, how normal or abnormal the performance was. Compared to more sophisticated high tech assessments, these sets of tasks are easy to perform, require virtually no equipment or testing time, and generally are valid. These sets of tasks provide a specific functional evaluation that is relevant to walking and may give clues to deficits in specific areas that are critical to level of dependency and that are amenable to physical therapy. A major issue is whether the low-tech measures are reliable and stable, particularly in diseased populations with potentially unstable clinical status. These scales are noted to be reliable in smaller, selected published samples but perhaps less reliable in larger epidemiologic settings [e.g., see Ref. 10 for critique of timed up and go (TUG) test]. Furthermore, as with any timed test, increased performance time may indicate more impairment or disability but may be the desired adaptation to maintain safety, particularly in someone at risk for falls. As far as the patient may be concerned, completion of the task, albeit slowly, safely, and without undue exhaustion, may still be preferable to being unable to perform the task at all.

A. Gait Speed

Gait speed has become a powerful assessment and outcome measure. Gait speed measured as part of a timed short distance (e.g., 8 ft) walk or as measured in terms of distance walked over time (such as 6 min) predicts disease activity (such as in arthritis), cardiac and pulmonary function (particularly in congestive heart failure) and ultimately mobility—and ADL—disability, institutionalization and mortality. Gait speed is affected by a number of factors, including disease (such as cardiopulmonary), leg function (such as strength), and other factors such as falls and physical activity. For a full review, see Alexander et al. (11), and also Chapter 7.

1. Usual and Maximal Gait Speed

Over relatively short distances (e.g., 11 m), usual walking speed may predict subsequent functional disability for the old–old (aged 75 and over) (12). However, maximal walking speed (walking as fast as possible such as on a 30 ft walk which includes one turn) is one of the factors that can independently predict cognitive decline prospectively in healthy older adults (13). In a recent study, Studenski et al. (9), in studying the impact of gait speed on functional outcomes, excluded the extremely fit (gait speed >1.3 m/sec) and the very impaired (<0.2 m/sec) and identified values of <0.6 and >1.0 m/sec as slow and fast walking status, respectively. These latter speeds are useful in predicting hospitalization and functional decline. Of note, while test–retest comparison of gait speed between clinic and a home visit one-week later was good (intraclass coefficient, ICC = 0.84), there is a suggestion that some of the slow walkers walked more quickly in the clinic (9). Overall, gait speed test–retest reliability (ICCs) tends to be high for short periods, such as in: Parkinson's disease, for usual gait speed and stride length, 1-week test–retest ICCs >0.9 (14); knee osteoarthritis, for usual and fast walk speed, 1-week test–retest ICCs generally >0.9 (15); stroke patients measured at home one year poststroke, for usual 10-m walk speed, 1-week ICC = 0.97 (16); and mildly functionally impaired older adults, usual walk speed, 2-week test–retest ICC = 0.79 (17). In a large epidemiological sample tested two to three weeks apart, the test–retest ICC for usual gait speed is lower (0.72) (18). Comfortable gait speed over a 5-m distance, as compared to TUG (see below) or fast walk speed, is thought to be most responsive to change (i.e., to detect clinically relevant change) following one month of stroke rehabilitation (19). Differences in walking speed may relate to whether average speed is determined from gait initiation, or if the speed is determined while the subject is already at constant velocity (see Chapter 1).

   2. 6-Minute Walk Test

Self-paced 6-minute walking distance is particularly useful in patients with cardiopulmonary disease (20). For example, the six-minute walk test (SMWT) discriminates between NYHA levels of congestive heart failure, and predicts hospitalization rates and mortality attributable to congestive heart failure (21). The SMWT correlates with age and self-reported physical functioning as well as performance on a number of other balance, gait speed over short distance, and leg strength measures in mildly mobility-impaired older adults (22–24). When applied in a rehabilitation setting, the SMWT is also sensitive to changes occurring during post-total knee arthroplasty (25) and as a result of an exercise program to improve function in knee osteoarthritis (26). Reliability is excellent: one-week test–retest Pearson's $r = 0.95$ in community-dwelling older adults of varying function (22), ICC $= 0.94$ in peripheral vascular disease patients (27), and ICC $= 0.93$ in mobility-impaired patients (28). A number of studies have noted small improvements in consecutive test–retest distances, e.g., approximately 6% in patients undergoing cardiac rehabilitation (29). An important concern with the SMWT is the motivation to perform maximally, i.e., some subjects will "pace" themselves to be able to complete the test instead of trying to cover as much distance as possible. Given the relatively good relationships between SMWT and self-assessment of functional limitations (e.g., Ref. 29), this "pacing" may thus reflect what the subject feels that he/she is able to perform on a daily basis (i.e., usual behavior) rather than their capacity. While designed to be a test of exercise endurance, in some patients with heart failure, the peak oxygen uptake during SMWT may approach peak values attained by standard treadmill testing, i.e., the test may also be considered a test of peak performance (30). Peak oxygen uptake during SMWT may approach 80% of the peak oxygen uptake during treadmill testing (31), suggesting that the SMWT is a near maximal exercise even for some healthy older adults.

   3. Long-Distance Corridor Walk

The long-distance corridor walk (LCDW) allows measurement of walking speed over 20 m, the distance covered in 2 minutes and the time taken to walk 400 m. The 2 minute walk serves as a warm-up for any practice effects and the subsequent 400 m portion gives a goal of distance, rather than time, and thus helps to better maintain a higher speed instead of "settling in" to a comfortable pace (32). The LCDW has been used among relatively high functioning older adults (without apparent walking difficulty or disability) as a measure of health status and fitness, in that performance correlates with measures of clinical and subclinical disease, heart rate and blood pressure response, and physical activity (33). The LCDW can help further delineate functional performance decrement, i.e., 26% of these high functioning older adults did not complete the full test because: (i) of cardiac-related abnormalities, 13% were excluded from participation; (ii) of those eligible, 2%, could not complete the 20 minute walk, 2% did not begin the 400-m walk, and 9% could not complete the full distance, making another 13% of those eligible who could not complete the full test (33,34). This leads to an important concern regarding how to provide a meaningful score in lower functioning older adults, many of whom cannot complete the full 400-m walk. For example, the mean SMWT distance in mildly mobility-impaired community older adults in one study is 448 m (23) and 374 m in congestive heart failure patients, with over 50% of those Class II and over 75% of those Class III–IV unable to walk more than 375 m (21). In a more recent study, nearly 1/3 (32%) of participants were unable to complete the 400-m walk, and although test–retest distances were nearly identical, no reliability coefficient was reported in regards to distance (35).

B. Sets of Multiple Tasks

The gait assessments described below among the most common found in the literature. For the sake of brevity, other important assessment batteries that focus on postural control under various conditions and that have limited gait-related items, such as the Berg Balance Scale (36), are not included.

1. Dynamic Gait Index

The dynamic gait index (DGI) was developed to evaluate gait alterations in response to changing task demands, including changing gait speed, head turns, turning, clearing an obstacle, and stair climbing. Inter-rater and test–retest reliability has been reported as >0.96 (after rater training), and as with a number of scales (including the performance-oriented mobility assessment, POMA), the DGI was responsive to change with exercise (37). In community-dwelling samples, using a cut-off score of 19 or less, sensitivity and specificity were fair in predicting falls: 59% and 64%, respectively (38) and 85% and 38% in older adults with dizziness (39). Subsequent inter-rater reliability was variable in individual items (kappa 0.35–1.0), and good for total score (kappa 0.64, Spearman's $r = 0.95$) in a vestibular-impaired sample of varying age and with a possible ceiling effect in the total score (40). A shortened version of the DGI with three new items thought to be particularly challenging to vestibular patients (walking backwards, with eyes closed, or on a narrowed support) has recently been reported (41).

2.   Emory Functional Ambulation Profile

The Emory Functional Ambulation Profile (EFAP) measures the time to walk under five environmental circumstances, with and without the use of an assistive device in stroke patients: (a) 5-m walk on hard floor; (b) 5-m walk on short pile carpeted floor; (c) TUG (as below); (d) step over a brick and then around a trash can; and (e) walk up four steps, turn around, and return (using hand rail if needed) (42). A modified version (mEFAP) incorporated manual assistance (contact guard, minimal assist, and moderate assist) in stroke patients undergoing day rehabilitation (43). In these small samples, both EFAP and mEFAP inter-rater and test–retest reliability are excellent (>0.99), both correlate with other balance and functional measures, and the mEFAP is sensitive to change over time.

3.   Short Physical Performance Battery

The SPPB is a short battery of the ability to maintain stance (e.g., tandem stance), the time to walk 8 ft at usual gait speed, and the time to rise from a chair five times. The SPPB predicts self-reported disability, nursing home admission, and mortality (44,45). However, a subsequent study reported that usual gait speed alone predicted ADL and mobility-related disability almost as well as the full SPPB battery (46). In a primary clinic sample, however, while usual gait speed predicted outcomes such as hospitalization and functional decline, the full SPPB battery provided additional predictive value, particularly in a VA cohort (9). A related battery (the MOBLI index) includes 3-m walk time, time to rise from a chair five times, and peak expiratory flow rate, three factors that predicted changes in self-reported inability or difficulty in walking a medium (e.g., quarter mile) distance (47). The MOBLI battery also predicts mortality (48) and was better than gait speed alone in predicting walking difficulty (49).

4.   Functional Ambulation Classification

The functional ambulation classification (FAC) (50) uses a five-point scale to rate the extent of human assistance (stand-by, intermittent touch, and continuous support) required to walk varying surfaces (level, nonlevel, stairs, and inclines) while using an assistive device if necessary (50,51) in patients with neurological impairment. While no reliability data are reported, the FAC does correlate with temporal-distance measures such as step length and velocity.

5.   Functional Obstacle Course

In the functional obstacle course (FOC), the subject must traverse a series of 12 simulations of functional mobility tasks or situations commonly encountered in and around the home environment (52,53). The subject walks approximately 100 m across flooring of different textures, as well as up and down ramps and stairs and over and around small obstacles. Outcomes include the time taken to complete the course as well as the quality of performance, i.e., the degree to which assistance and observed difficulty or unsteadiness was observed. Based on videotape ratings of subject perfor- mance, inter-rater and intrarater reliability was excellent for both time and quality scores (correlations, presumably Pearson's $r > 0.98$) and test– retest coefficient of variation for completion time was 5% (52,53). Fallers have poorer time and quality scores than nonfallers and the scores correlate with factors such as neurological impairment (53) as well as POMA score (see below) (54). Practice on the FOC as a part of an exercise program did not help reduce falls (55). In another version of an FOC (56), subjects walk in tandem, on foam, up and down a ramp and stairs, after picking up a box, under blinds suspended from the ceiling, and over a styrofoam block. Inter-rater reliability for video-rating quality scores (e.g., need for adaptive behaviors, steadiness, etc.) was high (kappa >0.95) and while test–retest quality scores were highly correlated (ICC >0.9), there were small improvements in mean scores (11%). Similar reliability and changes were noted with completion time. Both quality score and time correlated with measures such as the POMA and gait speed, and both quality score and time improved as a result of an exercise program, particularly in those with poorer scores initially. Note that one of the interesting issues not well addressed in these studies is the concept of time-accuracy trade-off, in that faster performance may occur at the expense of errors or poorer quality score. It appears that all subjects were instructed to walk at a comfortable pace, and were generally not instructed regarding the quality score, although there was probably an implicit assumption that the goal was safe performance without use of assistance.

6. Gait Abnormality Rating Scale

The Gait Abnormality Rating Scale (GARS) utilizes a videotaped four-level assessment of 16 individual gait descriptors with a focus on the lower extre- mity, trunk, and upper extremity (57). Items in the scale that best distinguish a group of nursing home fallers from nonfallers include limitation in shoulder extension, arm–heel-strike asynchrony, and guarded stepping and arm swing. Inter-rater reliability (Spearman's r) for total score was >0.95 but per item ranged from 0.5 to 0.9 (57). The modified GARS (GARS-M), a seven-item version, includes the items noted above plus varia- bility in stepping and arm movements, staggering (partial losses of balance), the degree to which the heel-strike occurs before forefoot impact, and loss of hip extension during gait (58). This seven-item version was analyzed in frail ambulatory veterans and had moderate inter-rater and intrarater reliability (kappa 0.6 for individual items, ICC >0.9 for total score, when done by trained physical therapists), good test–retest reliability (ICC >0.9), and correlated with gait speed and a history of falling. Using a cut-off score of nine in this same cohort resulted in a modest sensitivity of 62% and specificity of 87% in predicting two or more falls in the past year (59), compared to 72% and 74%, respectively for comfortable gait speed of 0.6 m/sec. Thus, these changes in gait may be more predictive of falls than simple gait speed.

7. Performance-Oriented Mobility Assessment

The POMA, also known as the Tinetti Balance and Gait Scale, is one of the earliest and most widely used batteries designed to assess balance, gait, and fall risk in older adults. The POMA includes an evaluation of balance under perturbed conditions (such as while rising from a chair, after a nudge, with eyes closed, and while turning) as well as an evaluation of gait characteristics (including gait initiation, step height, length, continuity and symmetry, trunk sway, and path deviation) (60). Lower scores on the POMA have been associated with increased falls (61) and with increased cerebral white matter disease, possibly related to cerebrovascular disease (62). A score less than 19 out of 28 has a sensitivity of 68% and a specificity of 88% for predicting an individual who will have two or more falls (60). A later amended version suggests that a score of 36 out of 40 identified single fallers with 70% sensitivity and 52% specificity (63). Initial reports suggest more than 90% inter-rater agreement on individual items (64). Note that a ceiling effect might be noted in the POMA, even in moderately disabled Parkinson's patients, while gait speed will continue to differentiate subtle changes in functional ability (65). This ceiling effect may have accounted for the sharp drop in sensitivity on a ROC curve to detect fall risk or it may also be a sign that other factors significant in fall causation (e.g., vision or environmental hazards) are not captured by the test (63).

8. Timed Up and Go Test

The TUG is a measure of the time taken to stand up from a chair with armrests, walk 3 m, turn, walk back to the chair and sit down. Difficulty and/or unsteadiness in TUG performance is recognized as an important part of fall risk assessment (66). In small community functionally impaired samples, ICCs for short periods are good: ICC > 0.9 for less than one week (67) and ICC = 0.74 for two weeks (17). Sensitivity and specificity for a history of falls is good (87%) (68). A cut-off score of 14 seconds or greater has been proposed as 80% sensitive and 100% specific for a history of falls (68). Reliability was found to be modest (ICC < 0.6) in a large ($n = 2305$) sample of which 63% were found to have cognitive impairment and 29% were unable to complete the test due to immobility, safety concerns, or refusal (10). Note that a shorter version (a walking distance of 2.44 m or 8 ft) has also been proposed with similar predictive value for a history of falls; this same study also found a substantially lower cut-off score for TUG in those with a history of falls, i.e., 10 seconds (69). Other studies suggest a cut-off of 12 seconds for older adults (77% were below 10 sec) (70), and 20 seconds for independence on most (but not all) ADLs (67). With its simplicity in administration and scoring, the TUG is among the most widely used of the measures noted here.

C. Dual Task Walking

Recently, dual task performance has been linked to an increased risk of falls based on walking performance while performing a simultaneous cognitive (dual) task. The risk of falls, measured prospectively, increases in assisted living residents who stop walking while talking (71). This simple "stops walking while talking" test, however, may be only useful in subjects who are very impaired in the ability to walk anyway (72). Adding an additional task to be performed simultaneously with the TUG may, however, add clinical utility. Lundin-Olsson et al. (73) compared TUG performance time either without or with a simultaneous upper extremity (carrying a full glass of water) task. Followed prospectively, those subjects with a difference of 4.5 seconds or greater between the two TUG tests had nearly a five times higher risk of falling. Note that the upper extremity task involves some attentional demand, and the outcome given, that no subjects spilled any water, reflects mastery of the dual task. Given that the task was to carry the glass during walking only and that the water level was 5 cm from the top of the glass, the motor and attentional demands seem modest. Shumway-Cook et al. (68) also compared TUG performance time either without or with a simultaneous cognitive (counting backwards by threes) or upper extremity (carrying a full glass of water) task. When comparing community-dwelling older adults either with or without a history of falls, both simultaneous cognitive and upper extremity tasks increased TUG time equally (over 20%), but did not provide additional predictive value (i.e., sensitivity or specificity) for a history of falls. One of the main issues in dual task studies is how the subject prioritizes walking versus the additional cognitive/motor task; is the subject instructed to prioritize one over the other, or does the subject self-prioritize, thereby adding an additional element of variability? Another related issue is the level of performance of the dual task; does the subject maintain a certain level of performance on the dual task or does the dual task performance decrease in the presence of the walking task? In general, in these studies, information regarding dual task performance outcomes or prioritization is not given. In a community sample followed prospectively, Verghese et al. (74) found that older adult fallers (vs. nonfallers) took longer to walk 20 ft, turn, and return while reciting the letters of the alphabet (walking while talking-simple, WWT-S) or alternate letters of the alphabet (walking while talking-complex, WWT-C). Inter-rater reliability, given only for the WWT-S, was fair for a timed task of a single trial ($r = 0.6$). Both WWT tests had good specificity (89–96%) but only modest sensitivity (39–46%). No score was given for either cognitive task, but the authors note that a number of subjects who slowed down also made errors in the alternate letter task. Had the subjects been forced to perform the alternate letter task without errors, walking might have slowed even more, suggesting that there may have been an underestimation of the effect of divided attention. In one prospective study in 85 years olds (75), fallers had slower walk time and poorer performance on verbal fluency, and, without prioritization of either task, poorer walk time and verbal fluency performance in a dual task situation. In contrast to previous studies of a dual task effect, no disproportionate dual task effect and no difference in the percentage who stopped walking while "talking" was seen in fallers vs. nonfallers, suggesting no benefit from using a dual task to predict falls. Thus, the dual task effect did not differ between different levels of fallers and nonfallers. This finding may have more to do with the fall classification scheme, in that one-year recollection and surrogate reports were used and may not be reliable, although the faller group was more functionally impaired (such as in depressive symptoms). Another possibility has to do with the complexity of the tasks (walking plus three 180 degree turns), which was likely to be difficult in all three groups, and because of this complexity, the relatively preserved verbal fluency had little differential group dual task effect. For further discussion on the effects of cognition on gait and mobility see Chapter 6.

D. Tests of Volitional Stepping

In reacting to a postural disturbance, a foot-in-place response is frequently not sufficient, necessitating a compensatory stepping response. Laboratory-based protocols designed to induce compensatory stepping (using, for example, a waist pull) frequently show that older and more balance-impaired individuals, compared to young controls, take more steps and have biomechanically less effective response strategies (76,77). These compensatory steps may differ from volitional steps, the latter triggered by a verbal or sensory (light or sound) command. Compared to compensatory steps, volitional steps are executed more slowly, and thus may underestimate the true compensatory stepping ability (78). Volitional stepping studies have found age- and impairment-associated declines in reaction time (the time of foot activation), but also describe declines in step completion time, the time taken to complete a step. Simple step completion time is generally slowest in older adult fallers (vs. healthy old and young controls) when stepping laterally onto instrumented pads in response to a simple light stimulus (79). Choice step completion time (stepping laterally or forward onto a switch with either foot in response to a light cue) is also prolonged in fallers versus nonfallers, correlates strongly with other immobility and fall risk factors (such as Trails B score and leg strength) and is an independent predictor for falls (80). While there may be prolongation of step completion time with increasing age, there may be no disproportionate increase in simple vs.

choice step completion time (81). One problem with stepping tests is that subjects may not have to substantially transfer their weight to complete a "step," thereby making the outcome a partial step, transferring just enough weight to activate the switch. This may occur because the step distance to switch activation is not individualized, i.e., to account for differences according to leg length and severity of the balance impairment. In order to encourage weight transfer and to provide a more individualized assessment of stepping ability, Medell and Alexander (82) instructed subjects to step out as far as possible and still successfully return to the original stance position in one step, the maximal step length (MSL). MSL declines with age and balance impairment and correlates strongly with measures of balance, fall risk, mobility performance, and self-reported function in balance-impaired older adults (82,83). Allowing more than one step in returning to stance (an altered version of the MSL) showed greater decline from the third to the ninth decade of life than other gait and balance measures (84). Test–retest reliability of the MSL is high (ICC = 0.86) and while the MSL was originally tested in three directions with either foot, a simplified version more appropriate for clinical settings (right foot forward only) is equally predictive of the functional outcomes above (83). Tests requiring steps in multiple directions with different feet have also been proposed. In the rapid step test (RST) (82), subjects are timed as they take 24 steps in three directions with either foot in response to verbal commands. The time required to step into contiguous squares in a sequence of forward, sideways, and backward steps, each step needing to clear a low-lying obstacle (a set of canes), is called the foursquare step test (FSST) (85). Both the RST and FSST are prolonged in balance-impaired or frequent falling older adults, correlate with other measures of mobility, balance, and fall risk measures, and are reliable (test–retest ICC >0.9) (82,85).

III. SUMMARY

The advantage of these no- and low-tech gait assessment measures are the low cost, lack of need for expensive equipment and facilities, relative ease of and minimal time needed for administration, potential for acceptance by older adults who might fear technology-based assessments, and potential to simulate more typical challenges incurred during day-to-day living. As is described more fully in Chapters 3 and 4, high tech measures utilize highly quantifiable measures that assess more subtle phenomena, especially underlying pathological mechanisms, not readily detectable by the clinician. Frequently a set of multiple tasks is proposed because gait disorders have multifactorial etiologies and may manifest themselves differently under different postural (or environmental) challenge situations. These sets of multiple tasks may provide additional sensitivity for changes in performance beyond the simpler performance or questionnaire tests. The simple sets may be most useful in more impaired individuals because of ceiling effects in the more able participants (see also Chapter 1). Sometimes the sets may require additional equipment or space, such as in the obstacle courses, that defeat the purpose of the simplicity of the measure and make the test more complex and less portable. Which measure is thus best to use? Selection of the proper instrument will depend on level of participant ambulation impairment (e.g., community ambulator vs. home bound) and the need for simple (e.g., busy clinic or hospital setting) vs. more time consuming but informative multiple task assessments (e.g., rehabilitation setting).

REFERENCES

1. Toro B, Nester CJ, Farren PC. The status of gait assessment among physiotherapists in the United Kingdom. Arch Phys Med Rehabil 2003; 84: 1878–1884.
2. Smith LA, Branch LG, Scherr PA, et al. Short-term variability of measures of physical function in older people. J Am Geriatr Soc 1990; 38:993–998.
3. Alexander NB, Guire KE, Thelen DG, et al. Self-reported walking ability predicts functional mobility performance in frail older adults. J Am Geriatr Soc 2000; 48:1408–1413.
4. Pine AM, Gurland B, Chren MM. Report of having slowed down: evidence for the validity of a new way to inquire about mild disability in elders. J Gerontol 2000; 55:M378–M383.
5. Guralnik JM, Ferrucci L, Balfour JL, et al. Progressive versus catastrophic loss of the ability to walk: implications for the prevention of mobility loss. J Am Geriatr Soc 2001; 49:1463–1470.
6. Jylha M, Guralnik JM, Balfour J, et al. Walking difficulty, walking speed and age as predictors of self-rated health: the Women's Health and Aging Study. J Gerontol 2001; 56A:M609–M617.
7. Tager IB, Swanson A, Satariano WA. Reliability of physical performance and self-reported functional measures in an older population. J Gerontol 1998; 53:M295–M300.
8. Mendes de Leon CF, Guralnik JM, Bandeen-Roche K. Short-term change in physical function and disability: the Women's Health and Aging Study. J Gerontol 2002; 57:S355–S365.
9. Studenski S, Perera S, Wallace D, et al. Physical performance measures in the clinical setting. J Am Geriatr Soc 2003; 51:314–322.
10. Rockwood K, Awalt E, Carver D, et al. Feasibility and measurement properties of the functional reach and timed up and go tests in the Canadian Study of Health and Aging. J Gerontol 2000; 55A:M70–M73.
11. Alexander NB. Gait disorders in older adults. J Am Geriatr Soc 1996; 44: 434–451.
12. Shinkai S, Watanabe S, Kumagai S, et al. Walking speed as a good predictor for the onset of functional dependence in a Japanese rural community population. Age Ageing 2000; 29:441–446.

13. Marquis S, Moore MM, Howieson DB, et al. Independent predictors of cognitive decline in healthy elderly persons. Arch Neurol 2002; 59:601–606.
14. Urquhart DM, Morris ME, Iansek R. Gait consistency over a 7-day interval in people with Parkinson's disease. Arch Phys Med Rehabil 1999; 80:696–701.
15. Fransen M, Crosbie J, Edmonds J. Reliability of gait measurements in people with osteoarthritis of the knee. Phys Ther 1997; 77:944–953.
16. Green J, Forster A, Young J. Reliability of gait speed measured by a timed walking test in patients one year after stroke. Clin Rehabil 2002; 16:306–314.
17. Jette AM, Jette DU, Ng J, et al. Are performance-based measures sufficiently reliable for use in multicenter trials. J Gerontol 1999; 54:M3–M6.
18. Ostchega Y, Harris TB, Hirsch R, et al. Reliability and prevalence of physical performance examination assessing mobility and balance in older persons in the US: data from the Third National Health and Nutrition Examination Survey. J Am Geriatr Soc 2000; 48:1136–1141.
19. Salbach NM, Mayo NE, Higgins J, et al. Responsiveness and predictability of gait speed and other disability measures in acute stroke. Arch Phys Med Rehabil 2001; 82:1204–1212.
20. Guyatt GH, Thompson PJ, Berman LB, et al. How should we measure function in patients with chronic heart and lung disease. J Chronic Dis 1985; 38:517–524.
21. Bittner V, Weiner DH, Yusuf S, et al. Prediction of mortality and morbidity with a six-minute walk test in patients with left ventricular dysfunction. J Am Med Asssoc 1993; 270:1702–1707.
22. Harada ND, Chiu V, Stewart AL. Mobility-related function in older adults: assessment with a 6-minute walk test. Arch Phys Med Rehabil 1999; 80: 837–841.
23. Bean JF, Kiely DK, Leveille SG, et al. The 6-minute walk test in mobility-limited elders: what is being measured? J Gerontol 2002; 57:M751–M756.
24. Lord SR, Menz H. Physiologic, psychologic, and health predictors of 6-minute walk performance in older people. Arch Phys Med Rehabil 2002; 83:907–911.
25. Parent E, Moffet H. Comparative responsiveness of locomotor tests and questionnaires used to follow early recovery after total knee arthroplasty. Arch Phys Med Rehabil 2002; 83:70–80.
26. Ettinger WH, Burns R, Messier SP, et al. A randomized trial comparing aerobic exercise and resistance exercise with a health education program in older adults with knee osteoarthritis. J Am Med Assoc 1997; 277:25–31.
27. Montgomery PS, Gardner AW. The clinical utility of a six-minute walk test in peripheral arterial occlusive disease patients. J Am Geriatr Soc 1998; 46: 706–711.
28. King B, Judge JO, Whipple R, et al. Reliability and responsiveness of two physical performance measures examined in the context of a functional training intervention. Phys Ther 2000; 80:8–16.
29. Hamilton DM, Haennel RG. Validity and reliability of the 6-minute walk test in a cardiac rehabilitation population. J Cardiopulm Rehabil 2000; 20:156–164.
30. Faggiano P, D'Aloia A, Gualeni A, et al. Assessment of oxygen uptake during the 6-minute walking test in patients with heart failure: preliminary experience with a portable device. Am Heart J 1997; 134:203–206.

31. Kervio G, Carre F, Ville NS. Reliability and intensity of the six-minute walk test in healthy elderly subjects. Med Sci Sports Exer 2003; 35:169–174.
32. Simonsick EM, Montgomery PS, Newman AB, et al. Measuring fitness in healthy older adults: the Health ABC Long Distance Corridor Walk. J Am Geriatr Soc 2001; 49:1544–1548.
33. Newman AB, Haggerty CL, Kritchevsky SB, et al. Walking performance and cardiovascular response: associations with age and morbidity—the Health, Aging, and Body Composition Study. J Gerontol 2003; 58A:715–720.
34. Simonsick EM, Newman AB, Nevitt MC, et al. Measuring higher level physical function in well-functioning older adults: expanding familiar approaches in the Health ABC Study. J Gerontol 2001; 56A:M644–M649.
35. Rolland YM, Cesari M, Miller ME, et al. Reliability of the 400-m usual-pace walk test as an assessment of mobility limitation in older adults. J Am Geriatr Soc 2004; 52:972–976.
36. Berg K, Wood-Dauphinee S, Williams JI, et al. Measuring balance in the elderly: preliminary development of an instrument. Physiother Can 1989; 41:304–311.
37. Shumway-Cook A, Gruber W, Baldwin M, et al. The effect of multidimentional exercises on balance, mobility and fall-risk in community-dwelling older adults. Phys Ther 1997; 77:46–57.
38. Shumway-Cook A, Baldwin M, Polissar NL, et al. Predicting the probability for falls in community-dwelling older adults. Phys Ther 1997; 77: 812–819.
39. Whitney SL, Hudak MT, Marchetti GF. The dynamic gait index relates to self-reported fall history in individuals with vestibular dysfunction. J Vestib Res 2000; 10:99–105.
40. Wrisley DM, Walker ML, Echternach JL, et al. Reliability of the dynamic gait index in people with vestibular disorders. Arch Phys Med Rehabil 2003; 84:1528–1533.
41. Wrisley DM, Marchetti GF, Kuharsky DK, et al. Reliability, internal consistency, and validity of data obtained with the Functional Gait Assessment. Phys Ther 2004; 84:906–918.
42. Wolf SL, Catlin PA, Gage K, et al. Establishing the reliability and validity of measurements of walking time using the Emory Functional Ambulation Profile. Phys Ther 1999; 79:1122–1133.
43. Baer HR, Wolf SL. Modified Emory Functional Ambulation Profile: an outcome measure for the rehabilitation of poststroke gait dysfunction. Stroke 2001; 32:973–979.
44. Guralnik J, Simonsick EM, Ferrucci L, et al. A short physical performance battery assessing lower extremity function: association with self-reported disability and prediction of mortality and nursing home admission. J Gerontol 1994; 49:M85–M94.
45. Guralnik J, Ferrucci L, Simonsick EM, et al. Lower extremity function in persons over the age of 70 years as a predictor of subsequent disability. N Eng J Med 1995; 332:556–561.
46. Guralnik JM, Ferrucci L, Pieper CF, et al. Lower extremity function and subsequent disability consistency across studies, predictive models, and value

of gait speed alone compared with the short physical performance battery. J Gerontol 2000; 55A:M221–M231.

47. Lan TY, Melzer D, Tom BDM, et al. Performance tests and disability: developing an objective index of mobility-related limitations in older persons. J Gerontol 2002; 57:M294–M301.

48. Melzer D, Lan TY, Guralnik JM. The predictive validity for mortality of the index of mobility-related limitation—results from the EPESE Study. Age Ageing 2003; 32:619–625.

49. Lan TY, Deeg DJH, Guralnik JM. Responsiveness of the index of mobility limitation: comparison with gait speed along in the Longitudinal Aging Study Amsterdam. J Gerontol 2003; 58:721–727.

50. Holden MK, Gill KM, Magliozzi MR, et al. Clinical gait assessment in the neurologically impaired: reliability and meaningfulness. Phys Ther 1984; 64: 35–40.

51. Holden MK, Gill KM, Magliozzi MR. Gait assessment for neurologically impaired patients: standards for outcome assessment. Phys Ther 1986; 66:1530–1539.

52. Means KM. The obstacle course: a tool for the assessment of functional balance and mobility in the elderly. J Rehabil Res Dev 1996; 33:413–428.

53. Means KM, Rodell DE, O'Sullivan PS. Use of an obstacle course to assess balance and mobility in the elderly. Am J Phys Med Rehabil 1996; 75:88–95.

54. Means KM, Rodell DE, O'Sullivan PS, et al. Comparison of a functional obstacle course with an index of clinical gait and balance and postural sway. J Gerontol 1998; 53A:M331–M335.

55. Means KM, Rodell DE, O'Sullivan PS, et al. Rehabilitation of elderly fallers: pilot study of a low to moderate intensity exercise program. Arch Phys Med Rehabil 1996; 77:1030–1036.

56. Rubenstein LZ, Josephson KR, Trueblood PR, et al. The reliability and validity of an obstacle course as a measure of gait and balance in older adults. Aging Clin Exp Res 1997; 9:127–135.

57. Wolfson L, Whipple R, Amerman P, et al. Gait assessment in the elderly: a gait abnormality rating scale and its relation to falls. J Gerontol 1990; 45:M12–M19.

58. VanSwearingen JM, Paschall KA, Bonino P, et al. The modified gait abnormality rating scale for recognizing the risk of recurrent falls in community-dwelling elderly adults. Phys Ther 1996; 76:994–1002.

59. VanSwearingen JM, Paschall KA, Bonino P, et al. Assessing recurrent fall risk of community-dwelling frail older veterans using specific tests of mobility and the physical performance test of function. J Gerontol 1998; 53A:M457–M464.

60. Tinetti ME, Williams TF, Mayewski R. Fall risk index for elderly patients based on number of chronic disabilities. Am J Med 1986; 80:429–434.

61. Tinetti ME, Speechley M, Ginter SF. Risk factors for falls among elderly persons living in the community. N Engl J Med 1988; 319:1701–1707.

62. Whitman GT, Tang T, Baloh RW. A prospective study of cerebral white matter abnormalities in older people with gait dysfunction. Neurology 2001; 57:990–994.

63. Raiche M, Hebert R, Prince F, et al. Screening older adults at risk of falling with the Tinetti Balance Scale. Lancet 2000; 356:1001–1002.

64. Tinetti ME. Performance-oriented assessment of mobility problems in elderly persons. J Am Geriatr Soc 1986; 34:119–126.

65. Behrman AL, Light KE, Miller GM. Sensitivity of the Tinetti Gait Assessment for detecting change in individuals with Parkinson's disease. Clin Rehabil 2002; 16:199–405.

66. American Geriatrics Society. Guideline for prevention of falls in older persons. J Am Geriatr Soc 2001; 49:664–672.

67. Posiadlo D, Richardson S. The timed "Up & Go": a test of basic functional mobility for frail elderly persons. J Am Geriatr Soc 1991; 39:142–148.

68. Shumway-Cook A, Brauer S, Woollacott M. Predicting the probability for falls in community-dwelling older adults using the timed get up and go test. Phys Ther 2000; 80:896–903.

69. Rose DJ, Jones CJ, Lucchese N. Predicting the probability of falls in community-residing older adults using the 8-foot up-and-go: a new measure of functional mobility. J Aging Phys Activity 2002; 10:466–475.

70. Bischoff HA, Stahelin HB, Monsch AU, et al. Identifying a cut-off point for normal mobility: a comparison of the timed 'up and go' test in community-dwelling and institutionalized elderly women. Age Ageing 2003; 32:315–320.

71. Lundin-Olsson L, Nyberg L, Gustafson Y. Stops walking while talking as a predictor of falls in elderly people. Lancet 1997; 349:617.

72. Hausdorff JM, Balash Y, Giladi N. Effects of cognitive challenge on gait variability in patients with Parkinson's disease. J Geriatr Psych Neurol 2003; 16:53–58.

73. Lundin-Olsson L, Nyberg L, Gustafson Y. Attention, frailty, and falls: the effect of a manual task on basic mobility. J Am Geriatr Soc 1998; 46:758–761.

74. Verghese J, Buschke H, Viola L, et al. Validity of divided attention tasks in predicting falls in older individuals: a preliminary study. J Am Geriatr Soc 2002; 50:1572–1576.

75. Bootsma-van der Wiel A, Gussekloo J, de Craen AJM, et al. Walking and talking as predictors of falls in the general population: the Leiden 85-plus study. J Am Geriatr Soc 2003; 51:1466–1471.

76. Luchies CW, Alexander NB, Schultz AB, Ashton-Miller JA. Stepping responses of young and old adults to postural disturbances: Kinematics. J Am Geriatr Soc 1994; 42:506–512.

77. Schulz BW, Ashton-Miller JA, Alexander NB. Compensatory stepping in response to waist pulls in balance-impaired and unimpaired women. Gait Posture. In press.

78. Luchies CW, Wallace D, Pazdor R, et al. Effects of age on balance assessment using voluntary and involuntary step tasks. J Gerontol Med Sci 1999; 54A:M140–M144.

79. White KN, Gunter KB, Snow CM, et al. The quick step: a new test for measuring reaction time and lateral stepping velocity. J Appl Biomech 2002; 18: 271–277.

80. Lord SR, Fitzpatrick RC. Choice stepping reaction time: a composite measure of falls risk in older people. J Gerontol 2001; 56A:M627–M632.

81. Luchies CW, Schiffman J, Richards LG, et al. Effects of age, step direction, and reaction condition on the ability to step quickly. J Gerontol Med Sci 2002; 57A:M246–M249.
82. Medell JL, Alexander NB. A clinical measure of maximal and rapid stepping in older women. J. Gerontol. 2000; 55A:M429–M433.
83. Cho B, Scarpace D, Alexander NB. Maximum step length: an indicator of mobility and dynamic balance in at-risk older adults. J Am Geriatr Soc 2004; 52:1168–1173.
84. Lindemann U, Bauerle C, Muche R, et al. Age-related differences in balance, strength, and motor function. Eur J Geriatr 2003; 5:15–22.
85. Dite W, Temple VA. A clinical test of stepping and change of direction to identify multiple falling older adults. Arch Phys Med Rehabil 2002; 83: 1566–1571.

3

Laboratory-Based Evaluation of Gait Disorders: High-Tech

Patrick O. Riley and D. Casey Kerrigan

Department of Physical Medicine and Rehabilitation, School of Medicine, University of Virginia, Charlottesville, Virginia, U.S.A.

I. INTRODUCTION

Chapter 2 dealt with "low-tech" approaches to evaluation of gait disorders. This chapter will focus on the "high-tech" approach, the clinical gait laboratory, and its place in the evaluation process. A pioneer in clinical gait analysis, Gordon Rose (1), confronted the issue of what constituted gait analysis 20 years ago. He suggested that the term "gait assessment" should be applied to the whole process of evaluating a patient's gait. The term "gait analysis," he suggested, should be reserved for the high-tech component of gait evaluation. In the diagnostic triad of history, physical examination, and laboratory tests, gait analysis is a laboratory test. Like all laboratory tests, gait analysis should provide answers to specific questions. This chapter will explain the technology used in gait analysis, the testing a patient undergoes, the parameters measured and their interpretation. We will then survey the application of gait analysis in various pathologies affecting gait. Finally, we will explore the potential for expanding the clinical relevance of the gait laboratory. While there is interest in applying the technology to evaluating human movements other than gait, gait analysis will be the focus of this discussion.

II. GAIT ANALYSIS LABORATORY METHODS

In the last decade, gait analysis technology improved significantly, resulting in a potential for wider clinical application. The development of powerful and inexpensive microcomputers reduced the time and labor cost of gait analysis (2). At the same time, commercial vendors developed standard packaged gait analysis systems that integrated the basic technologies required for gait analysis, motion capture, ground reaction force measurement, and muscle activity monitoring. With the standardization of technology, there arose a standardization of methodology. Gait laboratories developed a consistent set of parameters for describing gait and gait pathology.

Two recent developments promise even more significant advances. First, the entertainment industry began using motion capture technology to churn out blockbuster action movies and hot selling video games, where unnatural creatures move naturally. The entertainment industry brought to the field of motion capture high-performance demands and the money to finance technology development, producing a quantum improvement in the technology. The motion capture systems developed to meet these demands track the motion of a large number of very small markers at high data rates and with great precision. The research community is beginning to take advantage of these developments and it is reasonable to expect that clinical gait laboratories will follow suit.

Second, recent advances in computer modeling are likely to advance the usefulness of gait analysis. It is useful not only to sort through the gait analysis and identify the patient's specific impairments but also to be able to define how the measured impairments affect the patient's overall function, and predict the effectiveness of clinical interventions. While this task inherently requires a significant amount of clinical knowledge and judgment, computer modeling can potentially facilitate the process.

Later in the chapter, we will consider how these developments will affect the future of clinical gait analysis. First, let us examine the current state of the art in gait analysis and its potential for clinical application. We will examine the technology used in the gait laboratory and the parameters measured by that technology. We will then look at how that information is used to assess a patient's gait.

A. Technology

A clinical gait laboratory will usually have four systems for evaluating gait:

1. A video system records images of the patient walking.
2. A motion capture system tracks the patient's movements digitally.
3. Force plates are used to measure the ground reaction force.
4. An electromyography system is used to record the activity of the muscles in gait.

The information from these components is integrated to provide an understanding of the physiology and mechanics of the patient's gait.

These four systems may be augmented by other technologies to provide more specific or complete information. Foot plantar pressure measuring devices are used to measure the contact pressure between the feet and ground if the subject is walking barefoot, or between the feet and shoes if worn. Indirect calorimetric devices are used to measure the patient's oxygen consumption and/or carbon dioxide production, and infer the energy cost of ambulation.

1. Video

At least two cameras are used, usually viewing the subject from one side and the front/back. Additional cameras may be used to view both sides simultaneously, or from above. All cameras are synchronized and usually multiple camera views are integrated into a single image using a frame splitter. Although video media are still in use, it is becoming more common to record the images digitally.

Video recordings are used to augment observational gait analysis and provide a degree of quality control for the motion capture data. Slow motion and even frame-by-frame playback can be used as an adjunct to observational gait analysis, enabling quick or subtle movements to be more readily detected. Viewing the patient from multiple angles simultaneously can also be helpful in understanding the patient's movement patterns.

2. Motion Capture System

The motion capture system is the central and most complex technology used in the gait laboratory. The purpose of the system is to capture a more or less complete description of the gait kinematics in digital form that can then be analyzed and related to other measurements. This process uses the mathematics of photogrammetry, a science related to surveying that owes its origins to the fields of aerial and satellite mapping. In principle, if one has multiple images of the same object and knows the three-dimensional positions, orientations, and optical characteristics of the imaging devices, one can solve for the three-dimensional position of the object from the positions of the object in the two-dimensional pictures. Measuring the camera characters and positions with sufficient accuracy is a challenge. Today a combination of inverse photogrammetry and mathematical optimization techniques is used to define the camera configuration using smaller relatively simple, but still precise, calibration objects. Using these techniques, camera configurations can be optimized for the patients and protocol as frequently as needed.

A state-of-the-art gait laboratory will have a motion capture system consisting of a special purpose computer, interface boxes, and an array of video motion capture cameras. The motion capture system must be integrated with the force plates and EMG systems, and synchronization with video capture is desirable. Although the motion capture cameras are based on video technology, they have been tuned for the marker illumination and detection function, and produce no useable video image. The number of cameras will vary depending on the size, configuration, and use of the laboratory; a large number of cameras does not necessarily indicate a superior laboratory or higher quality data. The laboratory should have a viewing volume sufficient to capture full strides bilaterally. It should also have sufficient space so that the patient is walking at steady state in the viewing volume, not accelerating from the starting position or decelerating to stop just out of the volume.

3. Force Plates

Force plates measure the force applied to the ground by the feet as the patient walks over them. They may be thought of as a precision scale, but keep in mind that a force is three-dimensional. The force plates measure not only how hard the person is pushing down on the ground, but also braking and acceleration force, and force directed mediolaterally. This information is integrated with the body kinematics defined by the motion capture system to assess the mechanics of movement. The force plate data are acquired in synchrony with the motion capture data at the same or at a multiple of the motion capture frame rate.

The number of force plates varies according to the function of the laboratory. At least two plates are required if both limb functions are to be analyzed from a single walk, a desirable but not always achievable goal. If the force plates are not rigidly mounted, they may move when struck or due to floor vibrations producing false signals that can corrupt the biomechanical analysis. This issue arises most frequently in the high-energy dynamics of sports, but can manifest its presence in gait analysis.

While modern force plates are precision instruments, they do require some attention. Strain gage force plates, e.g., AMTI force plates, are temperature sensitive and should be adjusted frequently. Piezoelectric force plates, e.g., Kistler force plates, are subject to drift, especially if moisture is allowed to affect their cables and connectors. While the motion capture system will attempt to automatically compensate for offsets in force plate data, it is best to keep the instruments themselves well tuned.

4. EMG

The electromyography (EMG) system is used to record the activity of muscles during gait, a process referred to as dynamic EMG. EMG is generally recorded using either passive or active surface electrodes. Active electrodes have a built-in amplifier and are less susceptible to artifacts due to wire motion. They are rigid and have a bit of mass, and, unless securely mounted, are more susceptible to artifacts due to electrode motion relative to the skin.

EMG electrodes are usually interfaced with the data collection system via an umbilical cable. Telemetered systems are used with some success, replacing the umbilical with a small radio transmitter and power pack. The EMG system will typically be set up to monitor a number of muscles simultaneously. Eight- and 16-channel systems are common, and 32-channel systems are available.

Surface electrodes cannot readily be used to detect the activity of deep muscles, e.g., the tibialis posterior. In addition, surface EMG is subject to cross-talk, particularly when a rather small muscle is adjacent to larger muscles with overlapping firing patterns, e.g., the rectus femoris. If the EMG of such muscles is required, fine wire electrodes are used. Proper electrode placement and the absence of cross-talk in the fine wire electrodes should be verified by electronic muscle stimulation. While the process is relatively safe and effective, the procedure adds significantly to the complexity of gait analysis. Physicians desiring fine wire EMG should specifically request it in their referral, and indicate the reason for so requesting.

Like video recording, EMG may be captured simultaneously with motion capture or separately. Analysis of EMG can be done on several levels. The most basic level is asking if the activity of a muscle is phasic with clear on and off periods, or is nearly constant, either on or off, indicating absence of useful control. The next level of analysis asks if the muscle activity occurs at the normal time in the gait cycle. As we will see, this level of analysis lacks a sound theoretical basis and should only be used with caution and when supported by substantial clinical information. Examining only the timing of muscle activity assumes that the patient's gait is normal, in which case they should not be undergoing gait analysis. If the patient's posture or movement dynamics are abnormal, it follows that the mechanics of movement are altered; hence, the activity of the muscle driving their movement will also be altered. EMG analysis should first assess whether or not the muscle activity is appropriate to produce the forces acting at that instant to produce the existing gait pattern, and second, ask if the manifest forces are contributing to or inhibiting the desired movement. Muscle activity can only be effectively assessed from the logical interpretation of these two questions; i.e., it can only be assessed in conjunction with the kinematics and kinetics of gait. Hence, the closest possible coupling between EMG and motion capture and force plate data is desirable.

5. Metabolic Function

It may be desirable to assess the energy cost of walking. The amount of energy consumed while walking can be determined using indirect calorimetry, that is, by measuring the patient's oxygen consumption and carbon dioxide production. The ratio of carbon dioxide production to oxygen consumption also indicates if the patient has exceeded their anaerobic threshold. There is ample evidence that patients adjust their gait to avoid exceeding their maximum aerobic capacity (VO_{2max}). These measurements can be used to determine if the patient may benefit from conditioning, or if an intervention improves gait efficiency.

Historically, these measurements were made by collecting exhaled gasses over a period. Recently, instrumentation has become available to measure these parameters on a breath-by-breath basis. This instrumentation is more compact, portable and comfortable than the older equipment. To determine the metabolic cost of walking, it is necessary to subtract the average resting oxygen consumption from the average obtained during steady-state ambulation. Walking at constant speed on a clear track or treadmill for several minutes is required for the latter measurement. These requirements are not consistent with normal motion capture procedures and metabolic measurements are usually made independently of gait analysis trials. The results are affected by the patient's level of fatigue, recent diet and general condition.

6. Treadmills

Treadmills can be used to allow gait to be observed for prolonged times and at higher speeds than can be achieved on a gait laboratory walkway. Kinematics may be obtained if the treadmill is positioned in the motion capture system viewing volume. Treadmills with instrumentation to measure the vertical component of the ground reaction force are commercially available. Recently, treadmill force plates have been developed, which may permit analysis of both the kinematics and kinetics of treadmill gait.

7. Foot Pressure Analysis

Force plates measure the total force due to the foot contacting the ground, but do not measure how the load is distributed over the plantar surface of the foot. This information is of interest in dealing with patients with neuropathies and in defining the extent of and risks associated with foot deformities.

Two technologies are used to measure the plantar surface load distribution. The first is a floor-mounted device similar in appearance to a force plate, but divided into many small regions. The vertical force applied to each region is measured and used to calculate the pressure on the portion of the plantar surface above that region. As with a force plate, the measurement is made only when the foot is on the plate. These systems have high resolution and are quite repeatable.

The second technology uses flexible inserts between the foot and the shoe. The insert is again subdivided into a number of regions and each region is instrumented to measure the local force. The resolution of these devices is generally lower than that of the fixed plates. The measurements are affected by how the foot, shoe, and insert fit, and the load sensors tend to be less precise and less uniform than those used in the floor-mounted platforms. However, measurements for a number of steps may be obtained, and orthotics may be evaluated under conditions of actual use.

B. Terminology

The basic unit of walking and running is one *gait cycle*, or *stride*. Perry (3) described various functional elements of the gait cycle (Fig. 1), which have formed a standard frame of reference to describe normal and abnormal gait. At an average walking velocity, the stance period comprises about 60% of the gait cycle, while the swing period comprises 40%.

Time–distance parameters are used to quantitatively describe gait. *Gait velocity* is simply the speed of gait. *Stride time* is defined from the time of initial contact of one limb with the ground to the next initial contact of the same limb. *Step time* is the duration of time from initial contact of one limb

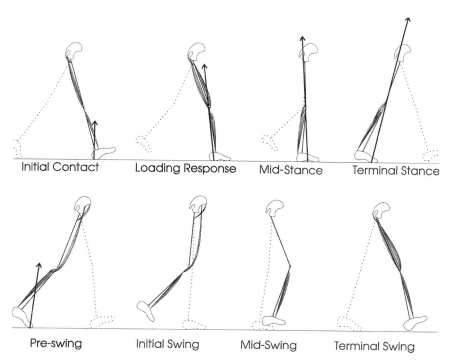

| Initial Contact | Loading Response | Mid-Stance | Terminal Stance |

| Pre-swing | Initial Swing | Mid-Swing | Terminal Swing |

Figure 1 The eight phases of the gait cycle include initial contact, loading response, mid-stance, terminal stance, pre-swing, initial swing, mid-swing, and terminal swing. The involved limb is shown as solid lines; the uninvolved limb is shown with dotted lines. The ground reaction force (GRF) vector is represented by a heavy solid line with an arrow. The major active muscles are shown during each phase of the gait cycle. *Source*: From Ref. 4.

to the time of initial contact of the contralateral limb. *Stride length* and *step length* refer to the distances covered during their respective times. The *cadence* of gait can be expressed in either strides per minute or steps per minute.

III. BIOMECHANICAL CONCEPTS PERTINENT TO GAIT

Kinematics describes the motions of limb segments and the angular motions of joints. Kinetics describes the moments and forces that cause motion. Similarly, the firing patterns of muscles can be determined with the aid of dynamic EMG. The principal advantage of gait analysis over observational gait evaluation is that the gait laboratory measures the kinetics, the link between EMG and kinematics.

To appreciate the insight provided by kinetics, it is necessary to consider the basic physics of motion. In quantitative gait analysis, we compute the net joint moments. A moment about a joint occurs when a force acts at a distance from the joint. For instance, a weight in the hand produces an externally applied extensor moment about the elbow. In this example, the lever is the forearm and the external moment is the product of the weight of the object and the length of the forearm. The concept of static equilibrium dictates that, in order for the joint angle to remain constant, all the moments acting about the joint must sum to zero. Thus, in our example, for the elbow angle to remain constant, an internal force from the biceps, acting through its muscle lever arm, must provide a resisting internal flexor moment that matches the external extensor moment due to the weight. Small deviations from equilibrium allow stable movement, a condition of dynamic equilibrium. Depending on the magnitude of the biceps force, the elbow joint angle will extend in a controlled fashion (eccentric contraction), stay the same (isometric contraction), or flex (concentric contraction). The controlled accelerations of the body segment masses produce inertial forces, which together with the internal and external moments, sum to zero, a condition of dynamic equilibrium.

These basic biomechanical concepts are pertinent to gait analysis. During walking, the joints and limb segments are in a state of dynamic equilibrium. The net joint moments match the externally applied forces, include gravity and the body's ground reaction force (GRF), defined as the force exerted by the ground at the point of contact (our feet) and the inertial forces from limb segments. During the stance period the inertial forces are extremely small, the net joint moments establish equilibrium with the external forces, gravity and the GRF. During swing, there is no ground reaction force but the inertial forces, although still small, are significant. The joint moments are in equilibrium with the gravitational and inertial forces.

The importance of knowing the direction and magnitude of the GRF and its relationship with muscle behavior and maintenance of equilibrium is

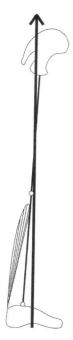

Quiet Standing

Figure 2 Quiet standing. The GRF, represented by the heavy solid line and arrow, is located anterior to the knee and ankle and posterior to the hip. The soleus muscle is active to stabilize the lower limb. *Source*: From Ref. 4.

best illustrated by the example of quiet standing (Fig. 2). In quiet standing, the GRF vector extends from the ground through the foot, passing anterior to the ankles and knees, and posterior to the hips. At the hip, passive ligamentous forces transmitted through the iliofemoral ligaments usually are sufficient to counteract the external extensor moment. Similarly, at the knee, the external knee extensor moment is counteracted by the passive forces transmitted through the posterior ligamentous capsule. At the ankle, the external dorsi flexion moment is usually counteracted with an internal ankle plantar flexor moment provided by the ankle plantar flexors. Thus, the only lower extremity muscles that are consistently active during quiet standing are the plantar flexors.

When we walk, the GRF is a function of the position of the body segments and their velocity and acceleration. Knowing where the line of the GRF lies with respect to the hip, knee and ankle joints gives us a reasonable approximation of the external moments occurring about each of these joints. The GRF can be directly measured with a force plate. Visualizing where the GRF lies with respect to a joint provides a means of approximating the internal moments that must be generated in order to stabilize that joint. For instance, if the GRF line is posterior to the knee, it produces an external knee flexor moment, which is the product of the ground reaction force multiplied by the distance of the GRF line from the axis of the knee joint. In order to maintain stability so that the knee does not collapse into flexion, an internal knee extensor moment must occur. This moment, provided by the knee extensors, is equal in magnitude to the external flexor moment.

During walking, the GRF vector changes position as the body progresses forward (Fig. 1). In early stance, the vector is anterior to the hip and posterior to the knee and ankle. In midstance, the vector passes through the hip and knee joints and is anterior to the ankle. During terminal stance, the vector moves posterior to the hip, anterior to the knee joint and maximally anterior to the ankle. With these dynamics in mind, normal gait function is easier to interpret. The muscles fire in response to the need for joint stability. In quantitative gait analysis, one can determine whether a muscle group is firing concentrically or eccentrically using the joint power, which is mathematically the product of the joint moment and the joint angular velocity. A positive joint power implies that the muscle group is firing concentrically while a negative joint power implies that the muscle group is firing eccentrically.

IV. NORMAL KINEMATIC AND KINETIC PARAMETERS

The following descriptions of normal sagittal plane kinematics and kinetics are based on data collected from the Spaulding Rehabilitation Hospital Gait Laboratory (Fig. 3) and are similar to those reported elsewhere. The general patterns of movement are representative of adults and nondisabled children older than 3 years of age (5). Figure 1 illustrates the chief actions occurring in each phase with a visual representation of the limb and joint positions, the GRF line, and the muscles that are active during that phase.

A. Initial Contact

Initial contact with the ground typically occurs with the heel. The hip is flexed at 30°, the knee is almost fully extended, and the ankle is in a neutral position. As the GRF is anterior to the hip, the hip extensors (gluteus maximus and hamstrings) are firing to maintain hip stability. At the knee, the GRF creates an external extensor moment, which is counteracted by hamstring activity. The foot is supported in the neutral position by the ankle dorsi flexors.

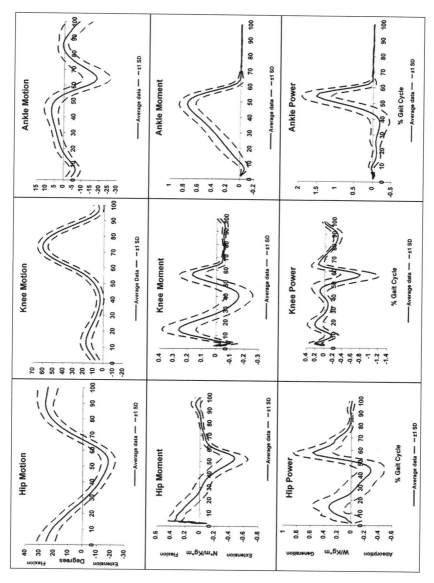

Figure 3 Sagittal plane kinematics and kinetics of the hip, knee, and ankle. *Source*: From Ref. 4.

B. Loading Response

During this phase, weight acceptance and shock absorption are achieved while maintaining forward progression. The hip extends and will continue to extend into the terminal stance phase. The GRF is anterior to the hip and the hip extensors must be active to resist uncontrolled hip flexion. Active hip extension implies that the hip extensors are concentrically active. With the location of the GRF now posterior to the knee joint, an external flexor moment is created. This external moment is resisted by an eccentric contraction of the quadriceps allowing knee flexion to approximately 20°. With the GRF posterior to the ankle, an external plantar flexion moment occurs which rapidly lowers the foot into 10° of plantar flexion. This action is controlled by the ankle dorsi flexors, which fire eccentrically. At the end of loading response, the foot is in full contact with the ground.

C. Midstance

During midstance, the limb supports the full body weight as the contralateral limb swings forward. The GRF vector passes through the hip joint, eliminating the need for hip extensor activity. At the knee, the GRF moves from a posterior to an anterior position, similarly eliminating the need for quadriceps activity. Knee extension occurs and is restrained passively by the knee's posterior ligamentous capsule, and is possibly actively restrained as well by eccentric popliteus and gastrocnemius action. At the ankle, the GRF is anterior to the ankle, thus producing an external ankle dorsi flexion moment. This moment is counteracted by the ankle plantar flexors, which eccentrically limit the dorsi flexion occurring during this phase.

D. Terminal Stance

In terminal stance, the body's mass continues to progress over the limb as the trunk falls forward. The GRF at the hip is now posterior, creating an extensor moment countered passively by the iliofemoral ligaments. The hip is maximally extended. At the knee, the GRF moves from an anterior to a posterior position. As the heel rises from the ground, the GRF moves further anterior to the ankle joint, generating an external dorsi flexion moment that is balanced by ankle plantar flexors activity. During this phase, the ankle is plantar flexing, and thus the action of the ankle planar flexors has switched from eccentric to concentric.

E. Pre-swing

During pre-swing, the limb begins to be propelled forward into swing. This phase is occurring as the contralateral limb advances through initial contact and loading response. From maximal hip extension, the hip begins flexing due to the combined activation of the iliopsoas, hip adductors, and rectus femoris, which are concentrically active. The knee quickly flexes to 40° as the GRF progresses rapidly posterior to the knee. Knee flexion may be controlled by rectus femoris activity. The ankle plantar flexes to approximately 20° due to continued concentric activity of the ankle plantar flexors.

F. Initial Swing

During initial swing, the limb is propelled forward. Hip flexion occurs because of the hip flexion momentum initiated in pre-swing and because of continued concentric activity of the hip flexors. The rectus femoris and vastus lateralis work independently during initial swing phase, with the rectus femoris activity directly correlated to walking speed (6). The rectus femoris is active during both loading response and pre- and initial-swing phases, regardless of walking speed, with much variability in patterns of muscular activity. Some subjects exhibit greater activity during late stance, while others have higher EMG amplitudes during early stance (7). The knee continues to flex to approximately 65°. Knee flexion occurs passively as a combined result of hip flexion and the momentum generated from pre-swing. The ankle dorsi flexors are concentrically dorsi flexing the ankle to provide toe clearance.

G. Mid-swing

In Mid-swing the limb continues to advance forward, primarily passively as a pendulum, from inertial forces generated in pre- and initial swing. The momentum generated in initial swing passively flexes the hip. The knee begins to extend passively because of gravity. The ankle remains in a neutral position with the continued activity of the ankle dorsi flexors.

H. Terminal Swing

In terminal swing, the previously generated momentum is controlled to provide stable limb alignment at initial contact. At the hip and knee joints, strong eccentric contraction of the hamstrings decelerates hip flexion and controls knee extension. The ankle dorsi flexors remain active allowing a neutral ankle position at initial contact.

I. Coronal Plane Motion

While lower extremity motion during gait occurs primarily in the sagittal plane, coronal plane motion is also of clinical interest. At initial contact, the pelvis and hip are in neutral positions in the coronal plane. During much of the stance period, the GRF passes medial to the hip, knee, and ankle joint centers as the opposite limb is unloading. This medial GRF about the hip causes an external adductor moment that allows the contralateral side of the pelvis to drop slightly. This motion is controlled by eccentric contraction of the hip abductors. During stance, the GRF position medial to the knee imposes an external varus moment about the knee, which must be counteracted by lateral ligament and tendon tension, eccentric muscle activity, and compression forces to the medial compartment of the knee. The presence of a varus moment throughout most of stance contributes to osteoarthritis of the knee, which most typically occurs in the medial compartment of the knee. The varus moment can be affected by external biomechanical factors such as shoe-wear (8).

V. CLINICAL APPLICATION OF LABORATORY GAIT ANALYSIS

A. Abnormal Gait Patterns Associated with Upper Motor Neuron Pathologies

Upper motor neuron (UMN) pathologies frequently produce hemiparetic, paraparetic, or diplegic impairments affecting gait (9–14). Atypical gait patterns associated with these impairments include, but are not limited to, reduced knee flexion in swing, also referred to as stiff-legged gait; equinus or excessive ankle plantar flexion occurring during one or more phases in either stance and/or swing; and knee hyperextension or recurvatum occurring in one or more phases of stance.

1. Spastic Paretic Stiff-Legged Gait

Spastic paretic stiff-legged gait is a classic atypical gait pattern observed in patients with UMN pathology (15–17). Stiff-legged gait can be functionally significant for several reasons. From an energy standpoint, lack of knee flexion in swing creates a large moment of inertia that significantly increases the energy required to initiate the swing period of the gait cycle. Additionally, associated compensatory actions to clear the stiff limb, such as vaulting on the unaffected side (18) and excessive pelvic motion (18), can increase the vertical COM displacement, thereby increasing energy expenditure. From a biomechanical standpoint, the same compensatory actions could place the unaffected knee at risk for posterior capsule damage, or the lower back to injury. Finally, lack of knee flexion may cause toe drag during swing, which increases the risk of falling.

One cause of stiff-legged gait is inappropriate activity in one or more bellies of the quadriceps during the pre- and/or initial swing phases of gait (15,20–22). Reduced knee flexion may also be caused by weak hip flexors, inappropriate hamstring activity and/or insufficient ankle plantar flexor muscle action (15–17). For many patients with spastic paretic stiff-legged gait who undergo a quantitative gait analysis, the cause of the stiff-legged gait is not obvious from the static or observational gait evaluations. For instance, patients with increased knee extensor tone often can be found to have quiescent quadriceps EMG activity during pre- and initial swing.

Conversely, a patient with normal knee extensor tone can have inappropriate activity during these phases in one or more of the quadriceps muscles. In the latter case, if the inappropriate activity is limited to just one quadriceps muscle, an intramuscular neurolytic procedure would be a reasonable treatment to improve the gait pattern. On the other hand, quantitative gait analysis may point to dynamically significant weak hip flexors, indicated by slow progression into hip flexion and poor hip power generation in preswing. These findings commonly are not correlated with hip flexion strength evaluated by static testing. In this case, hip flexion strengthening would be the optimal prescription. Gait analysis also can help provide information about the functional significance of the atypical gait pattern. For instance, the risk for injury to the posterior capsule and ligaments of the unaffected knee can be assessed by measuring the extensor moment during that limb's stance period. Finally, a follow-up gait analysis may be useful in quantifying the improvement in knee flexion as well as confirming that the treatment itself did not cause any new problems.

2. Dynamic Knee Recurvatum

Hyperextension of the knee during the stance period, referred to as dynamic knee recurvatum, is common in patients with UMN pathology. This atypical gait pattern may be caused by one or more of the following impairments: quadriceps weakness or spasticity, ankle planar flexor weakness or spasticity, dorsi flexor weakness, and heel cord contracture (5,23). A primary functional concern for patients with dynamic knee recurvatum is that the hyperextension may produce an abnormal external extensor moment across the knee, placing the capsular and ligamentous structures of the posterior aspect of the knee at risk for injury. Injury to these tissues may cause pain, ligamentous laxity, and eventual bony deformity. Not all patients with recurvatum have an abnormal knee external moment; in which case, the risk for injury is probably less (24). In such cases, dynamic recurvatum may be advantageous by providing a control mechanism for an otherwise unstable limb during the stance period of the gait cycle. If the associated knee extensor moment is small, then attempts to improve this atypical pattern may not be the appropriate treatment plan. Thus, quantitative gait analysis provides information, which can help assess the functional significance of the atypical gait pattern, as well as information, which can help delineate the pattern's underlying impairment(s).

3. Equinus Gait

Excessive ankle plantar flexion occurring in either stance or swing is common in patients with neurologic lesions. As in other atypical gait patterns, the functional significance of the pattern needs to be determined. Kerrigan et al. (25) recently reported, using biomechanical analyses, that toe walking can have biomechanical advantages for individuals with distal lower extremity weakness. Toe walking can require less knee extensor, ankle plantar flexor and ankle dorsi flexor strength than walking heel-to-toe. Thus, for patients with UMN injury who typically have greater distal than proximal weakness, toe walking may be a more efficient means of ambulation. On the other hand, during swing, excessive planar flexion may place an individual at increased risk for tripping and falls. Dynamic EMG is useful in identifying the presence of inappropriate soleus, gastrocnemius, or posterior tibialis activity as a cause of the excessive planar flexion. For equinus in swing, the lack of ankle plantar flexor activity suggests either a heel cord contracture or weak ankle dorsi flexors as a cause. Each patient also deserves evaluation for functionally significant compensatory mechanisms as well, such as increased hip flexion and hip hiking in swing.

B. Gait Patterns Associated with LMN and Orthopedic Disorders

Unlike that seen in most patients with UMN pathology, the atypical gait patterns associated with specific peripheral nerve injuries cause discrete patterns of muscle weakness and associated characteristic atypical gait patterns. The following examples illustrate atypical gait patterns, which arise from weakness of a specific functional muscle group. In order to determine the underlying impairment and functional limitation responsible for the atypical gait pattern, static evaluation and observational analysis are usually adequate. Kinetic assessment is often useful, however, in helping to determine the functional significance of an atypical gait pattern.

1. Gait Associated with Femoral Neuropathy

Selected quadriceps weakness, which can occur in femoral neuropathy in diabetes, femoral nerve entrapment, or poliomyelitis, impairs weight-bearing stability during stance. Normally, the quadriceps contract eccentrically to control the rate of knee flexion during the loading response of the limb with weakness, the knee tends to "buckle." The effective compensatory action is to position the lower extremity such that the GRF lies anterior to the knee joint, imparting an extension moment during stance phases. This is first achieved during initial contact by planar flexing the ankle. Contraction of the hip extensors can also help to hold the knee in hyperextension. As noted previously, gait analysis may be useful in evaluating the associated knee extensor moment which, if excessive, could place the posterior ligamentous capsule at risk for injury.

2. Atypical Gait Patterns Associated with Weak Ankle
Dorsi Flexors

Dorsi flexor weakness also has a characteristic gait pattern. Clinical conditions in which this is seen are peroneal nerve palsy occurring because of entrapment at the fibular head, or more proximally as an injury to a branch of the sciatic nerve, or in an L-5 radiculopathy. If the ankle dorsi flexors have a grade of 3 or 4/5, the characteristic clinical sign is "foot slap" occurring soon after initial contact, due to the inability of the ankle dorsi flexors to eccentrically contract to control the rate of planar flexion after heel contact. If the ankle dorsi flexors have less than 3/5 strength, a toe drag or a steppage gait pattern with excessive hip flexion in swing is likely. The cause of these patterns can usually be determined with a careful history, physical examination, and standard electrodiagnostic procedures, rather than a dynamic EMG assessment.

3. Atypical Gait Patterns Associated with Generalized LMN Lesions

More generalized LMN lesions commonly involve variable weakness patterns and thus often have unpredictable and often complex associated gait patterns. Poliomyelitis and Guillian Barre' syndrome are examples. For these diagnoses, kinetic assessment can be particularly useful in determining excessive joint moments, implying excessive soft tissue strain or the need for increased compensatory muscle action in another muscle group.

4. Trendelenburg Gait

Trendelenburg gait, also known as gluteus medius gait, describes a pattern of either excessive pelvic obliquity during the stance period of the affected side, uncompensated Trendelenburg gait, and/or excessive lateral truncal lean during the stance period of the affected side, compensated Trendelenburg gait. Weakness of or reluctance to use the gluteus medius can cause this atypical gait pattern. The most common cause of Trendelenburg gait is osteoarthritis of the hip or other painful disorder. In this case, the gait pattern, regardless of whether or not it is compensated or uncompensated, occurs as a compensatory response to reduce the overall forces across the hip during stance. This can be seen as a reduction in the external hip adductor moment, which ordinarily occurs in the stance period.

C. Atypical Gait Patterns Associated with Aging

Gait analysis has been used to characterize gait pattern alterations that accompany aging (26,27). There have been three principle foci of investigation: alterations due to reduced strength, alterations due to impaired balance control, and alterations due to limited range of motion. We will briefly review the findings in each area. It is fair to say that, while subtle differences have been identified in the gait patterns of elders as a group compared to healthy young persons, there is no well-defined elder gait pattern. Nor have any clear-cut diagnostic parameters been found to identify impaired function among elders.

1. Gait Patterns Associated with Impaired Strength
and/or Power-Generating Capacity

It is widely documented that elderly persons tend to walk more slowly due to reduced step length. Gait analysis kinetic parameters have been examined to determine if reduced speed is the result of reduced strength or agility. The role of strength may be assessed by examining the maximum net moment developed at each joint in gait. The role of agility may be assessed by examining the maximum power generated at each joint. Judge et al. (28) and Riley et al. (29) found that elders, when asked to walk fast, did not increase their maximum ankle plantar flexor moment implying that impaired push-off might be a factor limiting gait speed. However, linear power-flow analyses (discussed later) indicate that there is not a direct link between push-off and propulsion (29–31). Further, Kerrigan et al., in a study of a larger group, found that healthy elderly subjects were able to increase their peak ankle plantar flexor moment and power in order to walk faster. There is evidence that improving lower extremity strength improves mobility and gait speed (32).

2. Gait Patterns Associated with Impaired Balance Control

While strength affects balance control (33), a number of other functions with known age-associated changes are also factors. Vision, which commonly deteriorates with age, is important to balance control. Somatosensory function also seems to degrade with age, particularly in the presence of diabetes and circulatory dysfunction. The vestibular system may be impaired with age, due to physical degradation of the otoliths and subtle changes in cerebellar function. These age-related impairments can impair gait and mobility (34).

Standing balance control may be assessed in the gait laboratory using the force plates and posturography (35). Dynamic balance control may be characterized using such parameters as gait speed, double-support time and base of support width (27,36). Winter noted that the righting moment for dynamic balance is given by the person's weight and the distance from the projection of the center of mass (CoM) on the support surface to the ground reaction force point of action, the center of pressure (CoP) (37). The CoM–CoP moment arm can be used to quantify dynamic balance control (38–40). Balance control may be impaired by poor coordination of movement (41) and/or slow reaction times. Experimental protocols requiring the subjects to avoid obstacles have been used to assess this function in the gait laboratory (42–44). Increased variability in gait parameters has been observed in the elderly (45,46). While these tests are useful in comparing populations or assessing the effectiveness of interventions, they are not sufficiently sensitive or specific to be useful in evaluating individual patients.

Further, while characterizing the effect of balance impairment on overall gait function, they do not define or quantify the fundamental impairment.

3. Alterations in Gait Due to Restricted Range
of Motion and Flexibility

The mobility of elders may be adversely affected by the loss of flexibility and range of motion. In particular, Kerrigan et al. (47) found that maximum hip extension was restricted in healthy elders compared to young persons and even more restricted in elders who tend to fall (48). Further, exercise programs that specifically increase hip extension range of motion improve gait speed and normalize pelvic kinematics (49). Gait analysis is more effective at determining the dynamic hip range of motion than the classic Thomas Test (50). These findings suggest that assessment of flexibility is important in elderly patients, and that dynamic measures such as gait analysis may be more sensitive and specific than the classic physical examination.

D. Orthotic Influence on Gait

Orthoses are commonly prescribed to improve the gait of patients with orthopedic or neurological disorders (51). A gait deviation or compensation may be caused by anatomic abnormalities or by the orthosis. In some instances, such as circumduction, the orthosis itself can cause the compensation; a knee–ankle–foot orthoses, which has a knee lock, interferes with the wearer's ability to flex the knee during swing phase. In other cases, a faulty orthosis hampers walking. For example, if the ankle control on an ankle–foot orthosis is eroded or malaligned, the patient may exhibit foot slap during loading response.

VI. GAIT ANALYSIS—CURRENT DEVELOPMENTS

As we stated earlier, gait analysis has reached a point where the fundamental technologies, procedures, and analysis techniques are in place, and "routine" clinical application is feasible. The consensus in the gait analysis community is that the highest priority for development in the field is research on the efficacy, outcomes, and cost-effectiveness of gait analysis (52). That said, there are ongoing advances in the technology and analysis techniques that are likely to significantly improve the usefulness of gait analysis in the near future. Two areas receiving attention in the community and among vendors are improved tracking of kinematics, and model-aided analysis.

A. Improved Tracking

Improvements in motion capture system sampling rate and resolution were chiefly motivated by the desire to automate kinematic marker identification and tracking. Now that that goal has been achieved, further improvements in the technology are enabling the use of a larger number of smaller markers. The availability of additional kinematic markers makes it possible to optimize estimates of body segment kinematics (53–55). Additional markers also make it possible to track more segments. One result of this line of development is the widespread use of whole body marker sets, which allow the acquisition of upper body as well as lower limb kinematics. Whole body kinematics will make gait analysis more relevant to pathologies that impair balance and posture control (41,56–58).

A second result of being able to use more and smaller kinematic markers is that it is now possible to treat the foot as a multi-segment structure rather than a single rigid body. This will improve gait analysis as a tool for detecting and quantifying foot deformities. It will also enhance analysis of the kinetics of gait. The inverse dynamics used to assess kinetics in gait analysis is known to be imperfect (59). Errors in the estimates of body segment mass and inertial properties (59) and body segment velocities and accelerations (60,61) limit the accuracy of inverse dynamics. However, the inadequacy of the single segment foot model for characterizing the foot–floor interaction is also an important source, perhaps the major source, of error in inverse dynamic analysis. While application of multi-segment foot models to kinetic analysis of gait is in a very early stage, it is already shedding light on the power absorption that goes on within the foot complex (62).

B. Model-Based Analysis

Computer models can be used to enhance the quality and information content of inverse dynamic analysis, and to implement forward dynamic analysis and predict the effects of interventions to alter and improve the patient's gait pattern. Musculoskeletal modeling packages and dynamic simulation software are being integrated into motion laboratory systems. It is becoming feasible to develop biomechanical and musculoskeletal models of individual patients based on measurements and data acquired in the gait laboratory.

1. Enhanced Inverse Dynamic Analysis

One use of model-based analysis is simply to improve the quality of motion analysis data. Classic motion analysis kinematic methods assume that the tracking markers are at specified anatomic locations and connect the dots to form a representation of the patients posture. The analysis does not consider whether the resulting configuration is anatomically or kinematically possible. Model-based analysis first develops an anatomical model of the patient. This model specifies the dimensions of the body segments and the feasible motion of the joints connecting the body segments. The analysis then finds the body configuration meeting the model constraints that provides a best fit for the measured marker positions. Data that cannot fit the model within reasonable limits are rejected. While it is difficult to quantify how much this process improves the analysis (63), it at least transfers some of the burden of identifying useless data from the gait laboratory personnel to the gait laboratory technology.

Model-aided analysis can also enhance the information content of gait analysis. Inverse dynamic analysis calculates the net forces and moments acting at a joint. Model-based analysis can provide the orthopedist or rheumatologist with estimates of the internal forces acting on the anatomical or orthotic components of the joint (64–70). Models that include muscle attachment points can be used to assess the contribution of muscle tightness to postural deformity (71,72). Power-flow analysis (29,30,73) supplements inverse dynamic analysis by revealing how energy generated at one joint is transferred to other body segments. Induced acceleration analysis (31,74) reveals how the kinetics of one joint affect the overall body kinematics. Together these techniques can be used to determine how specific impairments affect overall function, or how what appears to be a joint-specific impairment can be the result of more proximal or distal involvement (75).

2. Forward Dynamic Modeling

Inverse dynamics and the modeling methods described so far estimate the forces and moments producing a movement from the measured kinematics. Forward dynamic modeling estimates the kinematics of movement given known force and moments. Forward dynamic models may be driven by muscles and used to assess the roles of specific muscles in producing the motion patterns (76–79). In this role, it is highly complementary to power flow and induced acceleration analyses.

There has long been an interest in forward dynamic modeling as a predictive tool (80). Forward dynamic modeling can predict how an intervention will alter the physics of movement, but not how the patient will adapt to the altered dynamics. Thus, the frequently stated goal of being able to show patients how they walk after an intervention can only be achieved when the intervention also determines the available compensations (81) or specifically includes the motor control function (82). Future developments of the predictive aspects of forward dynamic modeling will likely be coupled with developments in the fields of functional electrical stimulation, and the development of active (powered) and smart (controlled passive) orthotics and prosthetics.

VII. SUMMARY

A modern gait analysis laboratory enables quantitative measurement of human walking. Such a laboratory provides the researcher with specialized tools with for investigating gait and movement. In certain cases, a modern laboratory may also be used to address important clinical questions, but generally today, routine assessment is not performed in the lab. In recent years, the technology has become easier to use and more reliable. As the cost goes down, ease of use increases, and the technology continues to improve, we may look forward to seeing more increased clinical application of the high-tech lab.

REFERENCES

1. Rose GK. Clinical gait assessment: a personal view. J Med Eng Technol 1983; 7(6):273–279.
2. Whittle MW. Clinical gait analysis: a review. Hum Mov Sci 1996; 15(3): 369–387.
3. Perry J. Gait Analysis: Normal and Pathological Function. Thorofare: SLACK, Inc., 1992.
4. Kerrigan, D., M. Schaufele, and M. Wen, *Gait Analysis*, in *Rehabilitation Medicine, Principles and Practice, Third Edition*, J. DeLisa and B. Gans, Editors. 1998, Lippincott-Raven: Philadelphia.
5. Sutherland DH, Olshen RA, Biden EN, Wyatt MP. The Development of Mature Walking. Philadelphia: Mac Keith Press, 1988.
6. Nene A, Mayagoitia R, Veltink P. Assessment of rectus femoris function during initial swing phase. Gait Posture 1999; 9(1):1–9.
7. Annaswamy TM, Giddings C, Della Croce U, Kerrigan DC. Rectus femoris: its role in normal gait. Arch Phys Med Rehabil 1999; 80:930–934.
8. Kerrigan DC, Todd MK, Riley PO. Knee osteoarthritis and high-heeled shoes. Lancet 1998; 351(9113):1399–1401.
9. Peat M, Dubo HI, Winter DA, Quanbury AO, Steinke T, Grahame R. Electromyographic temporal analysis of gait: hemiplegic locomotion. Arch Phys Med Rehabil 1976; 57(9):421–425.
10. Hirschberg GG, Nathanson M. Electromyographic recordings of muscular activity in normal and spastic gaits. Arch Phys Med Rehabil 1947; 33:217–224.
11. Knutsson E, Richards C. Different types of disturbed motor control in gait of hemiparetic patients. Brain 1979; 102(2):405–430.
12. Shiavi R, Bugle HJ, Limbird T. Electromyographic gait assessment, part 2: preliminary assessment of hemiparetic synergy patterns. J Rehabil Res Dev 1987; 24(2):24–30.
13. Kerrigan DC, Sheffler L. Spastic paretic gait: an approach to evaluation and treatment. Crit Rev Phys Med Rehab 1995; 7:253–268.
14. Winters TF, Gage JR, Hicks R. Gait patterns in spastic hemiplegia in children and young adults. Am J Bone Joint Surg 1987; 69:437–441.
15. Kerrigan DC, Gronley J, Perry J. Stiff-legged gait in spastic paresis. A study of quadriceps and hamstrings muscle activity. Am J Phys Med Rehabil 1991; 70(6):294–300.
16. Kerrigan DC, Roth RS, Riley PO. The modelling of spastic paretic stiff-legged gait based on actual kinematic data. Gait Posture 1998; 7:117–124.
17. Kerrigan DC, Bang MS, Burke DT. An algorithm to assess stiff-legged gait in traumatic brain injury. J Head Trauma Rehabil 1999; 14(2):136–145.

18. Kerrigan DC, Frates EP, Rogan S, Riley PO. Spastic paretic stiff-legged gait: biomechanics of the unaffected limb. Am J Phys Med Rehabil 1999; 78(4): 354–360.

19. Kerrigan DC, Frates EP, Rogan S, Riley PO. Hip hiking and circumduction: quantitative definitions. Am J Phys Med Rehabil 2000; 79(3):247–252.

20. Treanor WJ. The role of physical medicine treatment in stroke rehabilitation. Clin Orthop 1969; 63:14–22.

21. Sutherland DH, Santi M, Abel MF. Treatment of stiff-knee gait in cerebral palsy: a comparison by gait analysis of distal rectus femoris transfer versus proximal rectus release. J Pediatr Orthop 1990; 10(4):433–441.

22. Waters RL, Garland DE, Perry J, Habig T, Slabaugh P. Stiff-legged gait in hemiplegia: surgical correction. Am J Bone Joint Surg 1979; 61(6A):927–933.

23. Simon SR, Deutsch SD, Nuzzo RM, Mansour MJ, Jackson JL, Koskinen M, Rosenthal RK. Genu recurvatum in spastic cerebral palsy. Report on findings by gait analysis. Am J Bone Joint Surg 1978; 60(7):882–894.

24. Kerrigan DC, Deming LC, Holden MK. Knee recurvatum in gait: a study of associated knee biomechanics. Arch Phys Med Rehabil 1996; 77(7):645–650.

25. Kerrigan DC, Riley PO, Rogan S, Burke DT. Compensatory advantages of toe walking. Arch Phys Med Rehabil 2000; 81(1):38–44.

26. Imms FJ, Edholm OG. Studies of gait and mobility in the elderly. Age Age 1981; 10(3):147–156.

27. Winter DA, Patla AE, Frank JS, Walt SE. Biomechanical walking pattern changes in the fit and healthy elderly. Phys Ther 1990; 70(6):340–347.

28. Judge JO, Davis RB III, Ounpuu S. Step length reductions in advanced age: the role of ankle and hip kinetics. J Gerontol Ser A Biol Sci Med Sci 1996; 51(6): M303–M312.

29. Riley PO, Della Croce U, Kerrigan DC. Effect of age on lower extremity joint moment contributions to gait speed. Gait Posture 2001; 82:1251–1254.

30. Meinders M, Gitter A, Czerniecki JM. The role of ankle plantar flexor muscle work during walking. Scand J Rehabil Med 1998; 30(1):39–46.

31. Riley PO, Della Croce U, Kerrigan DC. Propulsive adaptation to changing gait speed. J Biomech 2001; 34(2):197–202.

32. Chandler JM, Duncan PW, Kochersberger G, Studenski S. Is lower extremity strength gain associated with improvement in physical performance and disability in frail, community-dwelling elders? Arch Phys Med Rehabil 1998; 79(1): 24–30

33. Kerrigan DC, Lee LW, Nieto TJ, Markman JD, Collins JJ, Riley PO. Kinetic alterations independent of walking speed in elderly fallers. Arch Phys Med Rehabil 2000; 81(6):730–735.

34. Duncan PW, Chandler J, Studenski S, Hughes M, Prescott B. How do physiological components of balance affect mobility in elderly men? Arch Phys Med Rehabil 1993; 74(12):1343–1349

35. Shepard NT. The clinical use of dynamic posturography in the elderly. Ear Nose Throat J 1989; 68(12):940.

36. Winter DA, Patla AE, Frank JS. Assessment of balance control in humans. Med Prog Technol 1990; 16(1–2):31–51.

37. Winter DA. Biomechanics and Motor Control of Human Movement. 2nd ed. New York: John Wiley and Sons, 1990.
38. Krebs DE, Gill-Body KM, Riley PO, Parker SW. Double-blind, placebo-controlled trial of rehabilitation for bilateral vestibular hypofunction: preliminary report. Otolaryngol Head Neck Surg 1993; 109(4):735–741.
39. Benda B, Riley P, Krebs D. Biomechanical relationship between center of gravity and center of pressure during standing. IEEE Trans Rehabil Eng 1994; 2: 3–10.
40. Tucker CA, Ramirez J, Krebs DE, Riley PO. Center of gravity dynamic stability in normal and vestibulopathic gait. Gait Posture 1998; 8(2):117–123.
41. Kaya BK, Krebs DE, Riley PO. Dynamic stability in elders: momentum control in locomotor ADL. J Gerontol Ser A Biol Sci Med Sci 1998; 53(2):M126–M134.
42. Patla AE, Prentice SD, Robinson C, Neufeld J. Visual control of locomotion: strategies for changing direction and for going over obstacles. J Exp Psychol Hum Percept Perform 1991; 17(3):603–634.
43. Eng JJ, Winter DA, Patla AE. Strategies for recovery from a trip in early and late swing during human walking. Exp Brain Res 1994; 102(2):339–349.
44. Eng JJ, Winter DA, Patla AE. Intralimb dynamics simplify reactive control strategies during locomotion. J Biomech 1997; 30(6):581–588.
45. Hausdorff JM, Mitchell SL, Firtion R, Peng CK, Cudkowicz ME, Wei JY, Goldberger AL. Altered fractal dynamics of gait: reduced stride-interval correlations with aging and Huntington's disease. J Appl Physiol 1997; 82(1): 262–269.
46. Hausdorff JM, Edelberg HK, Mitchell SL, Goldberger AL, Wei JY. Increased gait unsteadiness in community-dwelling elderly fallers. Arch Phys Med Rehabil 1997; 78(3):278–283.
47. Kerrigan DC, Todd MK, Della Croce U, Lipsitz LA, Collins JJ. Biomechanical gait alterations independent of speed in the healthy elderly: evidence for specific limiting impairments. Arch Phys Med Rehabil 1998; 79(3):317–322.
48. Kerrigan D, Lee L, Collins J, Riley P, Lipsitz L. Reduced hip extension during walking: healthy elderly and fallers versus young adults. Arch Phys Med Rehabil 2001; 82(January):26–30.
49. Kerrigan DC, Xenopoulos-Oddsson A, Sullivan MJ, Lelas JJ, Riley PO. Effect of a hip flexor-stretching program on gait in the elderly. Arch Phys Med Rehabil 2003; 84(1):1–6.
50. Lee LW, Kerrigan DC, Della Croce U. Dynamic implications of hip flexion contractures. Am J Phys Med Rehabil 1997; 76(6):502–508.
51. Edelstein JE. Orthotic assessment and management. In: O'Sullivan SB, Schmitz TJ, eds. Physical Rehabilitation Assessment and Treatment. Philadelphia: F. A. Davis, 2000.
52. Cooper RA, Quatrano LA, Stanhope SJ, Cavanagh PR, Miller F, Kerrigan DC, Esquenazi A, Harris GF, Winters JM. Gait analysis in rehabilitation medicine: a brief report. Am J Phys Med Rehabil 1999; 78(3):278–280.
53. Mann RW, Antonsson EK. Gait analysis—precise, rapid, automatic, 3-D position and orientation kinematics and dynamics. Bull Hosp Joint Dis Orthop Inst 1983; 43(2):137–146.

54. Andriacchi TP, Alexander EJ. Studies of human locomotion: past, present and future. J Biomech 2000; 33(10):1217–1224.

55. Alexander EJ, Andriacchi TP. Correcting for deformation in skin-based marker systems. Journal of Biomechanics 2001; 34(3):355–361.

56. Riley PO, Mann RW, Hodge WA. Modelling of the biomechanics of posture and balance. J Biomech 1990; 23(5):503–506.

57. Winter DA, MacKinnon CD, Ruder GK, Wieman C. An integrated EMG/biomechanical model of upper body balance and posture during human gait. Prog Brain Res 1993; 97:359–367.

58. Zachazewski JE, Riley PO, Krebs DE. Biomechanical analysis of body mass transfer during stair ascent and descent of healthy subjects. J Rehabil Res Dev 1993; 30(4):412–422.

59. Hatze H. The fundamental problem of myoskeletal inverse dynamics and its implications. J Biomech 2002; 25(1):109–115.

60. van den Bogert A, Read L, Nigg BM. A method for inverse dynamic analysis using accelerometry. J Biomech 1996; 29(7):949–954.

61. Ladin Z, Wu G. Combining position and acceleration measurements for joint force estimation. J Biomech 1991; 24(12):1173–1187.

62. MacWilliams BA, Cowley M, Nicholson DE. Foot kinematics and kinetics during adolescent gait. Gait Posture 2003; 17(3):214–224.

63. Meglan DA. Enhanced analysis of human locomotion. PhD thesis, in Mechanical Engineering, The Ohio State University, Columbus, OH, 1991:271.

64. Harrington IJ. A bioengineering analysis of force actions at the knee in normal and pathological gait. Bio-Med Eng 1976; 11(5):167–172.

65. Lehmann JF, Warren CG. Restraining forces in various designs of knee ankle orthoses: their placement and effect on the anatomical knee joint. Arch Phys Med Rehabil 1976; 57(9):430–437.

66. Andriacchi TP, Andersson GB, Fermier RW, Stern D, Galante JO. A study of lower-limb mechanics during stair-climbing. Am J Bone Joint Surg 1980; 62(5):749–757.

67. Czerniecki JM, Lippert F, Olerud JE. A biomechanical evaluation of tibiofemoral rotation in anterior cruciate deficient knees during walking and running. Am J Sports Med 1988; 16(4):327–331.

68. Mikosz RP, Andriacchi TP, Andersson GB. Model analysis of factors influencing the prediction of muscle forces at the knee. J Orthop Res 1988; 6(2):205–214.

69. Brand RA, Pedersen DR, Davy DT, Kotzar GM, Heiple KG, Goldberg VM. Comparison of hip force calculations and measurements in the same patient. J Arthroplasty 1994; 9(1):45–51.

70. Simonsen EB, Dyhre-Poulsen P, Voigt M, Aagaard P, Sjogaard G, Bojsen-Moller F. Bone-on-bone forces during loaded and unloaded walking. Acta Anatomica 1995; 152(2):133–142.

71. Delp SL, Ringwelski DA, Carroll NC. Transfer of the rectus femoris: effects of transfer site on moment arms about the knee and hip. J Biomech 1994; 27(10):1201–1211.

72. Delp SL, Arnold AS, Speers RA, Moore CA. Hamstrings and psoas lengths during normal and crouch gait: implications for muscle-tendon surgery. J Orthop Res 1996; 14(1):144–151.
73. McGibbon CA, Krebs DE, Puniello MS. Mechanical energy analysis identifies compensatory strategies in disabled elders' gait. J Biomech 2001; 34:481–490.
74. Kepple TM, Siegel KL, Stanhope SJ. Relative contributions of the lower extremity joint moments to forward progression and support during gait. Gait Posture 1997; 6(1):1–8.
75. Riley PO, Kerrigan DC. Kinetics of stiff-legged gait: induced acceleration analysis. IEEE Trans Rehabil Eng 1999; 7(4):420–426.
76. Zajac FE. Muscle and tendon: properties, models, scaling, and application to biomechanics and motor control. Crit Rev Biomed Eng 1989; 17(4):359–411.
77. Zajac FE, Gordon MS. Determining muscle's force and action in multi-articular movement. Exercise Sport Sci Rev 1989; 17:187–230.
78. Neptune RR, Kautz SA, Zajac FE. Contributions of the individual ankle plantar flexors to support, forward progression and swing initiation during walking. J Biomech 2001; 34(11):1387–1398.
79. Zajac FE, Neptune RR, Kautz SA. Biomechanics and muscle coordination of human walking. Part II: lessons from dynamical simulations and clinical implications. Gait Posture 2003; 17(1):1–17.
80. Brand RA, Pedersen DR. Computer modeling of surgery and a consideration of the mechanical effects of proximal femoral osteotomies. Hip 1984:193–210.
81. Tashman S, Zajac FE, Perkash I. Modeling and simulation of paraplegic ambulation in a reciprocating gait orthosis. J Biomech Eng 1995; 117(3):300–308.
82. Yamaguchi GT, Zajac FE. Restoring unassisted natural gait to paraplegics via functional neuromuscular stimulation: a computer simulation study. IEEE Trans Biomed Eng 1990; 37(9):886–902.

4

Age-Associated Changes in the Biomechanics of Gait and Gait-Related Falls in Older Adults

James A. Ashton-Miller

Biomechanics Research Laboratory, Department of Mechanical Engineering, University of Michigan, Ann Arbor, Michigan, U.S.A.

I. PREVALENCE OF GAIT PROBLEMS AMONG OLDER ADULTS

Problems with mobility in older adults are common. In the United States, among persons 65 years and older, approximately 19% receive help with walking, 10% have difficulty with bathing, and 8% receive help with bed or chair transfers (1). The rate at which these problems occur increases progressively after age 65 years and climbs sharply after age 80 years, so that, for example, more than 34% of non-institutionalized persons who are 85 years or older have mobility problems (see also Chapters 1 and 8). In this chapter, we shall first focus on how advancing age alters biomechanical capacities relevant to gait-related activities. Then we will review the biomechanics of gait as they apply to older adults, some of the reasons why falls occur during gait, and finally, when a fall occurs, the biomechanical factors that determine whether an injury will result from the fall.

II. AGE-RELATED CHANGES IN BIOMECHANICAL CAPACITIES

The biomechanical factors that underlie mobility impairments among older adults in general, and falling and fall injuries in particular, are not well understood. To come to that understanding, examination of the changes in biomechanical capabilities that occur with natural aging and with disease is merited. This section discusses the changes that occur in myoelectric latencies, reaction times, proprioception, joint ranges of motion (ROM), and muscular strengths and the rapid development of those strengths.

A. Muscle Strength and Power

The loss of strength with age, even in healthy and physically active older adults, has long been recognized. Isometric strengths peak at about age 25 years and then decline. The loss is approximately one-third by age 65 years. Isometric strength is more reliably measured, and considerably greater values are recorded, when the patient exerts force on a fixed force transducer, rather than one held by an examiner. To express the strength developed about the joint in units of torque, the force (in newtons) developed by the limb segment against a force-measuring transducer is multiplied by its lever arm (in meters) about the joint being tested. Mean strengths of female adults of any age are about one-third lower than those of male adults. However, when those strengths are normalized by body size (for example, by dividing by the body weight times body height), then there is often no longer a significant gender difference in normalized strengths. Reports of strength values vary widely because they depend on many factors: for example, substantially on which subjects are measured, at which joint angles, whether under isometric or constant velocity conditions, and, at constant velocity, whether muscle shortening or lengthening is occurring. Thus, for the hip flexor muscles, which are needed to recover balance after tripping by swinging a leg forward rapidly, maximum hip flexor torque decreases linearly with increasing hip flexion angle, and, additionally, with increasing hip flexion speed. The capacity to move a limb segment or limb rapidly can best be measured by the maximum power developed about the relevant joint. Since power is defined as the product of torque and angular velocity, high hip flexion power values would be attained by being able to develop a large torque about the joint at a high rotational velocity. Maximum power usually occurs in a shortening muscle at about one-third of the maximum movement velocity. Older adults are particularly prone to loss of torque, and therefore power, at high velocities because of the irreversible loss of the largest (and fastest) motor units with age. The current methods for measuring maximum power developed at speeds over 250°/sec, however, leave much to be desired because of substantial measurement artifacts. Age differences in strength have been reported to be smaller when muscles lengthen than when they shorten.

The decline with aging in the ability of muscles to produce power is perhaps best illustrated by records of elite athletic performances. In short-distance races, male elite runners more than 70 years old run approximately one-third slower than do elite young adult male athletes. In long-distance races, male elite runners more than 70 years old run approximately half as fast as elite young adult male athletes. In rodent muscle, power outputs decline with aging approximately 30% in absolute terms and 20% on a per-unit-muscle-mass basis. Age-related changes in muscle morphology and physiology have been widely reported. The maximum speed of unloaded shortening and contraction times for specific fiber types do not seem to change significantly with aging, but fast/slow fiber innervation ratios do seem to do so. Muscle power reduction with aging may also be due to systemic factors, such as declines in cardiopulmonary function. It is thus likely that in order to maintain muscle function in older adults, the focus should be on the assessment and training of power in addition to isometric joint torques (2). With age-related declines, walking speed becomes more dependent on leg strength and power than aerobic capacity (3–6).

B. Rapid Development of Joint Torque Strengths

Upon a substantial perturbation of standing balance, fewer than 500 msec are often available for the critical initial phase of balance restoration; yet, 300–400 msec can be required to develop maximum joint torques. Even older adults who are healthy and physically active have diminished abilities to develop large joint torques rapidly, compared with young adults. More-over, older females have lower torque development rates than do older males. For example, in one study, the mean total time required to develop 60 Nm of ankle plantarflexion torque, when subjects were asked to develop maximum torque as fast as possible, was 311 msec in young adult females and 472 msec, or 161 msec (52%) longer, in older females (Fig. 1) (7). Corresponding times for males were 270 and 313 msec (16% longer), respectively. Maximum rate of torque development tends to correlate highly with maximum voluntary torque strength, with correlation coefficients of the order of 0.8. Owing to slowing in peak rate of joint torque development abilities, capacities of even healthy old adults to recover balance or to carry out other time-critical actions that require moderate-to-substantial strengths, such as those required to avoid obstacles that come suddenly to attention, may be considerably reduced.

C. Source of Age Differences in Rapid Strength Development

Measurements of myoelectric signals in ankle dorsiflexor and plantarflexor muscles during rapid isometric and isokinetic exertions have been used to explore the extent to which this age-related slowing in rapid torque develop-ment might be attributed to neural factors, that is, those processes that pre-cede the initiation of muscle contraction. In one study, latency times, muscle activation rates, and myoelectric activity levels of agonistic and antagonistic muscles were quantified (8). There were few marked age differences in the

Plantarflexion

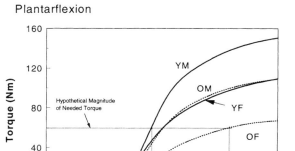

Figure 1 Mean age and gender differences in rapid development of ankle plantar-flexor torque. The subjects tested were healthy young and older (Y, O) females and males (F, M). Time is measured from a light flash cue signaling the subjects to push against a pedal as hard and as fast as possible. The four subject groups exhibited nearly the same mean reaction times, approximately 160 msec. However, the mean time needed to develop a given magnitude of torque varied substantially among the four age/gender groups. For example, with a plantarflexion torque of 60 Nm required to regain balance upon the initiation of a fall, YM would need approximately 275 msec to develop that torque, and OF would need approximately 475 msec. *Source*: Data from Ref. 7.

latencies or in the onset rates or magnitudes of agonistic or antagonistic muscle activities during maximum isometric and during isokinetic exertions. Myoelectric latency times were statistically associated with age, but in the mean, they were only approximately 10–25 msec longer in the old. Given the outcomes of this study, the differences observed in rapid torque development abilities in healthy elderly compared with healthy young adults seem due largely to differences in muscle contraction mechanisms once contraction is initiated, rather than to differences in the speeds of stimulus sensing or central processing of motor commands or to differences in the muscle recruitment decisions that precede contraction initiation.

D. Myoelectric Latencies

The myoelectric latency or premotor time is the delay from a test stimulus cue to the onset of the first measurable change in myoelectric activity in a muscle. Myoelectric activity refers to the electrical signals sent through the nerves to initiate or modify the muscle contraction process. At the latency time, the muscle will not yet have developed any significant contractile force or, if already contracted, changed that force.

Myoelectric latencies typically range from 30 to 50 msec for myotatic reflexes involving the muscle spindles; 50 to 80 msec when cerebellar or cortex neural pathways are involved; 80 to 120 msec when afferent receptors and higher motor centers are involved; and 120 to 180 msec for volitional actions.

E. Reaction Times

The term "reaction time" refers to the delay from a stimulus signaling a needed reaction to making a movement or developing a force. Reaction time is longer than myoelectric latency because it includes both the myoelectric latency and the finite time required for a muscle to develop or change its force magnitude after myoelectric activity begins. This additional time interval is called the motor time.

Researchers define reaction time in different ways. For example, in studies of postural control, reaction time is often defined as the delay between stimulus onset and the first measurable change in the forces exerted by the feet on the floor support. This reaction force is usually measured with an instrumented force plate. This force development reaction time incorporates the myoelectric latency and the motor time required for the muscles to contract in order to alter the body configuration enough to change the support force. This happens with little discernible foot movement or limb segment acceleration. Reaction time has also been defined to be the delay from stimulus onset until the first detectable acceleration of a body segment. This might be termed segment acceleration reaction time. Reaction time has also been defined as the delay from stimulus onset until a limb has been moved to a target. This movement-to-target reaction time incorporates myoelectric latencies, body segment acceleration reaction times, and body segment movement times. Movement reaction times depend on how far body segments have to be moved. Reaction times also depend on how many choices a subject has in responding to a cue. Simple reaction times are those exhibited when no choices are given the subject. Choice reaction times are those exhibited when the subject must decide between two or more courses of action, depending on which of two or more cues is presented. Choice reaction time increases in proportion to the logarithm of the number of choices to be made. Choice reaction times are typically considerably longer than simple reaction times. Speed–accuracy tradeoff is also found in reaction time measurements. As the accuracy requirement of the task is increased, reaction time increases. These differing definitions of reaction time and differing circumstances in which it is measured make it difficult to compare results from different studies of reaction times. Meaningful data on group differences in reaction times seem best obtained by comparing those times among different groups performing the same task, with the reaction time measure defined in the same way among the different groups.

F. Age and Gender Group Differences in Latencies and Reaction Times

Many studies report statistically significant age differences, but not gender differences, among healthy adults in myoelectric latencies. Myoelectric latencies are typically 10–20 msec longer in healthy old adults than in young adults.

Age systematically increases force development reaction times. Older, compared with younger, adults require perhaps 10–30 msec longer to volitionally develop from rest modest levels of ankle torque or to begin to take a step upon loss of balance. Systematic age differences in movement-to-target reaction times are often found. They increase on the order of 2 msec per age decade between the second and 10th decades. Age differences increase when subjects are not warned several seconds in advance of the cue that it is imminent. Much larger increases with age occur in choice reaction times than in simple reaction times. For example, in 10-choice button pushing tasks, where choices were identified by letter or color or both, choice reaction times increased 27–86% more in subjects aged 65 to 72 years compared with those aged 18 to 33 years. No notable gender differences in reaction times have been reported.

G. Biomechanical Effects of Age Differences in Latencies and Reaction Times Are Minor

These statistically significant age differences, of 10–20 msec in latencies and of 15–30 msec in some reaction times, are seldom critical to mobility function. Even rapid responses in time-critical situations take place over perhaps 200–500 msec, so these latency and reaction time differences are not large compared with the task execution times. For example, among healthy older adults, the time required to fully contract a muscle is of the order of 400 msec. The time to lift a foot in order to take a quick step is of the order of 200–400 msec. In Section IV.B, we shall see that warning times of the order of 400–500 msec are needed to be able to stop before reaching or to turn away from obstacles that come suddenly to attention.

Reaction times, which include muscle latencies, are task and strategy dependent. They are modifiable by central command. Reaction times of older adults are not always slower than those of the young. Moreover, reaction times do not necessarily predict performance on complex mobility tasks. For example, one of our studies found that simple reaction times in lifting a foot immediately upon a visual cue did not predict how well the same young or older subjects could avoid stepping on a suddenly appearing obstacle during level gait (9). In fact, age group differences in simple reaction times were substantially larger than age group differences in the response times needed to avoid the obstacles successfully.

H. Joint Ranges of Motion (ROM)

Body joint ROM have generally been found to diminish with age, but not all findings are consistent. For example, studies have reported approximately a 20% decline between ages 45 and 70 years in hip rotation and 10% declines in wrist and shoulder ROM. Comparisons of the ROM of lower extremity joints for young and middle-aged adults with those for older adults showed declines ranging from negligible to 57%. At age 79 years, one-fifth of a large group of subjects had restricted knee joint motion and two-thirds had restricted hip joint motion. Among more than 3000 blue-collar workers with ages ranging from 20 to 60 years, a 25% decline with age was found in ability to bend to the side and a 45% decline in shoulder motion. Declines of 25–50% have been found in various ROM of the lumbar spine between the ages of 20 and 80 years. However, a comparison between two groups with mean ages of approximately 65 and 80 years found no significant differences in 28 different joint ROM. At least one study suggests that passive or active stretching exercises can increase hip extension ROM in young adults by 8–17°, and another study suggested that exercises with a focus on stretching improve spine flexibility in older adults. In the absence of disease, age-related changes in ROM are not usually sufficient to alter comfortable gait. Neurologic and musculoskeletal diseases, however, can have profound effects on both ROM and gait.

I. Proprioception

The term "proprioception" describes awareness of body segment positions and orientations. Relatively few studies have examined changes with aging in proprioception. One study found joint position sense in the knee to deteriorate with age. Joint angles could be reproduced to within 2° by 20-year-olds, but only to within 6° by 80-year-olds. Twenty-year-olds could detect passive joint motions of 4°, but 80-year-olds could detect only motions larger than 7°. Other studies have found no major decline with age in motion perception in finger and toe joints but have found declines with aging in sensing vibration. Proprioceptive acuity at a joint is significantly better when muscles at the joint are active than when they are passive. Proprioceptive thresholds during weight bearing are at least an order of magnitude lower than those typically reported during non-weight-bearing tests. Recent studies exploring the effect of age on thresholds for sensing ankle rotations show that healthy adults can sense quite small rotations in the sagittal and frontal planes under the weight-bearing conditions of upright stance. The probability of successful detection of rotation increases with increasing magnitude and speed of imposed foot rotation (10,11). A 10-fold reduction in the angular threshold was observed on increasing the speed of rotation from 0.1° to 2.5° per second, but thresholds did not further reduce at higher speeds. In healthy adults between the third and eighth decades, age, rotation angle, and rotation speed also significantly affected the threshold for sensing the direction of foot rotation. Threshold angles were three to four times larger in older females than in young females (12).

Individuals with central or peripheral proprioceptive impairments can exhibit articular pathology. Examples include Charcot changes occurring in the upper or lower extremities due to central nervous system (CNS) damage by syringomyelia over several levels of the spinal cord, and changes in the foot or ankle due to lower extremity peripheral neuropathy often associated with diabetes. Peripheral neuropathy increases the proprioceptive threshold at the ankle nearly five-fold compared with age-matched healthy controls (13). This increased threshold adversely affects postural stability and raises the risk of obstacle contact during the swing phase of gait, suggesting one mechanism that might underlie the 20-fold increase in fall risk and the six-fold increase in fall-induced fractures that these patients have (14).

III. GAIT ON LEVEL SURFACES

The basic theoretical and experimental methods for studying human gait are reviewed in a classic textbook by Winter on the subject (15). The goal of gait analysis is usually to quantify the biomechanics of human locomotion in terms of variables such as its symmetry, stepping characteristics, stride variability, timing, metabolic cost, energetic efficiency, joint loading, and strength (moment) demands at each joint. Comparisons of one patient or patient group may be made to healthy age-matched controls in order to determine the biomechanical effects of a given pathology.

A. Gait Analysis Techniques

Human gait is a repeating gait cycle of two steps that comprise a single stride. Each cycle consists of two single (one leg) and two double (two leg) support phases. The cycle (and single support phase) starts at heel contact of the ipsilateral foot and extends through its foot flat, toe push-off, and finally toe-off phases until the first step (and ipsilateral leg single support phase) ends with heel contact of the contralateral foot. The second step then similarly starts with heel contact, foot flat, and toe-off phases of the contralateral foot until the ipsilateral foot heel contact. Each period of double support lasts from ipsilateral heel contact to toe-off. Each foot contacts the ground for about 60% of the stride cycle in normal gait: this decreases to 35% at the gait-to-run transition (16).

B. Classical Gait Biomechanics

Classic gait analysis usually involves 3-D measurements of body segment motions (kinematics), using one or more optoelectronic systems that track the 3-D locations of a standardized set of three or more markers on each body segment, foot–ground interaction (reaction) forces via one or more instrumented force plates embedded in the floor, and muscle myoelectric activity patterns via surface bipolar surface (and sometimes intramuscular wire) electrodes placed parallel to the fiber direction over the belly of each muscle of interest (see Chapter 3). In some patient groups (for example, diabetic neuropathics), it may also be instructive for orthotists to examine plantar pressure distributions under the foot using an array of tiny insole pressure sensors to check for unusually high-pressure regions. Foot–ground contact timing can be registered using portable equipment involving force sensing resistor switches placed beneath the heel and/or metatarsals, or body-mounted accelerometers.

Care should be taken to separate the concepts of the whole-body center of mass (often abbreviated as COM, the 3-D location of the weighted average of the mass distribution of the body), center of gravity (COG, the vertical location of the COM, with gravity acting downward along the vertical projection of the COM), and center of pressure (COP, the location of the center of the ground reaction force that is required to prevent the individual from sinking through the floor). In upright stance, ankle dorsiflexion moves the COP backward, thereby allowing the ground reaction force to apply a moment about the COM to accelerate it forward, while an ankle plantarflexion moment does the opposite. Similarly, in unipedal stance, active ankle inversion moves the COP laterally, while an eversion moment achieves the opposite. In asymmetric bipedal stance, the COM can initially be accelerated forward by moving the center of ground reaction posteriorly via retraction of the lead limb with dorsiflexion of its foot, backward via lead limb protraction and plantarflexion of its foot, to the left by protracting the right limb and inverting its foot, and vice versa. In quiet stance, Winter (17) has likened the COP to a sheep dog herding its flock, the COG; the vertical projection of the COG onto the floor must stay within the base of support represented by the feet, and more specifically within the functional base of support (the maximum possible area encompassing the locus of possible COP locations). When the vertical projection of the COG on the floor falls to the right, for example, the COP must move further to the right of the COG (i.e., "herd" it) in order for the ground reaction force to exert a moment about the COM that will restore balance, and vice versa to the left. During gait, the projection of the COG onto the ground is always being "herded" on its left by the COP under the left foot, and on its right by the COP under the right foot, as the COP passes from heel to toe under each stance foot.

From the kinematic (movement) and kinetic (force) measurements, calculations of each 3-D body segment position, velocity, and acceleration may be made. Once subject anthropometry is known, these data may be inserted into Newton's laws and the "inverse dynamics" method used to calculate the joint intersegmental forces and (turning) moment acting at each joint at any instant in time (18). By considering all the forces and moments acting on a segment, the moment acting at the joint of interest can be calculated by considering the dynamic equilibrium of the segment. The net "muscle" moment component (the sum of all the muscle and ligamentous moments acting at that joint) must equal a gravitational moment component (due to gravity acting at the COM of the segment) plus an inertial component (due to angular acceleration of the adjacent segment) plus a joint acceleration moment (due to the linear vertical and horizontal accelerations of the joint) plus a moment due to an external force(s) acting on the segment. An illustrative worked example of this type of analysis is given by MacKinnon and Winter (19) in their partitioning of the ankle moment required to control balance in the frontal plane during the single support phase of gait.

The Newton–Euler inverse dynamics calculation usually proceeds using a "bottom-up" (ground-up) approach starting with the location, magnitude, and orientation of the force-plate-measured ground reaction force under the foot, the first segment. (For simplicity, each body segment is assumed to be rigid.) It then proceeds to consider the joint intersegmental forces and moments acting at the first joint, the ankle, after taking into account the gravitational and inertial forces acting at the COM of the foot. Then because the foot exerts intersegmental forces and moments (equal and opposite to those just calculated) on its neighboring segment, the shank, via the ankle joint, the forces and moments acting at the next joint, the knee, are calculated after taking into account the gravitational and inertial forces acting at the leg COM. The process is then repeated for the thigh and then the head–arms–trunk (so-called "HAT" segment), and down the contralateral leg. The order of magnitude of sagittal plane ankle, knee, and hip moments required for level gait have been measured as being between 1 and 2 Nm/kg body weight, with plantarflexor moments being 12% less in elderly males than young males (15). For the elderly males, power generated and absorbed by the hip muscles at different points in the gait cycle peaked at about 0.75 and 0.5 W/kg, respectively; 0.5 and 1 W/kg at the knee, respectively; and 2.5 and 0.5 W/kg at the ankle.

The final step is to calculate the work done and power (rate of work) developed at each joint. Work (defined as force times distance moved) may be either positive- or negative-valued. By convention, when a muscle is activated and is allowed to shorten, it is defined as performing positive work; whereas if it is activated and forcibly lengthened, it is defined as doing negative work. For example, in the double support phase, the trailing leg muscles perform 97% of the positive external work, and the leading leg muscles simultaneously perform over 94% of the negative external work during that portion of the gait cycle (20). The instantaneous muscle power developed at a joint is the product of the net muscle moment times the segment angular velocity and, as with work, it can take a positive or negative value. Power is transferred from one segment to the next by muscle (21) acting in either a lengthening, isometric, or shortening contraction mode. Even when a muscle contracts isometrically, energy may be stored by stretching its endo- and exotendon, to be returned to the adjacent segment at a later stage in the gait cycle (22).

Using the inverse dynamics approach, it is possible to calculate the net muscle moment acting about a joint in any plane of interest, say. Andriacchi and co-workers have successfully used this approach to obtain clinically useful insights into how certain types of knee pathology affect gait: an example is how osteoarthritis affects knee adduction moments in patients before and after knee surgery (23,24). In the context of arthritis, it is worth making the point that muscle contractions, rather than body weight, are the major elements loading a joint. This is because the moment arm about a joint may be 5 to 10 times smaller than that of the gravitational force acting on a body segment about a joint. A simple example is the quadriceps muscle lever arm about the knee being approximately 5 cm, but body weight acting about the knee at a distance of 25 cm from the knee while ascending a step, necessitating a quadriceps force of at least five (25 cm/5 cm) times body weight.

Due to the multiplicity of muscles acting about any joint, it is not possible to calculate the individual muscle forces directly because there are more muscles than there are equations to solve for them. This is known to biomechanists as the muscle redundancy or indeterminacy problem. There are, for example, some 15 muscles responsible for the sagittal plane moments at the hip (iliopsoas, gluteus maximus, semitendinosus, semimembranosus, biceps femoris, sartorius, rectus femoris), knee (semitendinosus, semimembranosus, biceps femoris, sartorius, rectus femoris, vastus medialis, lateralis, and intermedius, gastrocnemius), and ankle (gastrocnemius, soleus and tibialis anterior and posterior, peroneus longus and brevis). Six equations of motion may be applied at each joint, but there are three (unknown) joint intersegmental forces and always more than three (unknown) muscle forces acting about the joint to solve for, as can be seen for any joint in the leg. Over the past 50 years, techniques have been developed to try to solve redundancy problems to calculate muscle forces, with varying degrees of success depending on the complexity of the movement or task. Each approach makes an assumption about how the central nervous system (CNS) might control the muscles in a given task.

For example, in the 1960s, J.P. Paul tried lumping agonists together to simplify the problem. In the 1980s, Crowninshield and others assumed that the CNS always optimized (maximized or minimized) one or more variables.

For example, it might minimize the sum of the joint forces, or the sum of the muscle forces, or the sum of the muscle forces raised to a power (in an effort to reduce muscle fatigue) (25). The difficulty with the optimization approach is that when an individual walks along a walkway, one can never be certain that his/her CNS is trying to optimize anything. While it is possible that someone walking at their comfortable speed may indeed be trying to minimize metabolic energy cost (see, for example, Ref. 26), especially over longer distances, there is no proof that this is so over the short 10 or 20 m walkways typically used for laboratory gait analysis. The difficulty is even greater if there is pathology of any sort, because now the patient may be trying to minimize discomfort or pain, maximize stability, or maximize symmetry of gait in order to appear as cosmetically normal as possible to the examiner. In the 1990s, an EMG-driven approach was pioneered by McGill and colleagues (22) in which the magnitude of EMG signals were used to estimate muscle forces by assuming a certain relationship, say linear, between EMG amplitude and muscle force.

A difficulty with the EMG-driven modeling approach to estimating muscle forces is that, because one cannot measure muscle force directly (without implanting a buckle force transducer on its tendon), the relationship between EMG activity and muscle force is never known exactly. So errors creep into the calculation. More recently, stochastic methods have been used to estimate muscle forces, again with mixed success. In general, the methods for calculating muscle forces work best when there is little doubt about the CNS goal or objective for the activity: as, for example, in a maximal height jump (27). In that example, it is clear what the CNS is trying to maximize. As mentioned above, this is not true of gait studied in the laboratory, or of any other mobility tasks performed in a submaximal manner, for that matter.

C. Simplified Gait Analysis Approaches

It is not always necessary to use full 3-D techniques or know exactly how the muscles act to develop useful insights about gait. Depending on the question to be answered, simpler and portable measurement techniques can suffice (28,29). One example is the insight obtained by Hausdorff and colleagues (16) that shows that subtle (<3%) increases in step time variability, as measured using a simple pressure switch under the plantar surface of each foot, over the several hundred steps taken in a 2-minute walk at comfortable speed, are a reliable predictor of injurious falls in a group of community-dwelling elderly. The advantage of this approach is the simplicity with which one aspect of gait is measured over longer distances and times than is possible in the gait laboratory. If other information, say on foot placement or step kinematics, is required for certain patient groups, then an alternative approach is required. However, the advent of microminiature linear accelerometers and angular rate gyroscopes, and ever better digital video recorders, may yield exciting new measurement approaches in the next few years.

D. Individual Muscle Contributions to Segmental Motions

It is important to first understand how the CNS coordinates muscles to achieve gait before one can analyze how a muscle impairment might affect gait. Zajac and colleagues (4) have pointed out the limitations of the inverse dynamics approach in this regard and have developed a novel theoretical technique for analyzing and comparing the segmental actions of individual muscles, such as the soleus and gastrocnemius, during gait. This enables one, for example, to estimate their contributions not only to moments about the ankle joint, but also to the horizontal and vertical accelerations of remote body segments (30). The knowledge that the soleus directly affects the dynamics of the torso several body segments removed is useful for analyzing and comparing the role of each lower extremity muscle during gait. For example, Zajac and colleagues estimated the contribution of soleus and gastrocnemius to forward progression (accelerates the trunk forward), trunk "support" (develops a vertical acceleration of the trunk), and swing initiation (develops positive power in the swing leg). Both muscles were found to provide trunk "support" during single leg stance. In mid-single limb stance, gastrocnemius accelerates the leg while soleus decelerates it; however, soleus accelerates the trunk while the gastrocnemius decelerates it. In late single leg stance, both muscles contribute to forward progression, while also helping to provide trunk support. However, the energy supplied by soleus mainly contributes to forward progression, while that of gastrocnemius goes into swinging the leg.

E. Energetics of Level Human Gait

If one thinks of gait as vaulting over each foot in the manner of an inverted pendulum whose lower end represents the foot and the upper end represents the whole-body COM, then energy is transferred back and forth between the potential energy of the body's COM at top-dead center and the kinetic energy of the COM as it reaches its lowest point until transitioning to the new step. At every point in time, the law of conservation of energy applies to any body structure during gait. This means that both work (a measure of energy flow from one segment to another as one segment does work on another—has the same units, J, as energy) and power (rate of energy change) can be tracked as they flow from one body segment to another during the cycle. Since muscles are the only source of mechanical energy generation during gait, metabolic energy (commonly measured by oxygen consumption) must flow into them in order for them to exert forces and do internal work on moving body segments. But since, during one gait cycle on the level, no net external work is performed (the body's COM ends up at the same height as it started, and the subject is not doing work on an external object, like pulling a sled, for instance), all the metabolic energy goes into moving the body segments, not doing external work. Energy can be transferred from one segment to the other by passive means, via one segment acting on its neighbor. For example, the energy lost by the swing leg toward the end of its swing is transferred upward through the thigh and converted into kinetic energy to accelerate the trunk forwards (31).

The energy cost of walking at a comfortable gait speed (1.5 m/sec) is least when the stride frequency is 0.95 Hz, and stride frequencies higher or lower than this will drive up the cost (26). Recent studies have used simple models to study the energetics of gait (20). These studies show that during the single support phase, the human body can be thought of as an inverted pendulum pivoting over the support foot that acts more or less as a circular roller (32). While mechanical energy is theoretically not required for that pendular motion, energy is required to transition the COM motion over to the contralateral inverted pendulum represented by the other limb. At a fixed cadence, the metabolic rate was highly sensitive to step length, in fact increasing with the fourth power of step length (i.e., thus a halving of step length decreased energy use 16-fold). Much of this metabolic cost was required for the step-to-step transition, while very little was required to swing the limbs forward. More complicated models have demonstrated that much of the mechanical work done by muscles during gait goes into lifting the whole-body COM during single support (33). This may partly explain why frail elderly tend to take steps that are shorter than overall foot length—they are energetically far less costly than a normal step length. (A shuffling gait also enables the user to maintain a larger quasistatic base of support, thereby increasing the margin of stability represented by the distance of the projected COG to the margin of the rhomboidal base of support, represented by the outline of the two feet.)

Recent studies have also shown that the mechanical and metabolic cost of gait increased by more than 50% when step widths wider than preferred values (0.15–0.45 step length) were used (34), again because of greater mechanical costs in the step-to-step transition phase. The authors concluded that since energy costs increased with extremely narrow foot widths, it appears as if humans normally select a step width to minimize energy cost. Pathologies such as peripheral neuropathy can often increase step width to cause wide-based gait (35), thereby decreasing the efficiency of the gait.

F. Motor Control of Gait

This topic is the subject of several books (31,36). Simple dynamical model analyses of gait conducted by Kuo and co-workers suggest that while the stability of human gait is essentially determined by the passive dynamical properties of the limbs in the sagittal plane, it requires active control to achieve stability in the frontal plane (37). This frontal plane control is mainly accomplished by the step-to-step adjustment of step width. Experimental evidence supporting this idea is the finding that lateral variability is 79% larger than sagittal variability. This variability was increased over 50% in the absence of vision. The step-width-to-step-length ratio was found to be 0.13.

The stride-to-stride and intersubject variability in the magnitude of the muscle activity, as measured by the temporal EMG profiles of 15 unilateral leg muscles along the erector spinae, have been quantified in healthy younger adults (38). Distal muscles were more active than proximal muscles. Most variability was found in the proximal muscles. Biarticular muscles were more variable than monoarticular muscles. Reliable EMG estimates of muscle firing patterns can be obtained by averaging EMG data from no more than three strides (39).

G. Gait Initiation and Termination

Gait is essentially triggered by initiating a forward fall in order to accelerate the whole-body COM forward (40). This is achieved by bilateral activation of the dorsiflexors and inhibition of the plantarflexors, and concurrent abduction of the swing hip, along with concurrent flexion of the stance limb hip and knee (41).

The energetics of gait initiation in healthy adults have been studied by Miller and Verstraete (42), who found similar, but diminished, amplitudes of energy flow compared to regular gait. The greatest energy cost was during the push-off phase from the stance limb in taking the second step, as the individual accelerated up to comfortable gait speed by the end of the third full step (42). Group differences have recently been noted between fallers and healthy older controls in that fallers took a smaller and more variable first step followed by a prolonged double support period (43).

Gait termination is characterized by the need to arrest the forward momentum of the whole-body COM using the frictional forces underfoot. Two steps are the minimum number of steps required to abruptly terminate gait from a comfortable walking speed in order to avoid a collision (44). This is achieved by increasing the extensor musculature activity in the lead limb (45), followed by deceleration of the swing limb (46). In healthy adults, gait termination behavior has been shown to be more variable in the absence of visual feedback or diminished proprioceptive information from plantar surfaces (47).

H. Effects of Age

In older adults free of overt neurological, musculoskeletal, cardiorespiratory, or cognitive problems, comfortable gait speed declines minimally until

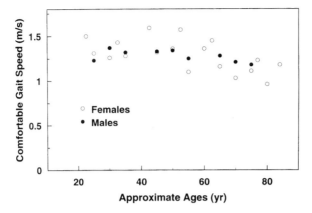

Figure 2 Age and gender differences in self-selected comfortable gait speeds. These data are graphed using those abstracted by Bohannon et al. (48), from seven earlier literature reports. The mean speeds reported vary substantially. Nonetheless, the general trend is for comfortable gait speed to decline minimally until approximately age 60 years and then to decline by 1–2% per year through age 80 years.

approximately age 60 years and then declines by 1–2% per year through age 80 years; however, there is substantial variability among studies of age-associated changes in comfortable gait speed (Fig. 2) (48–50).

The causes of gait slowing with age are a subject of controversy. They may be multifactorial, including subtle age-related changes in joint stiffness, leg strength, and energy conservation strategies. Independent of age, comfortable walking speed associates non-linearly with muscle strength (Fig. 3) (51) and maximum aerobic power. Much of the decline in speed has been attributed to reductions in step length. The earliest studies of gait in older adults found that men in their 60s demonstrated significantly shorter step and stride lengths and decreased ankle extension and pelvic rotation compared with younger males (for example, 52).

More recent studies have confirmed those findings, but not without exception. One concluded that increased variability in gait should not be regarded as a normal concomitant of old age (53). Still another study found that among older adults, more than 40% of the variance in normal walking speed can be accounted for by differences in height, calf muscle strength, and the presence of health problems such as leg pain (54). A recent prospective study in older women showed that those with the poorest knee strength and balance scores were five times more likely to develop severe walking disability than those with normal function (55). There is little evidence of an association between age-related reductions in stride length and gait speed and a tendency to fall (56). On the other hand, increased stride time

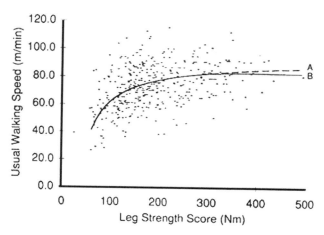

Figure 3 Comfortable gait speed is non-linearly related to leg muscle strength score in a population-based sample of over 400 adults between 60 and 96 years. The strength score was formed from the summed isokinetic right knee and ankle flexor and extensor muscle strengths. The regression curve represents the fit for an average age of 76 years. *Source*: Data from Ref. 51.

variability is associated with a five-fold increase in the risk of falling in community-dwelling elderly (16).

Age causes the hip extension measured during gait to decrease from a mean (SD) of 20(4) degrees in healthy young to 14(4) degrees in healthy old and 11(5) degrees in elderly fallers (57), suggesting tightness of the hip muscles in these individuals.

I. Turning in a Confined Space

It is often necessary to use the feet to turn through angles such as 90° or even 180° as one moves from one point to another (from a sink to a cupboard in bathrooms and kitchens, for example). Falling while walking and turning has been shown to be 7.9 times more likely to result in hip fracture than falling while walking straight (58). In an effort to understand why turning is linked to such a high rate of injury, my collaborators and I have studied how age affects the kinematics of foot placement in turning in healthy young and older women (Fig. 4). We found that subjects generally have a preferred direction of turning and that, in older women, the minimum foot separation distance during the turn was less when turning in the non-preferred direction than in the preferred direction, raising the probability of foot–foot collisions, and hence a trip (59). The minimum foot separation distance during the turns was generally 55% more variable in the healthy older women than

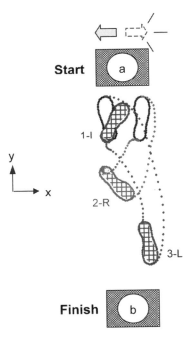

Figure 4 Overhead view of foot kinematics while an elderly female turns in a confined space to move a bowl from table (a) to table (b), starting from a symmetric stance. A common preparatory stepping pattern and foot trajectories for the 180° turn to the right are shown (cross-hatched pattern: 1-L = first step, left foot; 2-R = second step, right foot; etc.). Left and right arrows denote darkened and illuminated visual cues, respectively, showing the subject the desired turn direction. *Source*: From Ref. 59.

in young controls, despite the fact that they turned 20% slower. These results corroborate and extend those of Thigpen et al. (60).

J. Divided Attention During Gait

As detailed further in Chapter 6, cognitive demand relative to cognitive capacity substantially influences physical task performance. As mobility task complexity increases, so do the cognitive demands placed on the individual. For example, it has been noted that healthy elderly slow more than healthy young do when turning or performing a secondary task (61). The need to perform two tasks simultaneously or to divide attention degrades performances of healthy elderly significantly more than for healthy young. For example, in a study of abilities to step over suddenly appearing obstacles while walking, the attention of groups of healthy young and older adults was divided by having them simultaneously respond in two reaction time tasks (62). Both young and old adults had a significantly increased risk of obstacle contact while negotiating obstacles when their attention was divided, but attention division diminished obstacle avoidance abilities of the old significantly more than it did in the young. These results suggest that diminished abilities to respond to physical hazards present in the environment when attention is directed elsewhere may partially account for high rates of falls among the elderly. Many frail elderly are aware of the difficulty of dividing one's attention while walking, as demonstrated by the ability of the simple but effective "Stops Walking When Talking Test" to predict impending falls in certain groups of older adults (63). The effects of age on multitasking are discussed in greater detail in Chapter 6.

IV. OBSTACLE AVOIDANCE DURING LEVEL GAIT

A. Importance of Vision

The first line of defense in avoiding an obstacle is vision. Visual scanning for upcoming obstacles in the gait path allows the stride pattern to be altered in time to avoid the obstacle. Patla and colleagues have done considerable work in this area (64). Healthy individuals generally look two steps ahead (equivalent to 800–1000 msec before the foot would land) in order to land the foot at a specific location during gait (65). In addition, the authors showed that healthy individuals do not need to scan ahead continuously (66). Rather, they need to scan for less than 50% of the time available at a comfortable gait speed in order to avoid the obstacle (67). It has also been shown that 68% of eye saccades to the stepping target location have already been completed while the foot that would step on the obstacle is still on the ground (and the remainder are completed in the first 300 msec of the swing phase) (68); gaze fixation of just over 50 msec sufficed to fixate the target location. If gaze is disrupted or obstructed just prior to lift off of the foot that would eventually step on the obstacle, then stepping accuracy is impaired (69).

Additional experiments have been performed to determine where subjects look when they are cued to change gait direction through 30° or 60° to the right or left of their gait path (70). Before the turn cue, subjects made saccades within the plane of progression to the end of the original gait path. After the cue, subjects' gaze acquired the new heading followed by a head and body rotation to new gait direction.

Given the importance of vision, it is not surprising that both visual impairment (depth perception and distant-edge-contrast sensitivity) in one or both eyes is an independent risk factor for falls in community-dwelling elderly (71). More recently, multifocal glasses have been found to impair depth perception and distance-edge-contrast sensitivity and their use should be avoided in unfamiliar environments (72).

B. Stepping Over or Avoiding Obstacles by Turning or Stopping

1. Avoiding Obstacles by Stepping Over Them

The effect of age on the foot clearance normally used to step over a fixed obstacle ranging in height from 0 to 6 in. shows that both healthy young and older subjects adopt a similar (generous) foot clearance and keep the approach foot and toes a similar distance from the obstacle (73). The abilities of healthy and physically active young and older adults, who were walking forward at approximately 1.3 m/sec, to step over an obstacle that suddenly appeared at seemingly random times and locations in front of them has also been examined (9). The appearance of this obstacle was arranged to give the subjects available response times that varied from 200 to 450 msec before they would have stepped on it. This task is a time-critical one, but because avoidance requires relatively minor changes in stepping pattern and relatively minor redistributions among segments of kinetic energies and forward momentum, the strength requirements of the task likely are modest. Few young or older adults could avoid obstacles if only 200 msec was available. Most young and old adults reliably avoided obstacles that appeared with a 450 msec warning time. Over all available response times used, the older adults had statistically significantly lower avoidance success rates than the young, but in biomechanical terms, it was estimated that they would have needed only 30 msec more warning time to have the same success rates as the young. No significant gender differences in avoidance abilities were found. In a companion paper, my colleagues and I demonstrated that both healthy young and older subjects could fall unintentionally while walking on a flat surface (74). They did this when they felt obliged to abruptly change their stride pattern due to a perceived obstacle that actually was just a stripe of light on the floor. An important "take home" point is that even the perception of an obstacle that might cause a trip can cause a real trip and unexpected fall on a flat surface.

2. Avoiding Obstacles by Turning Away Before Reaching Them

In a study of abilities to make sudden turns to avoid previously unseen obstacles, healthy older adults were substantially less successful than young when available response times were short (75,76). For example, for an available response time of 450 msec, mean success rates in completing the turn without colliding with the obstacle were 68% in young and 27% in older adults. Moreover, males had substantially better success rates for given available response times than did females in corresponding age groups. This task is a time-critical one: avoidance requires complete arrest of forward momentum and quick development of lateral momentum, but relatively minor redistributions of kinetic energies among segments. Therefore, the strength requirements of the task likely are moderate.

3. Avoiding Obstacles by Stopping Before Reaching Them

In a similar study of abilities to make sudden stops to avoid previously unseen obstacles, healthy old adults again were substantially less successful than young when available response times were short (44,76). For example, for an available response time of 525 msec, mean success rates in stopping before passing forward of the obstacle were 58% for young females and male adults and 51% for older males, but only 23% for older females. This task is also a time-critical one: avoidance requires complete arrest of forward momentum but also total dissipation of body kinetic energy. Thus, the strength requirements of this task likely are substantial.

A comparison of the effect of how available response time affects the success rates of stepping over, turning away from, or stopping before reaching an obstacle are shown in Fig. 5.

V. GAIT ON SURFACES THAT ARE NOT LEVEL

A. Stepping One Step Up or Down

The effect of age has been studied on the kinematics and dynamics of stepping up onto or down from a raised surface in a small sample of healthy young and older women (77). The elderly afforded the leading edge of the step significantly less foot clearance than the young did when stepping up (9 cm vs. 11 cm). This finding has since been corroborated in men by McFadyen and Prince (78), who ascribed it to limited pelvic rotation in the frontal plane, and shorter stride lengths among other factors. The foot clearance used was generally similar to that used to step over a fixed obstacle of equivalent height to the step (73,78). When stepping down, the foot clearance was much less, of the order of 1–3 cm, with the elderly affording the larger foot clearances under the lead and trailing foot. Lark et al. (76) have stressed the importance of stance limb dynamic ankle stiffness as the subject prepares to lower their COM to the next level.

B. Stair Locomotion

One of the mechanisms for a fall while descending stairs is thought to be a slip between the foot and the stair tread (80) which can occur due to a poor choice of shoe tread or stair covering materials, poor lighting, or visual impairments, to name but a few factors. A recent study by Hamel and Cavanagh (81) showed that confidence may play a major role in determining risk-taking behavior on stairs, such as for example whether the individual uses a handrail. The biomechanics of stair locomotion have been reviewed by Startzell et al. (82). The mean sagittal plane ranges of motion of the hip, knee, and ankle have been reported in adult males as 42°, 88°, and 27°, respectively (83). The same study quantified the maximum hip moments

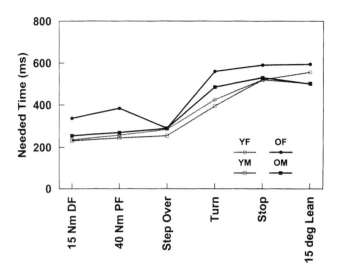

Figure 5 Summary of age and gender differences in times needed for various quick responses while walking. Mean values across groups of healthy older females (OF), older males (OM), young females (YF), and young males (YM) of the times required for six different responses are shown. The responses are indicated by the horizontal axis labels. Each of the situations being responded to is further described in the text of this chapter. From left to right, the responses are the development of, respectively, (1) 15 Nm of ankle dorsiflexor flexor torque, or (2) 40 Nm of ankle plantarflexor torque, as fast as possible; the achievement of a 50% rate of success in avoiding suddenly appearing obstacles by, respectively, (3) stepping over the obstacle, (4) turning away before reaching the obstacle, or (5) stopping before reaching the obstacle; and (6) the replacement of the stepped foot on the ground when recovering balance by taking a single step up on sudden release from a 15° whole-body forward lean. The data points are connected by lines only to help distinguish the four subject groups. *Source*: Replotted from Ref. 121.

required to ascend and descend stairs as being 124 and 113 Nm, respectively; knee moments as 57 and 147 Nm, respectively; and ankle moments as 137 and 108 Nm, respectively. Hence, the largest moments were developed by the knee extensors during descent, and by the ankle plantarflexors during ascent. As pointed out by Startzell et al. (82), the moments are large enough to exceed the functional reserve of some individuals.

C. Ramp Locomotion

The biomechanical demands of descending ramps of different inclinations have been investigated by Redfern and co-workers (84). With increasing ramp angle, step length and period decreased, while knee moment increased nearly four-fold to values of 1.5 Nm/kg body weight on a 20° ramp from values of 0.4 Nm/kg in level walking. Hip and ankle moments increased to a lesser extent. The peak foot–ground shear forces increased to 4.5 N/kg during heel contact, from +1.5 N/kg during heel contact and –1.5 N/kg on push-off while walking on the level. The required coefficient of friction (RCOF) to prevent the foot from slipping followed a similar pattern, increasing to 0.45 for the 20° ramp from a value of 0.2 on level ground.

D. Uneven Surface Locomotion

Many outdoor surfaces are irregular or uneven in nature. These include gravel, pebble, cobblestone, flagstone, and broken asphalt surfaces, and sand as well as frozen turf or snow surfaces, for example. Compared with the enormous body of literature on the mechanics and control of gait on flat level surfaces, relatively little is known about how humans negotiate uneven surfaces safely. Similarly, even less is known about the effect of age or disease on this capability.

That walking on an uneven or bumpy surface can pose a considerable challenge is evidenced by the fact that it was one of the two most frequent causes of falls in one study of community-dwelling elderly (85). One of the first studies of gait on uneven surfaces compared subjects with age-related maculopathy against controls while walking across level, compliant, and uneven surfaces (86). Moe-Nilssen (87) examined the reliability of trunk accelerometry while walking on uneven surfaces, while Menz and colleagues have used head and pelvic accelerometry to study healthy controls (88) and patients with peripheral neuropathy (89) walking on irregular surfaces. The patients had to slow their gait on the uneven surface. Li et al. (90) evaluated the effects of a walking intervention using cobblestone mats using the Medical Outcomes Study 120 item questionnaire and evaluations of instrumental activities of daily living, but did not study any kinematic or kinetic outcome variables. Most recently, Thies et al. (91,92) and Richardson et al. (93) have shown that an irregular surface increases step width variability in healthy young and old controls, and step time in peripheral neuropathic subjects who had to slow significantly on such surfaces. They showed that the irregular surface discriminated age and disease group differences in stepping pattern, as well as faller vs. non-faller group differences better than did similar tests on a level surface. They have also showed that the application of bilateral ankle braces improved the step width variability in neuropathics walking on uneven surfaces (35).

It is possible to "trip over one's own feet" when walking on uneven surfaces. This could be caused by narrowing the next step so much that it is placed across the midline, in what is known as a cross-over step (Fig. 6), thereby impeding the upcoming swing foot. My colleagues and I recently showed that a cross-over step is caused by stepping with a hard sole on a raised rigid perturbation of as little as 1.2 cm under the plantar surface of the medial forefoot (94).

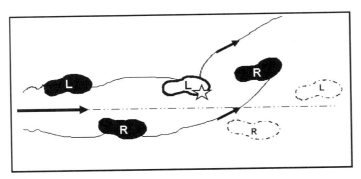

Figure 6 A cross-over step is caused by stepping on a single raised surface irregularity (indicated by the star) under the medial forefoot. *Source*: From Ref. 94. R and L denote right and left, respectively. The large arrow on the midline denotes the originally intended direction of progression, as do the dashed foot outlines. The smaller arrows on the foot marker trajectories connecting the solid black feet outlines show the actual direction of steps after the perturbation.

VI. TRIPS AND SLIPS

As already noted, the time available in which to recover from a substantial disturbance of upright balance or to safely arrest a fall is often less than 1 sec. For example, when walking forward at 1.3 m/sec, the comfortable walking speed typically self-selected by healthy young and old adults, only 200–300 msec may be available in which to make initial responses appropriate for balance recovery when tripping over an obstacle. If a large obstacle in the gait path, such as a moving vehicle, suddenly comes to attention 1 m ahead while walking at this speed, then a turn away from the obstacle or a stop before reaching it would have to be accomplished within approximately 750 msec. The term "time-critical" is used here to refer to such situations. Differences in abilities to respond appropriately in at least some time-critical situations may help explain age and gender differences in rates of falls and fall-related injuries.

A. Recovering from a Trip

A trip occurs when the swing foot encounters an obstacle, usually because the obstacle protrudes higher than the foot clearance afforded by the subject. The foot clearance used by young and old subjects to cross obstacles has been shown to be more than twice as much as the obstacle height and to increase with the height of the obstacle, and does not different with age (73). As long as the swing foot is not obstructed by an obstacle for longer than about 0.7 sec in a trip, then a healthy young subject can usually recover from the trip (95). Trips at any speed usually cause forward falls and frontal impacts, whereas slips and fainting while walking slowly are more likely to result in the individual landing on their hip (96).

Once a fall begins as a result of a trip, quick recovery of balance may be needed to avoid injury. In one set of studies by Grabiner and co-workers, forward falls were induced in healthy older adults by an unexpected trip or backward movement of the support surface (97). Factors associated with a failure to recover balance were one or more of the following: too short a recovery step, slower response time, greater trunk flexion angle at toe-off, greater trunk flexion velocity at recovery foot contact with the ground, and buckling of the recovery limb. In the case of an unexpected trip, Grabiner and colleagues have shown that there are two basic recovery strategies: a so-called "elevating" strategy and a "lowering" strategy (98). In the elevating strategy, the swing foot that is obstructed by the obstacle is directly lifted up and over the obstacle and then swung forward as quickly as possible as a (slightly delayed) recovery step. If it should prove difficult to disentangle the foot from the obstacle (thereby obviating use of the elevating strategy), then the subject can switch to a lowering strategy: the swing foot that is impeded by the obstacle is immediately placed onto the ground behind the obstacle to become the stance limb as the contralateral foot is lifted up and over the obstacle and used for the recovery step. Using a computer simulation of a simple inverted pendulum model to represent the forward fall of the body following the trip, this team found that the recovery foot placement must occur before the inclination of the COM exceeds a critical angle of 23–26° from the vertical (99). A faster response time was predicted to be more useful than a slower walking speed.

It has recently been shown that in the temporal domain there are two distinct phases of recovery from a trip in healthy adults: an early response and a later response. In the early response, a powerful stance limb plantar-flexion moment, knee extensor and hip extensor moment is used to slow the forward angular momentum (and rotation) of the whole body around the point of obstacle contact, as well as torso flexion about the hip joint (100). The powerful plantarflexion moment helps to achieve this by orienting the ground reaction force *in front of* the whole-body COM. The resultant slowing of forward angular momentum allows more time for the necessary second part of the response: the powerful hip and knee flexor moment required to swing the recovery limb forward fast enough and far enough to land its foot in front of the onward traveling whole-body COM. Finally, as the recovery limb impacts the ground, sufficient resistance must be generated by its knee and hip extensor muscles to resist flexion-buckling of the knee as the residual forward angular momentum of the body is attenuated. This resistance to buckling of the knee must come from the resistance of the knee extensor muscles to being forcibly lengthened. In other words the knee extensor muscles must first be adequately activated, and then there must be sufficient knee extensor muscle mass to generate adequate elastic and viscous resistance to the sudden stretch of the knee extensor muscles. Inadequate activation or inadequate knee extensor muscle mass will mean that the task demands will exceed the capacity of the knee muscles to handle the challenge, the knee will then buckle, and its owner will fall as the limb buckles under his/her weight.

It has recently been shown by Pijnappels et al. (101) that despite the fact that the initial reactions were not meaningfully slower, age adversely affects the ability of healthy individuals to generate an adequate stance limb ankle plantarflexor response and this caused the age-related increase in failure to recover from the trip.

My colleagues and I have studied the effect of age on the ability to recover from a forward fall by rapid step-taking (102). Subjects were released from a forward-leaning position and instructed to regain standing balance by taking a single step forward. Lean angle was successively increased until a subject failed to regain balance as instructed. This task is a time-critical one, likely requiring the use of maximal strengths. It was found that the mean maximum lean angle from which older males could recover balance as instructed, 23.9°, was significantly smaller than that for the young males, 32.5°. Corresponding angles for the females were 16.2° and 30.7°, but those numbers do not include five of the 10 older females, who could not recover balance from even the smallest lean angle at which they were tested, approximately 13° (103). Maximum lean angles were well correlated with the average forward step velocity and inversely correlated with the time required to unload the stepping foot, but were unrelated to myoelectric response latencies of ~70 msec in both young and elderly (104). A gender difference has been found in torques used for recovery of balance. None of the males needed to utilize their maximum ankle, knee, or hip torque capacities, but the young females utilized maximal hip flexion torques, and the older females utilized maximum plantarflexor, knee flexion, hip flexion, and extension torques (104).

From these studies, we can draw some lessons for planning future interventions. The results suggest that reduced abilities of healthy older adults to recover from forward falls result from an inability to generate adequate stance limb extensor torques and sufficiently rapid body segment movements, rather than from delayed initiation of response. This means that future interventions should target muscle training designed to increase hip, knee, and ankle extensor and flexion strengths, as well as the corresponding powers required to make sufficiently rapid movements.

B. Recovering from a Slip

An unexpected slip arguably demands the most physically challenging response required to recover balance during gait. Healthy young subjects walking onto a level slippery floor attempt to correct an ongoing slip between

25% and 45% of stance phase (190–350 msec after heel contact) (105). In healthy young adults, the initial response to an unexpected slip is an early flexor synergy (starting at about 146 msec) in the muscles of the perturbed limb, presumably serving to limit how far the slipping foot slips, bilateral shoulder muscle activation (143 msec) serving to produce bilateral arm elevation after about 288 msec, and rapid protraction of the trailing swing foot onto the ground in order to rapidly enlarge the base of support rearward (106,107) so as to be able to prevent a backward fall. They do this by slowing the acceleration of the whole-body COM by employing a flexor synergy of the trailing leg and decelerating the COM by using an extensor synergy of the leading leg (108). These authors found that the trailing leg takes an abbreviated step in order to be rapidly placed back on the ground to decelerate the descending COM. Arm elevation movements helped to dissipate forward momentum. After the first slip, healthy subjects exposed to successive slipping trials showed very rapid adaptation, with much less arm movement and more muscle co-contraction, often adopting a proactive "surfing" response whereby they slid forwards on both feet (106).

The physical characteristics determining the potential for a slip as well as the RCOF (ratio of the shear to the normal foot forces) on slippery surfaces have been reviewed by Gronqvist et al. (109) and Redfern et al. (84). Redfern and coworkers have demonstrated that on level floors and descending ramps healthy subjects make significant changes in gait (shorter stance phase duration, shorter normalized step lengths, and slower foot strike velocities) when anticipating the possibility of a slip (110).

C. Mechanisms Underlying Age and Gender Differences in Performance of Time-Critical Tasks With High Strength Demands

Some of the studies discussed here suggest that the source of both age and gender differences in performance of tasks that are both time critical and have high strength requirements lies primarily in strengths and speeds of muscle contraction, rather than in sensory processing or motor planning abilities. As pointed out earlier in this chapter, studies of myoelectric latencies for rapid ankle torque development have found no significant gender group differences. They have found statistically significant age group differences, but the differences in the mean latencies were only approximately 10–20 msec, whereas the total times needed to develop near-maximum torques were of the order of 400–600 msec. They showed that age group differences in the use of co-contraction were not responsible for the age group differences in torque development rates. Studies of mean reaction times have also found statistically significant age group differences in those times. However, those differences were only approximately 10–20 msec, whereas the total response times ranged approximately from 400 to 800 msec. No substantial gender differences were found in those reaction times. This suggests that among healthy older compared with young adults and among females compared with males, differences in rapid torque development abilities, noted earlier in this chapter, and differences in performance of tasks that are both time critical and have high strength requirements seem largely to be due to differences in strengths and speeds of muscle contraction once contraction is initiated, rather than to delays in initiating contraction.

The outcomes of the studies described, and those from other studies reported in the literature, suggest that healthy older compared with young adults, and healthy older females compared with older males, are more at risk for injury in tasks that are both time critical and have high strength requirements. Time-critical obstacle avoidance tasks involve rapid visual processing, rapid triggering of preplanned strategies, and rapid execution of movements, during which whole-body balance must be maintained. Among healthy adults, the times needed for the visual processing and response triggering phases are a few hundredths of a second longer for old than for young. In contrast, the times needed for movement execution are a few tenths of a second longer for old than for young. Almost exclusively because of these longer movement execution times, the warning times that older compared with younger adults need to successfully perform time-critical tasks with high strength requirements are a few tenths of a second longer. Although differences of a few tenths of a second in abilities to respond are not usually important, circumstances leading to needs for time-critical, high-strength responses probably combine at random. Sometimes the consequence of needing a few tenths of a second longer to execute avoidance or recovery maneuvers may not be small, and that need, when circumstances combine unfavorably, may substantially lower the probability of regaining balance or avoiding a fall-related injury.

VII. AGE AND GENDER DIFFERENCES IN FALLS AND FALL-RELATED INJURY RATES

The incidence of hip fractures rises much faster with age than that of falls. This increase in hip fractures with age is not fully accounted for by increases in the number of falls or decreases in bone mass of the hip with age. Therefore, other factors must increase susceptibility to hip fractures. The biomechanics of the fall arrest responses are likely to be among these factors. More than 85% of wrist fractures involve falls. The incidence of wrist fractures rises from age 50 to 65 years and then reaches a plateau after age 65 years, but why this occurs is not yet known.

Little is known about the changes with age in impending fall response biomechanics that must in part be responsible for these injury rate changes. For example, tripping during gait is commonly self-reported by older persons as a cause of falls. In a one year study of 1042 persons greater than 65 years of age, tripping was reported to be the cause of the fall in 53% of the 356 falls that were documented (111). Whatever the underlying neurological and physiological mechanisms, responses to trips are ultimately expressed in terms of biomechanical factors.

VIII. FALL-RELATED-INJURY BIOMECHANICS

A number of factors determine whether a fall will result in an injury: the initial conditions under which the fall begins, the biomechanics of the response during the fall, the passive and active mechanisms for dissipating energy upon impact with the ground or other surfaces, and the injury tolerance of the hard and soft tissues that are impacted. However, the biomechanics of fall arrests and of fall-related injuries have received little attention. Clear need exists to examine them, in order to improve assessments of risk and programs for both intervention and prevention.

A. The Biomechanics of Hip Fractures

The risk of bony fracture has been defined by Hayes and colleagues as the ratio, ϕ, of the magnitude of the force applied to the bone to the force necessary to cause fracture. When the value of ϕ exceeds 1.0, then fracture is inevitable. Ways of ameliorating fracture risk therefore include either finding fall strategies to decrease the impact load applied to the bone, using interventions to increase the fracture tolerance of the bone, or both. A fall from standing height directly onto the greater trochanter carries a 21-fold higher risk for hip fracture than landing on another body part (112,113). This is because the resulting loss in potential energy of the whole-body COM during such a fall is an order of magnitude greater than the average energy required to fracture the proximal femur in elderly cadaver specimens. Hence, falls in a lateral direction, which carry a higher risk for landing on the hip than other directions (114), must be avoided if possible. This is particularly true in an individual with reduced bone mineral density and reduced body mass index. Reductions in the latter are associated with less soft tissue over the hip to dissipate the impact energy (115). Hip pad protectors have been shown to be effective in reducing the risk of hip fracture in frail ambulatory elderly. By diverting the impact energy to adjacent tissues, the impact force on the hip may be more than halved. However, patient compliance has been problematic because the pads are uncomfortable to sleep with and the garment in which they are located can impede dressing and undressing.

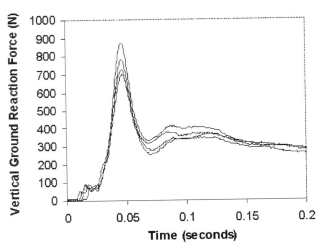

Figure 7 Example of the measured wrist impact force plotted versus time for one hand in four consecutive forward falls onto both arms for a young subject weighing 620 N. The subject fell onto a lightly padded surface from a shoulder height of 1 m. Note that (1) the time-to-peak-force is less than any upper extremity neuromuscular reflex, rendering reflexes unable to protect the wrist, and (2) the magnitude of the peak impact force on one hand exceeds as much as one body weight for a brief time in two of the four trials, mainly as a result of the ground arresting the downward momentum of the upper extremity over a relatively short distance. *Source*: Data from Ref. 117.

B.   The Biomechanics of Wrist Fracture

Once a fall is initiated, fall arrests have two post-initiation phases: a pre-impact phase and an impact phase. In a fall from standing height, the pre-impact phase lasts about 0.7 seconds as the body falls to the ground (116). The impact phase lasts only tens of milliseconds for structures near the impact site (Fig. 7) to a few tenths of a second at more proximal body sites further from impact. Thus, for structures near the impact site, like the hands and elbows in a forward fall, short- and long-loop neuromuscular reflexes are simply too long to be able to alter the fall arrest strategy during the impact phase.

The hands and arms are commonly used to protect the head and torso during a fall. The factors that determine the risk of Colles fracture, the most common upper extremity fall-related injury, include the height of the fall and the compliance of the surface. Moreover, at impact, the relative velocity of the hand as it strikes the surface, the elbow flexion angle, the angle of the lower arm with respect to the ground, and, of course, forearm bone mineral density status play a role (117). There is almost always time for older women or men to deploy their upper extremities in the event of a forward fall (118). But our research shows that a fall by an older woman from 25 cm or more onto a stiff surface, landing with a straight arm, will almost certainly break the wrist (119). However, falling onto a slightly flexed arm will reduce this risk (120), although triceps and shoulder muscle strength is required to prevent the elbow from buckling. This is one important justification to encourage maintenance of upper extremity muscle strength in older adults.

IX. CONCLUSIONS

Studies of the biomechanics of mobility and gait among healthy older adults suggest the following:

1. Comfortable gait speed is not usually affected by age-related changes in joint range of motion, joint flexibility, or reaction times.
2. Comfortable gait speed is relatively insensitive to age-related changes in muscle strength. Changes in comfortable gait speed usually only occur in association with larger declines in strength associated with age and disease.
3. There are substantial age and gender differences in abilities to develop joint torques rapidly. These differences generally only seem to be of importance when performing time-critical tasks requiring high strengths.
4. Recovery from trips and slips, and arresting a fall all require large joint torques and considerable strength. Inadequate strength is likely due to alterations in muscle contractile properties, suggesting promising avenues for intervention.
5. Even in healthy young and old adults, a fall can occur during gait on a perfectly flat surface if they suddenly feel compelled to abruptly change their stride pattern.
6. Gait tests performed on an irregular surface appear to discriminate age and disease effects better than gait tests conducted on a flat surface.

REFERENCES

1. Dawson D, Hendershot G, Fulton J. Aging in the Eighties: Functional Limitations of Individuals Age 65 Years and Over. Hyattsville, MD: National Center for Health Statistics, DHHS Publication, 1987:87–1250 (Advance Data No. 133).
2. Bean JF, Herman S, Kiely DK, et al. Increased velocity exercise specific to task (InVEST) training: a pilot study exploring effects on leg power, balance, and mobility in community-dwelling older women. J Am Geriatr Soc 2004; 52: 799–804.

3. Morley JE. Mobility performance: a high-tech test for geriatricians. J Gerontol A Biol Sci Med Sci 2003; 58:712–714.
4. Zajac FE, Neptune RR, Kautz SA. Biomechanics and muscle coordination of human walking. Part I: Introduction to concepts, power transfer, dynamics and simulations. Gait Posture 2002; 16:215–232.
5. Zajac FE, Neptune RR, Kautz SA. Biomechanics and muscle coordination of human walking. Part II: Lessons from dynamical simulations and clinical implications. Gait Posture 2003; 17:1–17.
6. Onder G, Penninx BW, Lapuerta P, et al. Change in physical performance over time in older women: The Women's Health and Aging Study. J Gerontol A Biol Sci Med Sci 2002; 57:M289–M293.
7. Thelen DG, Schultz AB, Alexander NB, Ashton-Miller JA. Effects of age on rapid ankle torque development. J Gerontol A Biol Sci Med Sci 1996; 51:M226–M232.
8. Thelen DG, Ashton-Miller JA, Schultz AB, Alexander NB. Do neural factors underlie age differences in rapid ankle torque development? J Am Geriatr Soc 1996; 44:804–808.
9. Chen HC, Ashton-Miller JA, Alexander NB, Schultz AB. Effects of age and available response time on ability to step over an obstacle. J Gerontol 1994; 49:M227–M233.
10. Gilsing MG, Van den Bosch CG, Lee SG, et al. Association of age with the threshold for detecting ankle inversion and eversion in upright stance. Age Ageing 1995; 24:58–66.
11. Thelen DG, Brockmiller C, Ashton-Miller JA, Schultz AB, Alexander NB. Thresholds for sensing foot dorsi- and plantarflexion during upright stance: effects of age and velocity. J Gerontol A Biol Sci Med Sci 1998; 53: M33–M38.
12. Ashton-Miller JA, Wojtys EM, Huston LJ, Fry-Welch D. Can proprioception really be improved by exercises? Eur J Knee Surg Sports Traumatol Arthrosc 2001; 9:128–136.
13. Van den Bosch CG, Gilsing MG, Lee SG, Richardson JK, Ashton-Miller JA. Peripheral neuropathy effect on ankle inversion and eversion detection thresholds. Arch Phys Med Rehabil 1995; 76:850–856.
14. Richardson JK, Ching C, Hurvitz EA. The relationship between electromyographically documented peripheral neuropathy and falls. J Am Geriatr Soc 1992; 40:1008–1012.
15. Winter DA. Biomechanics and Motor Control of Human Gait: Normal, Elderly and Pathological. 2nd ed. Ontario: University of Waterloo Press, 1991.
16. Hausdorff JM, Rios DA, Edelberg HK. Gait variability and fall risk in community-living older adults: a 1-year prospective study. Arch Phys Med Rehabil 2001; 82:1050–1056.
17. Winter DA. A.B.C. (Anatomy, Biomechanics, Control) of Balance during Standing and Walking. Waterloo: Graphic Services, 1995.
18. Vaughan CL, Davis BL, O'Connor JC. Dynamics of Human Gait.1st ed. Champaign, IL: Human Kinetics Publishers, 1992.
19. MacKinnon CD, Winter DA. Control of whole body balance in the frontal plane during human walking. J Biomech 1993; 26:633–644.

20. Donelan JM, Kram R, Kuo AD. Simultaneous positive and negative external mechanical work in human walking. J Biomech 2002; 35:117–124.
21. Neptune RR, Zajac FE, Kautz SA. Muscle force redistributes segmental power for body progression during walking. Gait Posture 2004; 19:194–205.
22. Cholewicki J, McGill SM, Norman RW. Comparison of muscle forces and joint load from an optimization and EMG assisted lumbar spine model: towards development of a hybrid approach. J Biomech 1995; 28:321–331.
23. Sharma L, Hurwitz DE, Thonar EJ, et al. Knee adduction moment, serum hyaluronan level, and disease severity in medial tibiofemoral osteoarthritis. Arthritis Rheum 1998; 41:1233–1240.
24. Prodromos CC, Andriacchi TP, Galante JO. A relationship between gait and clinical changes following high tibial osteotomy. J Bone Joint Surg Am 1985; 67:1188–1194.
25. Crowninshield RD, Brand RA. The prediction of forces in joint structures; distribution of intersegmental resultants. Exerc Sport Sci Rev 1981; 9:159–181.
26. Alexander RM. Energetics and optimization of human walking and running: The 2000 Raymond Pearl Memorial Lecture. Am J Hum Biol 2002; 14:641–648. Available from: medline. Accessed 2002.
27. Pandy MG, Zajac FE, Sim E, Levine WS. An optimal control model for maximum-height human jumping. J Biomech 1990; 23:1185–1198.
28. Menz HB, Latt MD, Tiedemann A, Mun San Kwan M, Lord SR. Reliability of the GAITRite® walkway system for the quantification of temporo-spatial parameters of gait in young and older people. Gait Posture 2004; 20:20–25.
29. Henriksen M, Lund H, Moe-Nilssen R, Bliddal H, Danneskiod-Samsoe B. Test–retest reliability of trunk accelerometric gait analysis. Gait Posture 2004; 19:288–297.
30. Neptune RR, Kautz SA, Zajac FE. Contributions of the individual ankle plantar flexors to support, forward progression and swing initiation during walking. J Biomech 2001; 34:1387–1398.
31. Winter DA. Biomechanics and Motor Control of Human Movement. New York: John Wiley & Sons, Inc., 1990.
32. Hansen AH, Childress DS, Knox EH. Roll-over shapes of human locomotor systems: effects of walking speed. Clin Biomech 2004; 19:407–414.
33. Neptune RR, Zajac FE, Kautz SA. Muscle mechanical work requirements during normal walking: the energetic cost of raising the body's center-of-mass is significant. J Biomech 2004; 37:817–825.
34. Donelan JM, Kram R, Kuo AD. Mechanical and metabolic determinants of the preferred step width in human walking. Proc R Soc Lond B Biol Sci 2001; 268:1985–1992.
35. Richardson JK, Thies SB, DeMott TK, Ashton-Miller JA. Interventions improve gait regularity in patients with peripheral neuropathy while walking on an irregular surface under low light. J Am Geriatr Soc 2004; 52:510–515.
36. Duysens J, Smits-Engelsman BCM, Kingma H, eds. Control of Posture and Gait. Amsterdam: Symposium of the International Society for Postural and Gait Research, 2001.
37. Bauby CE, Kuo AD. Active control of lateral balance in human walking. J Biomech 2000; 33:1433–1440.

38. Winter DA, Yack HJ. EMG profiles during normal human walking: stride-to-stride and inter-subject variability. Electroencephalogr Clin Neurophysiol 1987; 67:402–411.

39. Arsenault AB, Winter DA, Marteniuk RG, Hayes KC. How many strides are required for the analysis of electromyographic data in gait? Scand J Rehabil Med 1986; 18:133–135

40. Halliday SE, Winter DA, Frank JS, Patla AE, Prince F. The initiation of gait in young, elderly, and Parkinson's disease subjects. Gait Posture 1998; 8:8–14.

41. Elble RJ, Cousins R, Leffler K, Hughes L. Gait initiation by patients with lower-half parkinsonism. Brain 1996; 119(Pt 5):1705–1716.

42. Miller CA, Verstraete MC. A mechanical energy analysis of gait initiation. Gait Posture 1999; 9:158–166.

43. Mbourou GA, Lajoie Y, Teasdale N. Step length variability at gait initiation in elderly fallers and non-fallers, and young adults. Gerontology 2003; 49: 21–26.

44. Cao C, Ashton-Miller JA, Schultz AB, Alexander NB. Effects of age, available response time and gender on ability to stop suddenly when walking. Gait Posture 1998; 8:103–109.

45. Hase K, Stein RB. Analysis of rapid stopping during human walking. J Neurophysiol 1998; 80:255–261.

46. Crenna P, Cuong DM, Breniere Y. Motor programmes for the termination of gait in humans: organisation and velocity-dependent adaptation. J Physiol 2001; 537:1059–1072.

47. Perry SD, Santos LC, Patla AE. Contribution of vision and cutaneous sensation to the control of centre of mass (COM) during gait termination. Brain Res 2001; 913:27–34.

48. Bohannon RW, Andrews AW, Thomas MW. Walking speed: reference values and correlates for older adults. J Orthop Sports Phys Ther 1996; 24:86–90.

49. Bohannon RW. Strength deficits also predict gait performance in patients with stroke. Percept Mot Skills 1991; 73:146.

50. Bohannon RW. Comfortable and maximum walking speed of adults aged 20–79 years: reference values and determinants. Age Ageing 1997; 26:15–19.

51. Buchner DM, Larson EB, Wagner EH, Koepsell TD, de Lateur BJ. Evidence for a non-linear relationship between leg strength and gait speed. Age Ageing 1996; 25:386–391.

52. Winter DA, Patla AE, Frank JS, Watt SE. Biomechanical walking pattern changes in the fit and healthy elderly. Phys Ther 1990; 70:340–347.

53. Hausdorff JM, Edelberg HK, Mitchell SL, Goldberger AL, Wei JY. Increased gait unsteadiness in community-dwelling elderly fallers. Arch Phys Med Rehab 1997; 78:278–283.

54. Bendall MJ, Bassey EJ, Pearson MB. Factors affecting walking speed of elderly people. Age Ageing 1989; 18:327–332.

55. Rantanen T, Guralnik JM, Ferrucci L, et al. Coimpairments as predictors of severe walking disability in older women. J Am Geriatr Soc 2001; 49: 21–27.

56. Maki BE. Gait changes in older adults: predictors of falls or indicators of fear? J Am Geriatr Soc 1997; 43:313–320.

57. Kerrigan DC, Lee LW, Collins JJ, Riley PO, Lipsitz LA. Reduced hip extension during walking: healthy elderly and fallers versus young adults. Arch Phys Med Rehabil 2001; 82:26–30.

58. Cumming RG, Klineberg RJ. Fall frequency and characteristics and the risk of hip fractures. J Am Geriatr Soc 1994; 42:774–778.

59. Meinhart-Shibata P, Kramer M, Ashton-Miller JA, Persad C. Kinematic analyses of the 180° standing turn: effects of age on strategies adopted by healthy young and older women. Gait Posture. In press (available online 12 Oct 2004).

60. Thigpen MT, Light KE, Creel GL, Flynn SM. Turning difficulty characteristics of adults aged 65 years or older. Phys Ther 2000; 80:1174–1187.

61. Shkuratova N, Morris ME, Huxham F. Effects of age on balance control during walking. Arch Phys Med Rehabil 2004; 85:582–588.

62. Chen HC, Schultz AB, Ashton-Miller JA, Giordani B, Alexander NB, Guire KE. Stepping over obstacles: dividing attention impairs performance of old more than young adults. J Gerontol A Biol Sci Med Sci 1996; 51:M116–M122.

63. Lundin-Olsson L, Nyberg L, Gustafson Y. "Stops walking when talking" as a predictor of falls in elderly people. Lancet 1997; 349:617.

64. Patla AE. How is human gait controlled by vision? Ecol Psychol 1998; 10:287–302.

65. Patla AE, Vickers JN. How far ahead do we look when required to step on specific locations in the travel path during locomotion? Exp Brain Res 2003; 148:133–138.

66. Hollands MA, Marple-Horvat DE. Visually guided stepping under conditions of step cycle-related denial of visual information. Exp Brain Res 1996; 109:343–356.

67. Patla AE, Adkin A, Martin C, Holden R, Prentice S. Characteristics of voluntary visual sampling of the environment for safe locomotion over different terrains. Exp Brain Res 1996; 112:513–522.

68. Hollands MA, Marple-Horvat DE, Henkes S, Rowan AK. Human eye movements during visually guided stepping. J Mot Behav 1995; 27:155–163.

69. Di Fabio RP, Zampieri C, Greany JF. Aging and saccade-stepping interactions in humans. Neurosci Lett 2003; 339:179–182.

70. Hollands MA, Patla AE, Vickers JN. "Look where you're going!": gaze behaviour associated with maintaining and changing the direction of locomotion. Exp Brain Res 2002; 143:221–230.

71. Lord SR, Dayhew J. Visual risk factors for falls in older people. J Am Geriatr Soc 2001; 49:508–515.

72. Lord SR, Dayhew J, Howland A. Multifocal glasses impair edge-contrast sensitivity and depth perception and increase the risk of falls in older people. J Am Geriatr Soc 2002; 50:1760–1766.

73. Chen HC, Ashton-Miller JA, Alexander NB, Schultz AB. Stepping over obstacles: gait patterns of healthy young and old adults. J Gerontol 1991; 46:M196–M203.

74. Chen H-C, Ashton-Miller JA, Alexander NB, Schultz AB. Age effects on strategies used to avoid obstacles. Gait Posture 1994; 2:139–146.

75. Cao C, Ashton-Miller JA, Schultz AB, Alexander NB. Abilities to turn suddenly while walking: effects of age, gender, and available response time. J Gerontol A Biol Sci Med Sci 1997; 52:M88–M93.

76. Cao C, Schultz AB, Ashton-Miller JA, Alexander NB. Sudden turns and stops while walking: kinematic sources of age and gender differences. Gait Posture 1998; 7:45–52.

77. Begg RK, Sparrow WA. Gait characteristics of young and older individuals negotiating a raised surface: implications for the prevention of falls. J Gerontol A Biol Sci Med Sci 2000; 55:M147–M154.

78. McFadyen BJ, Prince F. Avoidance and accommodation of surface height changes by healthy, community-dwelling, young, and elderly men. J Gerontol A Biol Sci Med Sci 2002; 57:B166–B174.

79. Lark SD, Buckley JG, Bennett S, Jones D, Sargeant AJ. Joint torques and dynamic joint stiffness in elderly and young men during stepping down. Clin Biomech 2003; 18:848–855.

80. Christina KA, Cavanagh PR. Ground reaction forces and frictional demands during stair descent: effects of age and illumination. Gait Posture 2002; 15:153–158.

81. Hamel KA, Cavanagh PR. Stair performance in people aged 75 and older. J Am Geriatr Soc 2004; 52:563–567.

82. Startzell JK, Owens DA, Mulfinger LM, Cavanagh PR. Stair negotiation in older people: a review. J Am Geriatr Soc 2000; 48:567–580.

83. Andriacchi TP, Andersson GB, Fermier RW, Stern D, Galante JO. A study of lower-limb mechanics during stair-climbing. J Bone Joint Surg Am 1980; 62:749–757.

84. Redfern MS, Cham R, Gielo-Perczak K, et al. Biomechanics of slips. Ergonomics 2001; 44:1138–1166.

85. Berg WP, Alessio HM, Mills EM, Tong C. Circumstances and consequences of falls in independent community-dwelling older adults. Age Ageing 1997; 26:261–268.

86. Spaulding SJ, Patla AE, Elliott DB, Flanagan J, Rietdyk S, Brown S. Waterloo vision and mobility study: gait adaptations to altered surfaces in individuals with age-related maculopathy. Optom Vis Sci 1994; 71:770–777.

87. Moe-Nilssen R. Test–retest reliability of trunk accelerometry during standing and walking. Arch Phys Med Rehabil 1998; 79:1377–1385.

88. Menz HB, Lord SR, Fitzpatrick RC. Acceleration patterns of the head and pelvis when walking are associated with risk of falling in community-dwelling older people. J Gerontol A Biol Sci Med Sci 2003; 58:M446–M452.

89. Menz HB, Lord SR, St George R, Fitzpatrick RC. Walking stability and sensorimotor function in older people with diabetic peripheral neuropathy. Arch Phys Med Rehabil 2004; 85:245–252.

90. Li F, Harmer P, Wilson NL. Health benefits of cobblestone-mat walking: preliminary findings. J Aging Phys Act 2003; 11:487–501.

91. Thies SB, Richardson JK, Ashton-Miller JA. Influence of an irregular surface and low light on the step variability of patients with peripheral neuropathy during level gait. Gait Posture (available online 19 Aug 2004).

92. Thies SB, Richardson JK, Ashton-Miller JA. Effects of surface irregularity and lighting on step variability during gait: A study in healthy young and older women. Gait Posture (available online August 17, 2004).

93. Richardson JK, Thies SB, DeMott TK, Ashton-Miller JA. A comparison of gait characteristics between older women with and without peripheral neuropathy on smooth and unlevel surfaces. J Am Geriatr Soc 2004; 52:1532–1537.

94. Thies SB, Ashton-Miller JA, Richardson JK. What causes a crossover step when walking on uneven ground? A study in healthy young women. Gait Posture. Submitted for publication.

95. Smeesters C, Hayes WC, McMahon TA. The threshold trip duration for which recovery is no longer possible is associated with strength and reaction time. J Biomech 2001; 34:589–595.

96. Smeesters C, Hayes WC, McMahon TA. Disturbance type and gait speed affect fall direction and impact location. J Biomech 2001; 34:309–317.

97. Owings TM, Pavol MJ, Grabiner MD. Mechanisms of failed recovery following postural perturbations on a motorized treadmill mimic those associated with an actual forward trip. Clin Biomech 2001; 16:813–819.

98. Pavol MJ, Owings TM, Foley KT, Grabiner MD. Mechanisms leading to a fall from an induced trip in healthy older adults. J Gerontol A Biol Sci Med Sci 2001; 56:M428–M437.

99. van den Bogert AJ, Pavol MJ, Grabiner MD. Response time is more important than walking speed for the ability of older adults to avoid a fall after a trip. J Biomech 2002; 35:199–205.

100. Pijnappels M, Bobbert MF, van Dieen JH. Control of support limb muscles in recovery after tripping in young and older subjects. Exp Brain Res 2005; 160:326–333.

101. Pijnappels M, Bobbert MF, van Dieen JH. Changes in walking pattern caused by the possibility of a tripping reaction. Gait Posture 2001; 14:11–18.

102. Thelen DG, Wojcik LA, Schultz AB, Ashton-Miller JA, Alexander NB. Age differences in using a rapid step to regain balance during a forward fall. J Gerontol A Biol Sci Med Sci 1997; 52:M8–M13.

103. Wojcik LA, Thelen DG, Schultz AB, Ashton-Miller JA, Alexander NB. Age and gender differences in single-step recovery from a forward fall. J Gerontol A Biol Sci Med Sci 1999; 54:M44–M50.

104. Wojcik LA, Thelen DG, Schultz AB, Ashton-Miller JA, Alexander NB. Age and gender differences in peak lower extremity joint torques and ranges of motion used during single-step balance recovery from a forward fall. J Biomech 2001; 34:67–73.

105. Cham R, Redfern MS. Lower extremity corrective reactions to slip events. J Biomech 2001; 34:1439–1445.

106. Marigold DS, Patla AE. Strategies for dynamic stability during locomotion on a slippery surface: effects of prior experience and knowledge. J Neurophysiol 2002; 88:339–353.

107. Marigold DS, Bethune AJ, Patla AE. Role of the unperturbed limb and arms in the reactive recovery response to an unexpected slip during locomotion. J Neurophysiol 2003; 89:1727–1737.

108. Oates AR, Patla AE, Frank JS, Greig MA. Control of dynamic stability during gait termination on a slippery surface. J Neurophysiol 2005; 93:64–70.

109. Gronqvist R, Abeysekera J, Gard G, et al. Human-centred approaches in slipperiness measurement. Ergonomics 2001; 44:1167–1199.

110. Cham R, Redfern MS. Changes in gait when anticipating slippery floors. Gait Posture 2002; 15:159–171.

111. Luukinen H, Koski K, Hiltunen L, Kivela SL. Incidence rate of falls in an aged population in northern Finland. J Clin Epidemiol 1994; 47:843–850.

112. Robinovitch SN, Hayes WC, McMahon TA. Prediction of femoral impact forces in falls on the hip. J Biomech Eng 1991; 113:366–374.

113. Hayes WC, Myers ER, Morris JN, Gerhart TN, Yett HS, Lipsitz LA. Impact near the hip dominates fracture risk in elderly nursing home residents who fall. Calcif Tissue Int 1993; 52:192–198.

114. Nevitt MC, Cummings SR. Type of fall and risk of hip and wrist fractures: the study of osteoporotic fractures. The Study of Osteoporotic Fractures Research Group. J Am Geriatr Soc 1993; 41:1226–1234.

115. Lauritzen JB, Askegaard V. Protection against hip fractures by energy absorption. Dan Med Bull 1992; 39:91–93.

116. Hsiao ET, Robinovitch SN. Common protective movements govern unexpected falls from standing height. J Biomech 1998; 31:1–9.

117. DeGoede KM, Ashton-Miller JA, Schultz AB. Fall-related upper body injuries in the older adult: a review of the biomechanical issues. J Biomech 2003; 36:1043–1053.

118. DeGoede KM, Ashton-Miller JA, Liao JM, Alexander NB. How quickly can healthy adults move their hands to intercept an approaching object? Age and gender effects. J Gerontol A Biol Sci Med Sci 2001; 56:M584–M588.

119. DeGoede KM, Ashton-Miller JA. Biomechanical simulations of forward fall arrests: effects of upper extremity arrest strategy, gender and aging-related declines in muscle strength. J Biomech 2003; 36:413–420.

120. DeGoede KM, Ashton-Miller JA. Fall arrest strategy affects peak hand impact force in a forward fall. J Biomech 2002; 35:843–848.

121. Ashton-Miller JA, Alexander NB. Biomechanics of mobility in older adults. In: Hazzard WR, Blass JP, Halter JB, Ouslander JG, Tinetti ME, eds. Principles of Geriatric Medicine & Gerontology. 5th ed. New York: McGraw Hill, 2003:919–930.

5

Neuromuscular and Biomechanical Elements of Postural Equilibrium

Karen L. Reed-Troy and Mark D. Grabiner

Department of Movement Sciences, University of Illinois at Chicago, Chicago, Illinois, U.S.A.

I. INTRODUCTION

The study of postural control spans diverse disciplines that include computer science, engineering, mathematics, medicine, pharmacology, physiology, and robotics. The influence of the aging neuromuscular system on postural control and mobility lies at an intersection of these and other disciplines. The typical trajectories of the age-related anatomical and physiological changes have been well characterized. In some cases, these changes are compounded by pathology. Collectively, age-related changes give rise to postural and mobility problems that can exert a considerable impact on quality of life issues, in general, and fall-related morbidity and mortality, in particular.

The quantitative relationship between postural control and the incidence of falls by older adults has been of long-term interest clinically. Increased economic pressure on health-care systems has increased this interest. After all, decreasing the incidence of falls by older adults will decrease fall-related injuries and reduce the economic impact of these injuries. Nevertheless, questions still remain related to what the most appropriate data collection methods and variables used to represent postural control might be. Additionally, there are still questions regarding the extent to which these methods and variables may be generalized across sub-populations of older adults (e.g., frail, transitioning to frailty and healthy). Of primary importance is determining for older adults whose health and functional status may range from poor to excellent, those quantitative measures of postural stability that demonstrate a cause–effect relationship with falls, especially injurious falls, and that are sensitive to intervention. However, a generalized cause–effect relationship between measures of postural stability and falling has not yet been characterized.

The scientific and clinical study of postural control has a distinguished and long history. For example, in the introduction to their work, Vernazza-Martin et al. (1) referenced postural synergies during anterior and posterior trunk motion documented a century earlier (2). During the intervening 100 years, and particularly in the last 30 years, neuromuscular control of posture has been the focus of intense scrutiny, a testament to technological advances that have allowed entry and access to the structural and functional complexity of the neuromuscular system. This has given rise to greater appreciation of what the central nervous system monitors and controls, and when it does so. In addition, the extent of what is understood about the manner in which monitoring and controlling interacts with the biomechanical states of the body and the constraints placed upon the system by virtue of physiological capabilities of the person has broadened and deepened.

Figure 1 presents a generalized conceptual model of key factors that contribute to quasi-static and dynamic postural control. The model includes feed-forward and feedback control functions. Feed-forward postural control, which operates without the input of sensory feedback (upper left of Fig. 1) stabilizes the center of mass against postural disturbances that are anticipated. These anticipated postural disturbances arise from forces generated during the production of voluntary motion, or in anticipation of destabilizing external forces. This type of postural adjustment, referred to as anticipatory, involves estimation of the magnitude and direction of postural disturbance and initiation of a motor program by the central nervous system. The motor program is a set of neural commands that is selected based on an internal, or forward model, of the task to be performed. Once initiated, the motor program is executed in an open loop manner, i.e., without feedback (3), which circumvents the potentially deleterious processing delays inherent in feedback control (4). Ideally, the motor program activates the musculature that produces a set of appropriately scaled and timed pre-emptive muscle forces and joint moments that precede and negate the anticipated postural disturbance.

During feedback control, a postural disturbance, the origin of which may be either internal or external, causes a change in body kinematics (right side of Fig. 1). If the change in kinematics exceeds some threshold value to which the central nervous system has assigned importance, a corrective postural response will be generated. This type of postural adjustment is referred

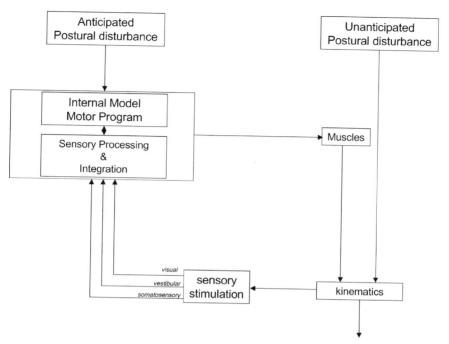

Figure 1 A generalized conceptual model of key factors that contribute to quasi-static and dynamic postural control. Elements of feed-forward postural control that occur in anticipation of a postural disturbance, which initially operate independently of sensory feedback, are stylized in the upper left-hand quadrant of the figure. Feed-back driven, or compensatory postural control, is driven by sensory feedback arising from kinematic changes induced by a disturbance.

to as compensatory. The postural disturbance is marked by a change in body kinematics reflecting the magnitude and direction of the destabilizing force, as well as the point of its application. The change in the kinematics stimulates visual, vestibular, and somatosensory system sensors that subsequently transmit the information to the central nervous system. Processing the sensory information involves comparing the detected state of the body to a desired state. Ideally, if the difference between the detected and desired states, that is, an error signal, is of sufficient magnitude, a corrective postural response consisting of muscle forces and joint moments will be executed. The muscle forces and joint moments subsequently affect body kinematics, generating a new set of sensory signals and another loop of the feedback process is initiated.

The realm of postural control ranges from quasi-static conditions, the most commonly studied of which is upright standing, to dynamic conditions during which balance must be maintained. Dynamic conditions include postural disturbances arising from voluntary motion, expected and unexpected external postural disturbances, and maintaining dynamic equilibrium during locomotion. During these dynamic conditions, the variables that are monitored and controlled by the central nervous system may generally be similar. However, given the large range over which the biomechanical states can vary the solution to the problem of postural equilibrium during dynamic conditions becomes more complex. The range over which the postural control system must operate is considerable. At one end postural control solutions are relatively simple. For example, for upright standing in the absence of external disturbances, the time available to select and execute postural control solutions is considerable. In contrast, for a person who trips or slips while walking, the postural control solution is complex, given that many interacting body segments must be appropriately controlled in a brief period of time. This operating range is central to explaining why a generalized cause–effect relationship between postural control and the incidence of falls by older adults has not yet been characterized. The remainder of this chapter will summarize some of the extant literature suggesting why such a relationship has been elusive.

A. Quasi-Static Posture

A sine qua non of postural control, during either quasi-static or dynamic conditions, is the relationship between the body's center of mass (center of gravity) and the center of pressure. In this relationship, the center of mass is considered to be the variable that is controlled. The means by which the center of mass is controlled is the center of pressure. The center of pressure is a single point that represents the forces between the feet and the ground. It is the point at which the ground reaction force is located. The magnitude, direction, and location of the ground reaction force reflect the net neuromuscular response which the central nervous system intends to control the center of mass (5).

During upright stance with the feet positioned parallel to and aligned with one another, if the center of mass is positioned vertically over the center of pressure, and the velocity of the center of mass is zero, then the system is in static equilibrium. However, a more common scenario is one in which the horizontal distance between the locations of the center of mass and the center of pressure, and their respective velocities, is not zero. These are the conditions that give rise to postural sway. The resulting sway in the saggital and frontal planes is generally maintained within the appropriate spatial boundaries using an ankle strategy. An ankle strategy controlling anteriorly and posteriorly directed sway is based on control of the ground reactions generated by plantarflexor and dorsiflexor muscle contractions, respectively. Similarly, the medially and laterally directed sway of the center of mass is controlled by the hip adductor and abductor muscles. These strategies are quite sensitive to the position of the feet. For example, during tandem stance, anterior–posterior motion of the center of mass is controlled from the hips rather than ankles and control of the medial–lateral motion of the center of mass arises primarily from the ankle joint invertor and evertor muscles (5).

The manner in which control of the center of mass is exerted by the center of pressure is illustrated in a plot of the anterior–posterior motions of each (Fig. 2, from Ref. 5). During the 7 seconds over which these data were collected the subject was asked to minimize postural sway. The difference between the position of the center of pressure and that of the center of mass, both of which are referenced relative to the ankle joint, is proportional to the horizontal acceleration of the center of mass. Thus, when the distance of the center of pressure from the ankle joint exceeds the distance between the center of mass and the ankle joint, the center of mass accelerates toward the ankle joint. A general pattern is evident in which the center of pressure moves through a greater distance and at a higher velocity (not explicitly illustrated) than the center of mass. What is not evident, however, is the complexity of the system that gives rise to this somewhat simple behavior.

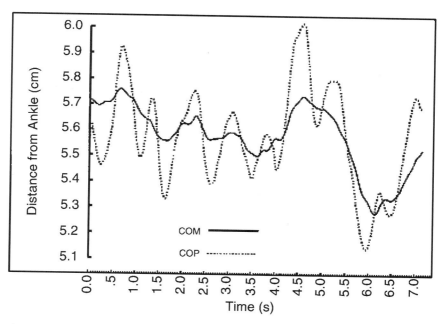

Figure 2 Illustration of the relationship between the controlled variable, the body center of mass, and the controlling variable, the center of pressure during 7 seconds of quasi-static upright standing (from Ref. 5). Acceleration of the center of mass is proportional to the difference between the position of the center of pressure and that of the center of mass.

During quasi-static postural control, the central nervous system is charged with a deceptively simple task. That is, to maintain the position of the body's center of mass within the boundaries of the base of support. Generally, during quasi-static posture, when normal subjects are asked to minimize postural sway, the center of mass does not approach the boundaries of the base of support. Furthermore, the velocity of the center of pressure does not approach its maximum voluntary value. As indicated earlier, feedback-driven responses to postural disturbances occur when kinematic variables exceed some threshold value to which the central nervous system has assigned importance. This implies that there are system states to which the central nervous system is sensitive, and other system states to which it is ambivalent, or chooses to disregard. System states that the central nervous system disregards implicitly suggest a small level of risk to equilibrium (6).

During quasi-static conditions such as quiet standing the anterior–posterior and medial–lateral displacement of the body center of mass is often represented by a stabilogram. The stabilogram qualitatively describes the anterior–posterior and medial–lateral motions of the center of pressure that are easily measured beneath the feet using a number of technologies

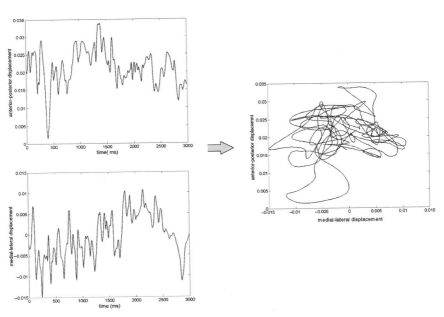

Figure 3 Individual time series of center of pressure motion in the medial–lateral and anterior–posterior directions during quasi-static upright standing are combined to create a stabilogram. The often used summary statistics from the stabilogram, such as the maximum distance over which the postural sway occurs, globally represent overall body sway but provide limited information related to the mechanisms of postural control.

such as force plates and capacitive mats (Fig. 3). The extent to which the body sways is often represented by various summary statistics. Examples include the maximum distance over which the postural sway occurs and the maximum velocity of the center of pressure during the excursion. Under conditions in which normal subjects have been asked to minimize postural sway, the excursion distance tends to be small relative to the maximum distance through which the center of pressure can be voluntarily controlled without having to take a corrective step. This is the case even in older adults. For example, the postural sway of healthy older adults in the anterior–posterior and medial–lateral directions was reported as $6.9 \pm 1.9\%$ and $7.8 \pm 2.3\%$ of the length of the foot and percent of the width of the feet, respectively (7). Furthermore, these sway distances represent only about 15% of the limit of stability, that is, the maximum anterior–posterior and medial–lateral distances through which the center of pressure can be voluntarily controlled without having to perform a corrective stepping response. Similarly, the average velocity of the center of pressure motion is less than 10% of the maximum velocity that may be achieved voluntarily. Nevertheless, although these distances are small compared to the maximum available distance, older adults generally demonstrate larger postural sway and smaller limits of stability than young adults using this type of center of pressure trajectory analysis.

Although widely used, summary statistics of center of pressure trajectory provide limited information about the underlying control of postural stability. For example, older adults generally have larger postural sway amplitudes compared to young adults. However, the age-related differences can be small relative to the between-group differences in age. In addition, and perhaps more importantly, these differences confer little insight about changes and various combinations of changes to the postural control system elements that underlie the difference. Larger sway amplitude and sway velocity during quasi-static conditions suggest, for example, that the application of an external force in the direction of the sway could result in a larger postural disturbance. If the external force caused the center of mass to move beyond the boundary of the base of support, summary statistics of center of pressure motion would not be informative with regard to the biomechanical qualities of the stepping response or the biomechanical outcome of the stepping response. Indeed, it has been demonstrated using healthy older adults that the success, or failure, of recovery efforts following very large postural disturbances requiring stepping responses could not generally be predicted from measures of quasi-static postural sway and limits of stability (7).

In contrast to various summary statistics, random walk analysis performed on center of pressure data has been reported to reflect the neuromuscular mechanisms underlying postural control (8). The basis of random walk analysis is the stabilogram–diffusion plot that is based on the explicit presumption that center of pressure trajectories reflect both stochastic and deterministic processes (9). The stabilogram–diffusion plot arises from a mathematical manipulation of the time-related center of pressure trajectory data that is based on the assumption of Brownian motion. In the first phase of the random walk analysis, two distinct regions in the stabilogram–diffusion plot are identified based on the slope of the function in the two regions. The two regions are separated at a transition point. The regions to the left and right of the transition point are thought to reflect short-term and long-term control mechanisms, respectively, that are used by the central nervous system to regulate the center of pressure motion (Fig. 4).

Random walk analysis of center of pressure trajectories provides insights that are not available from summary statistics of the center of pressure trajectory. Two of the variables that are calculated using random walk analysis describe the behavior of the center of pressure trajectory in terms of short- and long-term control exerted by the central nervous system. For example, the regions associated with short-term control have been

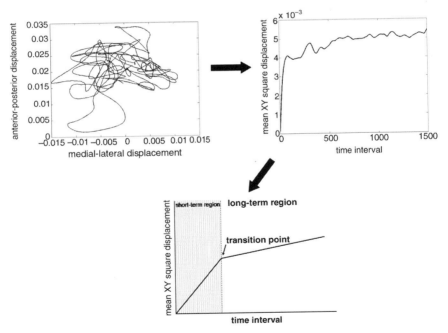

Figure 4 The stabilogram presented in the upper left quadrant of the figure is transformed to a stabilogram–diffusion plot (upper right-hand quadrant) using a random walk analysis (10). The distinctly different slopes of the stabilogram–diffusion plot separated by a transition point represent regions of short-term and long-term control processes. This type of information cannot be provided by simple summary statistics computed for stabilograms.

interpreted as reflecting the time intervals (which are related to excursion distances) through which the center of pressure can move without corrective action by the central nervous system. Indeed, the behavior of the center of pressure trajectory in the short-term region is described as positively corre-lated (persistent). This means that the center of pressure tends to increas-ingly move away from an equilibrium point. In contrast, regions associated with long-term control have been identified as time intervals dur-ing which the nervous system is exerting active control over the center of pressure. The behavior of the center of pressure trajectory in the long-term region is described as negatively correlated, or anti-persistent. Anti-persistent behavior reflects motion for which movement away from (or toward) an equilibrium point tends to be followed by movement toward (or away from) the equilibrium point.

One plausible interpretation of the persistent behavior in the short-term control region is that, since the center of pressure motion has not ele-vated the likelihood of an impending loss of balance, the movement of the center of pressure within this region does not require active regulation. An extension of this interpretation is that diminished and/or inaccurate sensory feedback signaling the location of the center of pressure would increase the unregulated region. Indeed, the increased drift of the center of pressure dur-ing the short-term control region reported for healthy older adults com-pared to young adults (10), in Parkinson's patients compared to normal controls (11), and in astronauts following exposure to microgravity (11), is consistent with this interpretation.

The random walk analysis of center of pressure data implicates the dynamics of excursion distance as the variable of concern to the central ner-vous system. Using available sensory feedback, the central nervous system decides on the nature of control of the center of mass. Compensatory responses are necessary if the center of mass drifts beyond the region around some equilibrium set point within which the central nervous system exhibits little physiological concern. It has been suggested that within this region the central nervous system controls sway in a feed-forward manner by specify-ing the requisite ankle joint muscle stiffness to constrain postural sway (6,13). Compensatory (feedback) adjustments occur after the center of mass has been sensed to have drifted from this region. The compensatory responses that bring the center of mass back toward the set point give rise to the anti-persistent behavior observed from the random walk analysis.

Sampling available sensory data to assess the position of the center of mass relative to the base of support does not actually appear to provide ade-quate information on which postural control decisions can unambiguously be made. For example, postural equilibrium is increasingly challenged as the position of the center of mass approaches the anterior boundary of the base of support. However, the extent of the challenge is somewhat ambiguous in the absence of information regarding the direction and magnitude of the horizontal velocity of the center of mass (14). Clearly, if the horizontal velocity is directed away from the anterior boundary of the base of support, the postural challenge established by the position of the center of mass relative to the boundary is considerably diminished. The central nervous system may use these state variables, i.e., position and velocity, in conjunction with a safety margin to assess the relative stability of the overall system. Indeed, a dynamic model that includes both the position and velocity of the center of mass relative to the base of support has been shown to be superior to a static model, which involves only center of mass position, in predicting the need for a corrective stepping response for waist-pull perturbations and support-surface translation (15,16). Conceptually, the safety margin, which may include both spatial and temporal components, is a metric reflecting the spatial and temporal proximity of the system to a destabilizing condition (17).

B. Perturbed Quasi-Static Posture

Postural disturbances arise from the forces and moments associated with voluntary movement, whether episodic or periodic. In addition to being the source of the postural disturbance, these forces and moments can also negatively influence the quality of voluntary movement. The central nervous system deals with these disturbances by predicting and neutralizing their effects using anticipatory postural adjustments that occur prior to expected postural disturbances. This type of response, the intent of which is to ameliorate the postural disturbances associated with the movement requirements, appear to be planned in detail by the central nervous system (18).

One of the first observations of anticipatory postural adjustment was that when instructed to rapidly flex the shoulder joint while in an upright standing position, activation of the anterior deltoid muscle, an agonist muscle, was preceded by activation of the muscles on the dorsal aspect of the body. Indeed, the anticipatory activation of the hamstrings occurred about 50–60 msec before that of the agonist deltoid muscle (19). Factors that influence anticipatory responses include the size of the predicted postural perturbation (20), the availability of mechanical support and perceptual information (21), the extent to which faulty adjustments can contribute to loss of balance (22); postural constraints imposed by the task (23), and the body configuration prior to the voluntary action (24).

Since the magnitude of the anticipated postural disturbance is smaller during slower movements, studies of anticipatory activation of older adults are complicated by the tendency of older adults to move more slowly during self-paced and reaction time conditions (25–27). The results of one study in which movement velocity was controlled for in younger and older adults suggested that age-related changes in anticipatory activation are, in fact, contributed to by the nervous system (28). Since anticipatory adjustments represent a neuromuscular skill that can be acquired, or learned (29,30), one would not be surprised if this family of responses could demonstrate improvement in older adults after practice.

Poorly timed anticipatory activation, that is, activation that is either delayed or advanced, might be expected to decrease quasi-static postural equilibrium. As mentioned above, it is also possible that anticipatory activation can be enhanced. However, given the specificity of practice-related improvement in anticipatory activation, it is questionable as to whether the improvement would bear any influence on the ability to perform stepping responses following large postural disturbances. Indeed, a cause–effect relationship between altered anticipatory activation and the predisposition to falls by older adults is not evident in the literature.

C. Perturbed Quasi-Static Posture Requiring Stepping Responses

During conditions in which stepping responses are initiated voluntarily from quasi-static conditions, older adults generally require more time to initiate the steps compared to young adults (31). Since delays as short as 100 msec in a response can lead to a fall following a forward-directed trip (32), the delay in voluntary stepping responses is notable. However, during conditions in which stepping responses are induced by an external perturbation, stepping responses by older adults can occur not only as fast but in some cases faster than younger adults (33). Thus, the interesting age-related differences between voluntary, triggered and reflexive stepping responses further complicates the identification of a unified method by which falls can be predicted and the predicted physiological causes targeted for intervention.

There is a growing literature related to the relationship between biomechanical states, such as center of mass position and velocity relative to the boundary of the base of support, and the likelihood of initiating a stepping response. Based upon Fig. 1, a compensatory stepping response is expected if the magnitude of the postural disturbance results in a change in body state that exceeds some threshold to which the central nervous system places importance. Interestingly, stepping responses induced in young and older adults by waist-pull perturbations appear to be triggered earlier than what is biomechanically necessary (34). Waist-pull experiments, in which motion of the subjects is in the forward direction, have revealed a threshold boundary, relative to the base of support, that when crossed always results in a stepping response (35). Similarly, there is a boundary behind which stepping never occurs. The former threshold boundary is not fixed. Rather, it shifts posteriorly, toward the ankle, as the waist-pull velocity increases. The threshold boundary for stepping responses in the forward direction is closer to the ankle for older subjects than for younger subjects. The triggering of a stepping response prior to its being biomechanically necessary is suggestive of a component of on-line predictive processing of sensory data and not simply a compensatory response to bio-mechanical states.

The extent to which biomechanical and physiological variables associated with corrective stepping responses elicited in a laboratory can predict falls by older adults, and the extent to which these variables can be effectively targeted for intervention has not yet been reported. The shared biomechanical similarities between stepping responses induced by a forward-directed waist-pull perturbation and the initial stepping response following a forward-directed trip may increase the extent to which the former may serve as a surrogate for the latter. However, there are numerous, and substantial between-task differences that may complicate comparisons. For example, the waist-pull experiments are initiated from a quasi-static condition. In contrast, a trip during locomotion is initiated from a dynamic condition. Therefore, the initial neural and biomechanical conditions represent potentially very different levels of physiological complexity. For example, immediately after a forward-directed trip the trunk rotates forward through a large range of motion (32,36,37). However, the initial rotation of the trunk following a waist pull can be backward albeit to a much smaller extent. Nevertheless, this between-task difference gives rise to considerable differences in the nature of visual feedback (i.e., optical flow) and somatosensory and possibly vestibular and otolith feedback. Another between-task difference relates to the ability to preplan the response. Waist-pull perturbations are delivered to subjects during quasi-static conditions. Prior to the delivery of the disturbance there is ample time for subjects to pre-plan the required motor response that will be performed in an area that may be completely surveyed. However, very little, if any pre-planning time is available immediately after a trip. Indeed, response delays of 100 msec can result in falls following trips induced during locomotion and large postural perturbations delivered using a motorized treadmill (32,38). Furthermore, in contrast with the surveyed environment of the waist-pull and treadmill experiments, a trip quite often will be induced by a previously unseen object. Following the trip, the properties, size, and location of the object that caused the trip is known only in the broadest terms. This imparts a substantial level of ambiguity about the area in which the stepping responses must be executed (39). The result is a stepping response that is biomechanically and statistically different than a stepping response performed over known terrain and with no obstacles.

Earlier in the chapter the challenge of establishing, for older adults whose health and functional status may range from poor to excellent, those quantitative measures of postural stability that demonstrate a cause–effect relationship with falls and which are sensitive to intervention were identified. This is a formidable challenge to scientists and clinicians. The extant literature provides pieces of the solution to the challenge, necessary pieces that now span the range of experimental control and physiological complexity from quasi-static postural conditions to dynamic conditions. The socioeconomic and demographic considerations of an aging population merit the vigorous and continued collaboration between laboratory and clinic to ultimately meet the challenge.

REFERENCES

1. Vernazza-Martin S, Martin N, Massion J. Kinematic synergies and equilibrium control during trunk movement under loaded and unloaded conditions. Exp Brain Res 1999; 128:517–526.
2. Babinski J. De l'asynergie cérébelleuse. Rev Neurol 1899; 7:806–816.
3. Schmidt RA. Motor control and learning: a behavioral emphasis (Second Edition). 1988 Champaign, IL,. Human Kinetics Publishers, Inc.
4. Miall RC, Wolpert DM. Forward models for physiological motor control. Neural Networks 1996; 9:1265–1279.
5. Winter DA, Prince F, Frank JS, Powell C, Zabjek KF. Unified theory regarding A/P and M/L balance in stance. J Neurophysiol 1996; 75:2334–2343.
6. Gatev P, Thomas S, Kepple T, Hallett M. Feedforward ankle strategy of balance during quiet stance in adults. J Physiol 1999; 514:915–928.
7. Owings TM, Pavol MP, Foley KT, Grabiner MD. Measures of postural stability are not predictors of recovery from large postural disturbances in healthy older adults. J Am Geriatrics Soc 2000; 48:42–50.
8. Priplata A, Niemi J, Salen M, Harry J, Lipsitz LA, Collins JJ. Noise-enhanced human balance control. Phys Rev Lett 2002; 89:238101-1–238101-4.
9. Collins JJ, DeLuca CJ. Open-loop and closed loop control of posture: a random-walk analysis of center-of-pressure trajectories. Exp Brain Res 1993; 95:308–318.
10. Collins JJ, DeLuca CJ, Pavlik AE, Roy SH, Emley MS. The effects of space-flight on open-loop and closed-loop postural control mechanisms: human neurovestibular studies on SLS-2. Exp Brain Res 1995; 107:145–150.
11. Mitchell SL, Collins JJ, DeLuca CJ, Burrows A, Lipsitz LA. Open-loop and closed-loop postural control mechanisms in Parkinson's disease: increased mediolateral activity during quiet standing. Neurosci Lett 1995; 197:133–136.
12. Collins JJ, DeLuca CJ, Burrows A, Lipsitz LA. Age-related changes in open-loop and closed-loop postural control mechanisms. Exp Brain Res 1995; 104:480–492.
13. Winter DA, Patla AE, Prince F, Ishac M, Gielo-Perczak K. Stiffness control of balance in quiet standing. J Neurophysiol 1998; 80:1211–1221.
14. Pai Y-C, Patton J. Center of mass velocity-position predictions for balance control. J Biomech 1997; 30:347–354.
15. Pai Y-C, Rogers MW, Patton J, Cain TD, Hanke TA. Static versus dynamic predictions of protective stepping following waist-pull perturbations in young and older subjects. J Biomech 1998; 31:1111–1118.
16. Pai Y-C, Maki BE, Iqbal K, McIlroy WE, Perry SD. Thresholds for step initiation induced by support-surface translation: a dynamic center of mass model provides much better prediction than a static model. J Biomech, 2000; 33:387–92.

17. Patton JL, Lee WA, Pai Y-C. Relative stability improves with experience in a dynamic standing task. Exp Brain Res 2000; 135:117–126.
18. Benvenuti F, Stanhope SJ, Thomas SL, Panzer VP, Hallett M. Flexibility of anticipatory postural adjustments revealed by self-paced and reaction-time arm movements. Brain Res 1997; 761:59–70.
19. Belen'kii VY, Gurfinkel VS, Pal'tsev YI. Elements of control of voluntary movements. Biophysics 1967; 12:154–161.
20. Aruin AS, Latash ML. Anticipatory postural adjustments during self-initiated perturbations of different magnitude triggered by a standard motor action. Electroencephal Clin Neurophysiol 1996; 101:497–503.
21. Slipjer H, Latash M. The effects of instability and additional hand support on anticipatory postural adjustments in leg, trunk and arm muscle during standing. Exp Brain Res 2000; 135:81–93.
22. Adkin AL, Frank JS, Carpenter MG, Peysar GW. Fear of falling modifies anticipatory postural control. Exp Brian Res 2002; 143:160–170.
23. Cordo P, Nashner LM. Properties of postural adjustments associated with rapid arm movements. J Neurophysiol 1982; 47:287–302.
24. Aruin AS. The effect of changes in the body configuration on anticipatory postural adjustments. Motor Control 2003; 7:264–277.
25. Inglin B, Woollacott M. Age-related changes in anticipatory adjustments associated with arm movements. J Gerontol Med Sci 1988; 43:M105–M113.
26. Stelmach GE, Populin L, Müller F. Postural muscle onset and voluntary movement in the elderly. Neuroscience Lett 1990; 117:188–193.
27. Rogers MW, Kukulka CG, Soderberg GL. Age-related changes in postural responses preceding rapid self-paced and reaction time arm movements. J of Gerontol Med Sci 1992; 47:M159–M165.
28. Woollacott M, Manchester DL. Anticipatory postural adjustments in older adults: are changes in response characteristics due to changes in strategy? J Gerontol Med Sci 1993; 48:M64–M70.
29. Friedli WG, Hallet M, Simon SR. Postural adjustments associated with rapid voluntary arm movements 1. Electromyographic data. J Neurol Neurosurg Psychiatry 1984; 47:611–622.
30. Pedotti A, Crenna P, Deat A, Frigo C, Massion J. Postura synergies in axial movements: short and long-term adaptation. Exp Brain Res 1989; 74:3–10.
31. Lord SR, Fitzpatrick RC. Choice stepping reaction time: a composite measure of falls risk in older people. J Gerontol 2001; 56:M627–M632.
32. Pavol MJ, Owings TM, Foley KT, Grabiner MD. Mechanisms leading to a fall from an induced trip in healthy older adults. J Gerontol: Med Sci 2001; 56A:M428–M437.
33. Luchies CW, Wallace D, Pazdur S, Young S, DeYoung AJ. Effects of age on balance assessment using voluntary and involuntary step tasks. J Gerontol 1999; 3:M140–M144.
34. Rogers MW, Hedman LD, Johnson ME, Martinez KM, Mille M-L. Triggering of protective stepping for the control of human balance: age and contextual dependence. Cognitive Brain Res 2003; 16:192–198.

35. Mille M-L, Rogers MW, Martinez K, Hedman LD, Johnson ME, Lord SR, Fitzpatrick RC. Thresholds for inducing protective stepping responses to external perturbations of human standing. J Neurophysiol 2003; 90:666–674.
36. Grabiner MD, Koh TJ, Lundin T, Jahnigen DW. Kinematics of recovery from a stumble. J Gerontol 1993; 48:M97–M102.
37. Grabiner MD, Feuerbach JW, Jahnigen DW. Successful recovery from a trip: control of the trunk during the initial phase following perturbation. J Biomech 1996; 29:735–744.
38. Owings TM, Pavol MJ, Grabiner MD. Mechanisms of failed recovery following postural perturbations on a motorized treadmill mimic those associated with an actual forward trip. Clin Biomech 2001; 16:813–819.
39. Troy KL, Grabiner MD. The presence of an obstacle influences the stepping response during induced trips and surrogate tasks. Exp Brain Res 2005; 161:343–50.

6

Neuropsychological Influences on Gait in the Elderly

Bruno Giordani and Carol C. Persad

Neuropsychology Section, Department of Psychiatry, University of Michigan, Ann Arbor, Michigan, U.S.A.

The incidence of falls rises sharply with age (1), and falls are now the leading cause of disability among older adults (2,3). Falls in older individuals are associated with severe outcomes, such as fractures and head injuries (4,5), as well as significant declines in adaptive functioning and immobility (6). Characterization and further understanding of falls risk factors, therefore, are important for the development of effective interventions to maintain adaptive independence in older adults (7).

Although falls in older individuals can come from sudden loss of postural stability (e.g., falling from a ladder, postural hypotension), the highest incidence of falls for older persons occurs while walking (8). This is especially true in more demanding or less familiar environments, such as settings with many distractions, environmental hazards, or obstacles (9–14). Gait changes and falls in the elderly have been associated with a range of biomechanical, vestibular/sensory, and disease-related mechanisms that accompany aging, including progressive degeneration of sensory systems and especially of sensory input from the lower extremities (15). These changes, however, are not enough to explain increases in balance and falls risk (16), implicating the role of additional factors. Indeed, studies have consistently demonstrated that cognitive skills independently contribute to this process (17).

Traditionally, postural control was considered an automatic process, though recent studies have shown that such basic neuropsychological or cognitive processes as attention are necessary for balance maintenance (18–20). Across the age range, increasing motor demand (e.g., from sitting to standing, to walking) has been shown to require increased attentional control (c.f., Ref. 21). Walking is even a more complex process than standing, with different postural and balance requirements (22). Specifically, walking has been described as essentially a series of episodes of loss of balance and recovery in a continually changing environment (23). Whereas aspects of attentional control may be critical for posture and balance, walking involves a range of cognitive systems for response selection, monitoring, and adjustment to environmental, as well as physical and other age-related changes.

The role of cognition becomes even more apparent during many activities of daily living, such as when people need to selectively attend to foot placement (e.g., stepping on an icy sidewalk, stepping up onto a curb), when performing actions simultaneously or quickly shifting attention and control from one task to another (e.g., walking while talking, walking across a busy intersection while watching for oncoming traffic). Central to such actions are the abilities to effectively monitor the environment, choose flexible response patterns to balance threats that may appear, and make appropriate motor responses in order to complete goals at hand (24).

Neuropsychology aims to describe how specific cognitive processes and other behaviors, including the role of emotional, family, and environmental factors, reflect basic brain–behavior relationships (25). A Life-Span Neuropsychological Model has been proposed that views such processes as ever-changing and adaptive throughout the course of life, representing a dynamic interplay of brain functioning, psychological capabilities, and environmental resources across a person's lifetime (26). Proficiencies or deficiencies in neuropsychological functioning can then be considered with regard to how they affect coping and adaptation in a number of situations including balance and gait, within the context of basic transitions in life and aging. This chapter will present a comprehensive Behavioral Control Model, incorporating a range of neuropsychological factors, which have direct influence both on the choice of motor output and the execution of the response. Central to the model is the integral role of executive control processes that are necessary for implementation of most complex motor programs. Factors affecting the system are outlined and research methods that can be used to test the model are presented. Finally, the clinical implications of the model, especially in relation to rehabilitation strategies are discussed.

I. BEHAVIORAL CONTROL SYSTEM

By drawing on available research, we present a comprehensive model of a Behavioral Control System that expands upon the model of attention as a factor in mobility and describes additional processes involved in complex motor performance. This model has drawn on the work of a number of researchers in the fields of neuropsychology and cognitive psychology (27–30). It is important to recognize that motor responses can occur with minimal participation of this system, such as those responses that are reflexive or overlearned (e.g., walking at a normal pace along an obstacle-free walkway). The actual amount of involvement on the part of the Behavioral Control System is determined by a variety of modulating factors. These include factors that are specific to the task, the individual, and/or the environment and are discussed in later sections.

The Behavioral Control System model is presented in Fig. 1. The overarching theme of this model is the role of the Executive Control Dimension in the evaluation of available information and the integration of resources to make a response. Although the focus of this chapter is on gait and ambulation, this model can be applied to any response, be it motor, cognitive, or emotional. At the first level of the model are the three basic components or dimensions that provide input into the system before a motor response is determined. These components reflect physiological, cognitive, and affective processes and will be briefly discussed below.

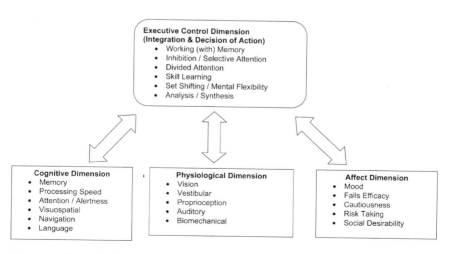

Figure 1 Behavioral control system.

A. Physiological Dimension

This component refers to the range of basic motoric/skeletal/sensory processes that are necessarily involved in movement. These include (but are not limited to) factors such as biomechanical processes (e.g., muscle strength, range of motion, nerve conduction velocity), sensory processes (e.g., vision and proprioception), and vestibular functioning. For a fuller discussion of these factors and their relation to ambulation, please refer to related chapters in this volume.

B. Cognitive Dimension

This component encompasses fundamental cognitive processes, including basic attention skills such as alertness and arousal, language, episodic and semantic memory, visual spatial skills and related navigation ability, and information processing speed. The degree to which any one of these domains is involved in a response is determined by the task itself, though attention has been shown to be involved in even the most basic postural stability tasks (31,32). Memory ability may be important in the recall of motor schemas and retention of task instructions, as well as recalling directions and routes while walking. Visual spatial skills and navigation are involved in maneuvering successfully in space, while language skills are important to understanding such things as the thread of concurrent conversations while walking, or verbal directions.

C. Behavioral/Affective Dimension

Tinetti et al. (2) have discussed the importance of studying the impact of both cognitive and emotional factors on gait and motor performance, especially in older individuals. Subjects' affective states at the time of completing tasks, as well as their perceptions of task demands and inherent risks, can be very important in understanding variability found across studies attempting to identify significant predictors of falls risk. Moreover, self-perception of motor abilities can have a direct influence on actual outcomes (33,34). One area that has been studied in some detail is the role of anxiety to balance impairment leading to falls (35,36). Even in healthy, younger controls, links between anxiety experienced in the laboratory setting, and balance and postural sway have been found (37,38). Cautiousness or hesitation in a response, often attributed to behavioral change with aging (21), also can affect motor outcome. For example, among older individuals, there is a strong link between fear of falling, and both mobility performance in the laboratory and falls risk in the community (9,39,40). In a study of older adults living in the community, our group also has found that scores on the Falls Efficacy Scale (FES), as well as self-ratings for anxiousness, depressed mood, and general willingness to take risks were significantly related to both self-report and performance-based measures of functional status (33,41,42). In addition, more global mood disturbances such as clinical depression have been shown to impact mobility-related factors, including gait speed, in older individuals (34).

Another factor of importance to be considered is social desirability. In general, this term refers to an individual's desire to perform in a manner felt to be acceptable to an observer, rather than how a person might actually perform without this self-perceived pressure. Social desirability can potentially affect performance in both a positive and negative manner. For example, a person who is very concerned with social desirability and wants to present the best possible image may exert more effort than usual during a laboratory mobility task in front of research observers. In the research setting, the use of a formal social desirability questionnaire or debriefing questions is important in evaluating underlying factors to inter-subject response variability and can provide useful information in the interpretation of unexpected results.

D. Executive Control Dimension

The Behavior Control System model includes the Executive Control Dimension, involved in the integration and execution of more complex motor responses. Although not an exhaustive list, Figure 1 presents skill areas under the purview of executive control that are more typically associated with motor control and gait. *Working memory* (43) or *working with memory* (44) has been operationalized as an active system that allows for temporary storage and on-line processing of information during action. As part of the Executive Control Dimension, working memory is regarded as important for the continual, on-line processing needed to execute an action and make continual corrections based on the response feedback that is received. In the work of Baddeley, working memory has three components—the visual spatial sketchpad and the phonological loop that hold visual spatial and verbal material, respectively, and a central executive component that processes and manipulates this briefly stored information. Although the central executive is very similar in nature to the Executive Control Dimension presented here, the currently proposed model (Fig. 1) encompasses additional aspects of cognition involved in integration, decision making, and response selection that are outside of the currently defined scope of working memory.

One of these additional aspects of executive control, *inhibition* represents the ability to: (a) prevent distracting information from entering working memory and causing interference, (b) suppress previously relevant information that is no longer necessary to the task at hand, and (c) prevent pre-potent (automatic) responses that may not be appropriate to the current situation (45–47). Examples of this can range from a situation that requires one to inhibit an activated stepping pattern and thus change the location of foot placement in order to avoid stepping on a suddenly appearing obstacle, to the need to inhibit distracting thoughts so that one can concentrate and carefully cross a busy intersection. The ability to *divide attention* between two tasks also is crucial to gait performance. In everyday life, we often complete two or more tasks simultaneously, such as walking down the street while talking to another person, crossing a busy intersection while watching for oncoming traffic, or carrying grocery bags while climbing a flight of steps. Effective allocation of attentional resources has been viewed as either a passive process in which multiple tasks compete for limited attentional resources and the setting exerts a strong influence on task selection (48) or as an active process in which some actions are selected and others either completely or partially blocked through the active control of the individual (49,50). Regardless on which viewpoint is held, it can be argued that the Executive Control Dimension is crucial to the process of prioritization of one action over another.

Processes, such as *set shifting* and *mental flexibility*, are important in effectively switching responses or making adequate compensatory adjustments based on new information or available feedback. These abilities also are crucial in problem solving in situations that are complex and require novel or modified movements to develop alternative strategies or responses. *Procedural* or "skill" *learning* is an indirect or implicit process leading to the acquisition of skilled responses. These responses, such as skipping or riding a bicycle, initially involve executive control during the learning phase, but as performance improves with practice, become essentially "automatic" with sufficient experience (51) and thus requires only minimal involvement of the Executive Control System.

Within the Behavioral Control System, *analysis and synthesis* of the available data from the cognitive, physical, and affective domains in the context of the situational demands allow a response selection to be made and a behavior executed. Related to this is the concept of risk analysis of a given motor response. An individual will assess a given situation based on an evaluation of the particular risk benefit ratio that takes into account the person's perceived ability to perform the motor response, as well as the salience of the goal. This analysis can help shape the type of response that is chosen as well as the amount of attention or effort placed into completing the response. It has been shown that under certain dual task conditions, subjects who generally emphasize performance on a cognitive task to the detriment of postural control, can alter that approach and prioritize postural stability under conditions that are viewed as more threatening to balance maintenance (52,53).

The Executive Control Dimension also is involved in the analysis of the effectiveness of the response after a behavior has been executed. As such, the model provides for feedback loops (double arrows in Fig. 1) between the executive control and the other dimensions to allow for this updating of information. These feedback loops provide for continual monitoring of the success of the response and can allow for compensation as factors change either internally or externally. In addition, this monitoring allows for recognition of when the chosen response is no longer appropriate to the current task.

Although it is likely that many brain regions are involved in executive control processes, the prefrontal cortex (PFC) has been particularly implicated (28). The executive control functions represented in Figure 1 are all involved to some degree in the necessary on-line processing of available data and can influence motor output to ensure that an optimal response has been made. Interconnections between the basal ganglia and the PFC facilitate the transfer of control from the PFC to the basal ganglia with increasing practice of a movement. This allows the PFC to divert attentional and/or other cognitive resources to other motor or cognitive tasks as necessary (54,55). In support of this, functional imaging studies have shown significant activation of the PFC and anterior cingulate during new learning that then disappears as a task becomes more automatic and thus requires less attention (56). Further, research has shown that the PFC is particularly affected by the aging process (57) and may be integral to understanding age-related changes in mobility.

II. INDIVIDUAL MODULATING FACTORS

The extent of involvement, as well as the overall performance of the Behavioral Control System, is determined not only by its individual dimensions, but also, in part, by additional modulating factors. These factors can be intrinsic to the individual completing the movement, environmental, and/ or reflective of the nature of the task itself (Fig. 2).

A. Aging

It is well documented that aging has detrimental effects on many aspects of the three basic dimensions that provide input into the Executive Control System. As sensory and other physiological systems decline with age, individuals demonstrate increased reliance on already limited sensory systems, such as vision. For example, older persons require longer periods of direct visual information (look down more often) when walking over simple or more complex walkways (58,59). As a result of this increased reliance on already taxed sensory systems, the cognitive control demands for completing even relatively simple tasks increase with age due to the need to compensate for these age-associated changes. For instance, increased attention is necessary in order to "heighten" the signal coming from peripheral sensory systems, and executive control processes are required to effectively interpret and combine what sensory information is available in order to gain the necessary information for proper motor planning to maintain postural control (60).

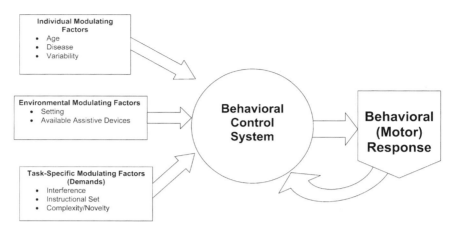

Figure 2 Response selection and general factors affecting behavioral control.

Concomitant with physical and sensory changes with aging, mechanisms related to cognitive control and supervision also decrease in efficiency, and some are disproportionately compromised by older age (61). Declines in executive functioning in older adults, including declines in processes such as inhibitory control, mental flexibility, problem solving skills, divided attention, and working memory, represent the very skills that the Executive Control Dimension relies upon to integrate information and compensate for age-related changes to other physical systems. Essentially, with advancing age, cognitive control mechanisms are more and more called for but less and less able to counteract wide-ranging adverse consequences of sensory, motor, basic cognitive, and affective changes (62). This can lead to inefficient interpretation and integration of already compromised incoming information and result in an impaired ability to efficiently allocate these resources, resulting in inappropriate motor programs that potentially lead to falls. Although the presence of multiple impairments across physical and neuropsychological domains frequently should lead to a disproportionate increase in disability and potentially a higher falls risk, little research has directly examined the combined effects of these impairments with aging.

Affective changes also occur with age, including a tendency to approach tasks in a more cautious way that often results in an altered response (63). Only minimal research has been specifically directed to characterizing differences in the approach that younger and older persons take when facing complex mobility tasks. Aging does appear to affect the selection of different responses in successfully adjusting to competing cognitive and motor demands while walking (64). Older persons' adjustments, however, although initially appearing to be more cautious, could actually lead to increased risk of tripping or falls (e.g., early step initiation to clear obstacles may increase risk of later foot contact with an obstacle during final foot placement) (65,66).

B. Disease

There are a number of diseases that can influence gait and other motor responses in all individuals, but can have the greatest impact on older adults. These include such disorders as arthritis, diabetes, peripheral neuropathy, heart disease, and visual disturbances (e.g., macular degeneration). These and other medical conditions are fully covered in other chapters and will not be discussed in detail here. However, studies have demonstrated an increased need for cognitive control during mobility tasks in patients with medical disorders. For instance, patients with diabetic peripheral neuropathies have been shown to increase their reaction times significantly as compared to controls when walking and responding to a simple auditory reaction time task. This demonstrates the increase in attentional resources needed by these patients in order to adjust to limits on the available gait-related sensory information (67). Turano et al. (68) have shown that patients with vision difficulties (e.g., retinitis pigmentosa; RP) had longer auditory reaction times compared with normal-vision controls when walking on a complex, but not a simple route. Reaction time on the complex route correlated with contrast sensitivity and log retinal area (walking speeds were maintained across all task conditions). Thus, increased cognitive control (corresponding to an increase in reaction time) is needed for RP patients only in more complex conditions that place a sufficiently high demand for attention and problem solving. Bowen et al. (69) asked patients recovering from strokes to walk at their comfortable pace alone and while completing an auditory choice reaction time task. Under dual task performance, stroke patients demonstrated an increased time in the dual-support phase of walking, reflecting the need for increased time in a more stable posture.

Alzheimer's disease (AD) patients, as compared to healthy controls, have a threefold increase in falls, causing hip fractures or hospitalization, and an increased rate of institutionalization following falls (70). Length of survival among AD patients also has been tied to falls (70a), and level of dementia has been shown to be a significant predictor in patients' ability to benefit from nursing home-based interventions (e.g., changes in chair design) (71). Other AD-associated complicating factors, in particular extrapyramidal symptoms and general health status, clearly play a role in increasing the risk of falls. Longitudinal studies, however, have consistently demonstrated that dementia severity contributes to falls risk independently of such factors (17,72,73). As executive function and control of attention are generally affected early on in AD (74), this suggests a link between decreased Executive Control and mobility for increased falls risk in this group.

Although few mobility studies have been completed with AD patients relative to healthy controls, AD patients' disproportionately greater difficulty completing divided attention tasks has been linked to impairments in balance (75), as well as gait speed and obstacle clearance (76,77). AD patients, even those without extrapyramidal signs, appear to be impaired in shifting and re-proportioning attention as needed. In AD patients with normal vestibular function, for example, falls and balance impairment have been related to problems in inhibiting previously learned responses under changing task demands and to an inability to effectively suppress visual distraction or shift visual attention (78). Parkinson disease (PD) patients also have been shown to have deficits in procedural learning and other executive functions that may place them at particularly high risk of falls and loss of balance. PD patients, for example, exhibit changes in velocity and step length regardless of whether dual-task conditions include all motor or both motor and cognitive tasks (54,79,80).

C. Variability

Deficits in attention, such as present in AD, can lead to variability in cognitive performance across time, increasing the risk of falls due to lapses of attention. Minimal research, however, has involved the relationship of other factors such as fatigue or endurance with cognition that can potentially lead to variable performance. Understanding variability can be important as mobility deficits may not arise in the laboratory setting due to the relatively short time period of most studies, whereas these very changes of interest may occur at home while completing a related movement after a long day of physical activity. In one study, regardless of age, poor sleepers reported more daytime difficulties across cognitive and motor domains than good sleepers (81). Variability in performance also has been tied in some tasks to gender issues. For example, when completing a computer-based navigation task with either an articulatory or spatial distracter, the articulatory interference affected women selectively, whereas performance of men was not affected differentially by either type of interference (82).

III. ENVIRONMENTAL MODULATING FACTORS

A. Setting

In addition to intrinsic factors related to the individual, external factors, such as features of the environment, can greatly impact the demand placed on the Behavioral Control System in determining a motor response. Institutional- and community-based studies report that falls tend to occur at times when activity on the ward is the greatest (83) or while a person is engaged in an activity or confronted by an obstacle (2,9). Low lighting conditions also have been shown to significantly impact mobility performance (84). Because tripping has been found to be so important in falls (9), several studies have incorporated obstacle avoidance in their walking components. For example, Chen et al. (65), asked young and older healthy controls to walk at their own pace and step over a "virtual" obstacle projected suddenly on the floor, while performing or not performing an auditory reaction time task. Although only very small reaction time changes were noted in the dual task situation, the risk of obstacle contact in the older patients disproportionately increased under dual task conditions as compared to young. Environmental situations that require an individual to quickly complete a task may also adversely impact performance. Persons who fall often attribute their accidents to "hurrying" or "rushing" (9,85). In a study looking at changes in gait under divided attention conditions, when asked to walk as fast as they could and step over an obstacle, older individuals had difficulty completing a simple number task at the same time (66).

B. Available Assisted Devices

The use of assistive devices, such as canes or walkers, has been shown to improve gait performance in individuals with mobility deficits, and may decrease the amount of cognitive control necessary for ambulation. For example, patients with peripheral neuropathy demonstrated improved performance on a gait task under three different intervention conditions (cane, ankle othoses, and touching a vertical surface) as reflected in decreased gait variability (86). Although an extensive literature does not exist related to the interaction of cognitive factors with use of available assisted devices for mobility, older patients with cognitive impairment have been shown to minimally, if at all, benefit from such nursing home-based interventions as changes in chair design to improve chair-rise prior to ambulation (71). In a study involving only younger, healthy controls, Wright and Kemp (87) found that walking with either rolling or standard walkers was highly attention demanding, with greater attentional demands actually found for the standard, as opposed to rolling, walker. Understanding how neuropsychological factors interact with an individual's ability to use assistive devices can lead to better designed products and more effective teaching strategies that can increase the benefits of these interventions.

IV. TASK-SPECIFIC MODULATING FACTORS

A. Task Interference

Two sources of interference have been proposed to explain decrements in performance noted when a person attempts to complete more than one task simultaneously (48). "Structural" interference occurs when two or more tasks share the same peripheral input or output systems, thus leading to greater interference effects in that particular system, thus reducing performance. "Capacity" interference assumes that a person has a "total," limited overall pool of attentional or other neuropsychological resources that can be drawn upon for completing any given task or set of tasks.

In a study by Sparrow et al. (88), performance of young and old subjects was contrasted while walking and stepping onto a specified target area marked on the walkway, while completing a reaction time task involving visual, auditory, or a combination of each stimuli. Performance on the visual reaction time or a combination of both visual and auditory reaction time tasks declined most during the dual task, but only for the older subjects. These findings were interpreted as reflecting structural interference effects associated with the visual demands, consistent with earlier findings that demonstrated an increased reliance on visual input while walking in older adults (58,89). Lundin-Olsson et al. (83) have shown that increasing the structural interference demands on mobility by having a person engage in two motor tasks at the same time (i.e., walking and holding a glass of water) better reflects differences between healthy and frail individuals than doing one task alone (i.e., walking). As a further example, Bond and Morris (54) demonstrated that PD patients can effectively perform more than one motor task at a time even while walking (i.e., carrying an empty tray). Increasing the motor demand to a certain point (i.e., carrying a tray with four glasses), however, resulted in a change in performance (i.e., slowing walking speed in order to complete the task appropriately). Although limited capacity models remain somewhat controversial and have not been specifically addressed in mobility research, it is hard to refute that there is a point in any system when the level of situational demand can be so high that an effective response cannot be generated by the Behavioral Control System.

B. Instructional Set

A careful consideration of the use of instructional sets to prioritize performance of one task over another is important in terms of understanding the outcome, especially in research paradigms when participants may be asked to complete more than one task simultaneously. For example, Courtemanche et al. (67) asked both healthy controls and diabetic peripheral neuropathy patients to maintain their preferred pace while doing a simple attention task (i.e., auditory reaction time). Consistent with the instructional set, neither patients nor controls changed their walking speed while doing the reaction time task. The reaction time of the patients as compared to controls, however, declined significantly more when walking as compared to when sitting. The authors interpreted these findings as consistent with the increased need for attention in the patient group while walking, in order to compensate for reduced peripheral sensory input. In most studies that involve this dual task approach, however, many research groups have not wished to prioritize either the walking or cognitive task, with interest more in a "naturalistic" setting of allowing the subject to decide. This can lead to significant difficulties in interpretation if performance in both tasks changes. These results could then be interpreted as related to the inherent difficulty of doing two tasks simultaneously or alternatively represent an intentional change in priority, such that subjects choose not to perform a task to their fullest ability due to factors such as increased cautiousness or fear of falling.

C. Novelty and Complexity

Novel or complex situations call for increased reliance on executive functioning and problem solving. When these executive skill areas are under greater strain based on age- or disease-related decrements, the ability to perform at a sufficient level can be compromised, as for instance on a crowded, active nursing care ward (83). It appears possible, however, to differentiate novelty from complexity demands. In one study in which novelty (with and without practice) and complexity (walking on oval or aperiodic tracks) were both manipulated, complexity of task demands appeared to be most salient (90), though older individuals may not benefit from practice as efficiently as do younger persons (91).

V. METHODOLOGICAL APPROACHES FOR CLARIFYING BEHAVIORAL CONTROL SYSTEM FACTORS IN WALKING

There are a number of approaches to examining the association between neuropsychological factors and mobility in older adults. Although each has limitations, the use of the multiple approaches can provide converging evidence that will lead to a more comprehensive model. Several examples are listed below.

A. Correlational Model

This type of design can be useful in providing regression-based information regarding factors that may impact an individual's fall risk, as well as assist in identifying the association between specific aspects of cognition and mobility task performance. As already mentioned, dementia severity has been shown to correlate with subsequent falls. The risk of major fall-related injuries also has been shown to be significantly higher with slowed performance on complex visual processing and set shifting tasks in older community-dwelling individuals (92,93). In addition, greater inefficiency in more complex walking tasks has been associated with performance on tests of focused attention and executive problem solving in community-dwelling elderly (94,95) and patients with both PD (96) and AD (77).

B. Patient Groups

The study of patients with well-characterized symptom profiles provides an opportunity for studying the effects of specific decrements in individual dimensions of the Behavioral Control System model on mobility. AD patients, for example, have clear cognitive difficulties, and in their earliest stages when there are at most very minimal mobility difficulties, provide an interesting contrast to healthy, older controls without cognitive compromise (77,97). Further, patients with RP provide a model for studying the role of visual difficulties in gait-associated paradigms, while patients with diabetic peripheral neuropathies assist in understanding the effect of restricting sensory input (68). Patients with stroke have been recruited for several studies, because they are considered a high risk group for falls associated with increased balance problems (69,98). The use of patients with well-circumscribed lesions known to affect specific neuropsychological systems can provide useful information regarding the role of cognitive factors to mobility performance. Patients with PD also are of interest, because they have known deficits in gait and balance, along with specific cognitive deficits (24,54,79,80,96,99). Severity effects also can be examined by studying longitudinal cognitive changes evident in either recovery from stroke or continued decline in dementia (100).

C. Challenge Studies

Experimental designs that directly challenge specific aspects of the Behavioral Control System, while controlling for other factors, provide valuable information in understanding the relationship between cognition and mobility in older adults. For instance, our group has examined response inhibition in both young and old adults while completing a turn (101). Subjects were required to make a 180° turn as quickly as possible while holding a bowl filled with balls. On some of the trials, a tone was sounded as a signal to suddenly switch the direction of the turn. On these "switch" trials requiring inhibition of the original motor program and initiation of a new one, the older adults experienced more difficulty (i.e., took more steps and were slower to complete the turn than younger adults). The risk of foot interference during a turn was higher for the older persons as measured by a decrease in foot distance. These findings related to age-associated declines in inhibition are particularly relevant, given the higher risk of both falls and more severe injuries noted in older individuals while turning (102).

To look at the effects of set shifting and mental flexibility on mobility performance in both healthy and cognitively impaired older adults, our laboratory has developed a walking version of a clinical neuropsychological, paper-and-pencil measure of visual scanning and mental flexibility, the Trail Making Test. In this mobility version of the task, participants are asked to walk along pathways of instrumented markers that showed either sequential numbers (as in Trails A) or an alternating sequence of numbers and letters (as in Trails B) amongst other number or letter distracters. Subjects are required to walk along the instrumented pathways by stepping on the numbers and/or letters in order, analogous to what is done in the standard paper-and-pencil Trails task. Comparing young and old adults on this task under high and low lighting, Alexander et al. (84) demonstrated that older adults exhibited greater difficulty than younger adults in the more cognitively demanding Trails B condition, requiring mental flexibility. This was especially true under conditions of low lighting. In another study using the Trails paradigm (103), three groups of subjects were studied—healthy, older adults, patients with Mild Cognitive Impairment (MCI) who presented with at least a memory deficit, and patients with mild AD. Preliminary results showed that the AD patients had significant difficulty on all of the walkways compared to the other two groups, as would be expected. Of particular interest, however, are the results of the MCI group. No differences in performance between the MCI and healthy old subjects were found on the Trails A walkways that required attention processing. However, variable performance was noted on the more complex Trails B walkways. In particular, those MCI patients with just a memory deficit only showed minimal slowing on Trails B, while those MCI patients with both memory and executive functioning deficits exhibited considerable slowing on the Trails B walkways with performance more closely resembling the AD patients. These results lend support to the theory that the mobility deficits in early AD are related to changes in executive control, rather than a decline in memory processes or other physical factors, alone.

D. Dual Task Paradigm

The Dual Task paradigm is a well-researched approach to challenge studies. The capacity to "dual task" or perform more than one task at the same time is conceptualized as the ability to complete a "primary" task, which is the major focus of attention and action, and a "secondary" or "distracter" task at the same time (104). In the cognitive psychology literature, this approach has been extremely fruitful in characterizing and clarifying the role of executive control of attention and has more recently been applied to motor skills. The literature on dual tasking, specifically with regard to gait, can be predominantly characterized as four separate approaches (Table 1) that provide different information dependent on particular instructional sets.

When the emphasis is on holding the mobility task as primary by maintaining constant performance across the single and dual task situations, two approaches can be taken in the selection of the secondary task. If tasks are chosen with low structural interference, that is, when the primary and secondary tasks do not compete for similar processing needs (e.g., both tasks do not depend on limited visual resources), then the variability in performance of the secondary task can be interpreted as reflecting the actual amount of attention and central processing needed to complete the motor task (104). Auditory simple "probe" or reaction time measures are usually chosen for these paradigms, because they represent a measure of focused attention and vigilance that usually has minimal physical overlap with mobility task demands. If a secondary task is chosen with high structural interference, such as, when another motor task is chosen as the secondary task, the information provided by variability in performance of the secondary task is less clear. In this case, declines in the secondary task performance can be interpreted as reflecting not only attentional needs, but potentially processing limits within the single modality involved with both the primary and secondary task.

If the cognitive task is considered primary, requiring the subjects to hold performance on the cognitive task constant while motor performance (e.g., gait speed or variability) is allowed to vary, then information about changes in mobility task performance may be used to identify what types of cognitive load most affect gait or mobility. Although this technique has not been specifically pursued in research on gait, it provides a unique methodology for evaluating underlying mechanisms for control of mobility. As part of an ongoing study in our laboratory, subjects are asked to keep their performance on a set of cognitive tasks constant while walking along a pathway. The cognitive tasks were chosen to examine more specifically working memory processes and executive control. These tasks also were equated for difficulty across subject groups and include measures associated with the executive control system, along with its component parts, the phonological loop and the visual–spatial sketch pad. Relative changes in walking speed and gait characteristics can then be compared when subjects perform specific types of cognitive tasks in order to examine various aspects of behavioral control.

By far, the majority of dual task studies involving gait and mobility have either instructed the subject to consider both tasks as primary (e.g., maintain optimal performance on both) or did not instruct the subjects about prioritization, in order to allow the subject to choose freely, much as they might within the natural setting. Schrodt et al. (66) asked subjects to walk as fast as possible and step over an obstacle simulating a door threshold alone and while completing a verbal working memory task. Under the dual task condition, subjects were instructed to complete both tasks as fast and accurately as possible at essentially the same performance level as the single task conditions. Gait speed was maintained in the dual task condition, though a decline in working memory accuracy was noted. Most interesting was the fact that older adults in this study also altered their step pattern in the approach and crossing over the obstacle, suggesting that they employed a more cautious approach to the dual task situation in order to

Table 1 Dual Task Methodology Approaches to Mobility Research

Primary task	Instruction	Secondary task	Instruction	Evaluation goal
Mobility task	Hold performance constant	Cognitive task (low structural interference)	Allow performance to vary	Determine attentional requirements of the primary (motor) task
Mobility task	Hold performance constant	Cognitive task (high structural interference) or mobility task	Allow performance to vary	Determine the limits of capacity in one modality
Cognitive task	Hold performance constant	Mobility task	Allow performance to vary	Compare effects of distracters on mobility
Mobility task Cognitive task	Equal emphasis or not addressed	None	None	Determine effectiveness of attentional shifting and/or adaptive prioritization

lower their risk of tripping. This demonstrates that even older individuals can employ a flexible approach to attentional resource allocation based on their evaluation of task demands. However, using the approach of equal or no prioritization for primary and secondary tasks can lead to difficulties in interpretation of obtained results. This is because it is often difficult to ascertain whether changes in performance are due to impairment in effectively allocating attention resources between two tasks or a result of an intentional decision to focus on one task to the decrement of the other. This decision choice also may fluctuate dependent on the situation at the time of the testing or vary across time points as tasks continue, resulting in increased variability of results. In order to improve the clarity of results, studies should report data on the accuracy of both the mobility and cognitive tasks and preferably report on change in performance over time when longer tasks or multiple trials are employed.

VI.   PRACTICAL CLINICAL IMPLICATIONS FOR A BEHAVIORAL CONTROL SYSTEM APPROACH

A fuller understanding of the contributing cognitive factors to mobility performance can provide critical data for a number of important questions in aging, including detection of persons at heightened risk of falling, as well as to assist in the development of more specific intervention strategies in rehabilitation. Understanding the interaction among environmental, physical, and cognitive factors impacting an individual's mobility performance and subsequent likelihood of falling will lead to a more comprehensive and inclusive theoretical model of falls in older adults (91).

   Approaches to predicting falls risk have often included a neuropsychological component. For example, in comparing the time a subject took walking on a measured walkway without distraction (Timed-Up-Go, TUG task) to walking while talking (i.e., answering questions, the Walking-While-Talking task), Lundin-Olsson et al. (105) demonstrated that persons who stopped walking while talking: (a) went on to experience a fall within the next six months, (b) had less safe gait characteristics, (c) were slower with basic mobility, and (d) were more dependent during ADLs. In a follow-up study, the same author (83) found that patients who walked slower while carrying a glass of water (TUG manual, a mobility-based, rather than cognitive, secondary task) were more frail and fell more often. Dual task conditions have not always proved successful in predicting increased difficulty or falls risk in aging, however. Shumway-Cook and Woollacott (106) reported that adding an oral subtraction task to the TUG did not increase the falls likelihood predictability of the task as compared to the basic TUG. Another study (107) also found no increased proficiency in predicting falls when adding a categorical fluency task to the TUG. On the other hand, Verghese and coworkers found that increasing the complexity and challenge of the TUG (i.e., by instructing the subject to recite alternate letters of the alphabet, rather than the alphabet sequentially) led to a progressive increase in positive predictive power.

The effectiveness of rehabilitation strategies also has been examined from a neuropsychological approach. Cockburn et al. (100) found that although simple walking speed improved following nine months of post-stroke rehabilitation, gait speed under dual task conditions (i.e. completing a verbal fluency task while walking) did not necessarily improve at the same rate. Because many everyday activities involve concurrent cognitive and motor components, dual task paradigms may provide a better index of functional ability than motor tasks performed under single task conditions (98). Understanding the relationship between attention and executive control to performance in dual task situations can lead to approaches to rehabilitation training that might direct patients to avoid or minimize situations involving dual task load or, alternatively, directly teach strategies to effectively conduct two tasks concurrently.

For older persons, providing information about safety concerns when doing two tasks simultaneously or directly teaching safety techniques for such situations (e.g., learning to minimize distraction when walking across a busy intersection) may represent important techniques in reducing falls risk. Gait-based training interventions also could incorporate the use of dual task paradigms, to better prepare older individuals for such situations (24), as well as provide a useful metric for measuring the efficiency or "automaticity" of a newly learned skill (104). Understanding the impact of age-related changes in other executive control processes such as inhibition and set shifting to mobility performance can also help identify those at greatest risk of falling as well as direct future intervention strategies. In addition, knowledge of those cognitive factors influencing mobility performance can affect the design and manufacture of assistive devices. Although many devices are designed to improve safety, they also seem to detract from travel because they require the user to process artificial input or make novel motor responses, thereby increasing cognitive load. It will be important to develop cognitive load-reducing mobility aids if such interventions expect to be successful.

REFERENCES

1. Lord SR, Ward JA, Williams P. An epidemiological study of falls in older community-dwelling women: The Randwick falls and ractures study. Aust J Public Health 1993; 17:240–245.
2. Tinetti ME, Speechley M, Ginter SF. Risk factors for falls among elderly persons living in the community. N Engl J Med 1988; 319(26):1701–1707.

3. Brauer SG, Woollacott M, Shumway-Cook A. The interacting effects of cognitive demand and recovery of postural stability in balance-impaired elderly persons. J Gerontol 2000; 56A:M489–M496.

4. Dargent-Molina P, Favier F, Grandjean H. Fall-related factors and risk of hip fracture. Lancet 1996; 348:145–149.

5. Kannus P, Palvanen M, Niemi S'. Time trends in severe head injuries among elderly Finns. J Am Med Assoc 2001; 286:673–674.

6. Marottoli RA, Berkman LF, Cooney LM. Decline in physical function following hip fracture. J Am Geriatr Soc 1992; 40:861–866.

7. Verghese J, Buschke H, Viola L, Katz M, Hall C, Kuslansky G et al. Validity of divided attention tasks in predicting falls in older individuals: a preliminary study. J Am Geriatr Soc 2002; 50(9):1572–1576.

8. Lipsitz LA, Jonsson PV, Kelley MM, Koestner JS. Causes and correlates of recurrent falls in ambulatory frail elderly. J Gerontol 1991; 46:114–122.

9. Hill K, Schwarz J, Flicker L, Carroll S. Falls among healthy, community-dwelling, older women: a prospective study of frequency, circumstances, consequences and prediction accuracy. Aust NZ J Public Health 1999; 23(1): 41–48.

10. Sehested P, Severinnielsen T. Falls by hospitalized elderly patients—causes, prevention. Geriatrics 1977; 32(4):101–108.

11. Tinetti ME, Williams TF, Mayewski R. Fall risk index for elderly patients based on number of chronic disabilities. Am J Med 1986; 80:429–434.

12. Nyberg L, Gustafson Y. Patient falls in stroke rehabilitation—a challenge to rehabilitation strategies. Stroke 1995; 26(5):838–842.

13. Blake AJ, Morgan K, Bendall MJ, Dallosso H, Ebrahim SBJ, Arie THD, et al. Falls by elderly people at home: prevalence and associated factors. Age Ageing 1988; 17:365–372.

14. Connell BR, Wolf SL. Environmental and behavioral circumstances associated with falls at home among healthy elderly individuals. Arch Phys Med Rehabil 1997; 78(2):179–186.

15. Calne DB. Age and complexity hypothesis. In: Poon L, ed. Aging in the 1980s. Washington, DC: American Psychological Association, 1980:332–339.

16. Alexander NB. Postural control in older adults. J Am Geriatr Soc 1994; 42: 93–108.

17. Buchner DM, Larson EB. Falls and fractures in patients with Alzheimer-type dementia. J Am Med Assoc 1987; 257(11):1492–1495.

18. Macpherson JM, Horak FB, Dunbar DC, Dow RS. Stance dependence of automatic postural adjustments in humans. Exp Brain Res 1989; 78(3): 557–566.

19. McIlroy WE, Maki BE. Changes in early automatic postural responses associated with the prior-planning and execution of a compensatory step. Brain Res 1993; 36(3):203–211.

20. Nashner LM, Woollacott MH. The organization of rapid postural adjustments of standing humans: an experimental conceptual model. Posture Mov 1979; 631(2):243–257.

21. Woollacott M, Shumway-Cook A. Attention and the control of posture and gait: a review of an emerging area of research. Gait Posture 2002; 16(1):1–14.

22. Lajoie Y, Teasdale N, Bard C, Fleury M. Upright standing and gait: are there changes in attentional requirements related to normal aging? Exp Aging Res 1996; 22:185–198.

23. Downtown JH, Andrews K. Postural disturbance and psychological symptoms amongst elderly people living at home. Int J Geriatr Psychiatry 1990; 5:93–98.

24. O'Shea S, Morris ME, Iansek R. Dual task interference during gait in people with Parkinson disease: effects of motor versus cognitive secondary tasks. Phys Ther 2002; 82(9):888–897.

25. Giordani B. Intellectual and cognitive disturbances in epileptic patients. In: Sackellares JC, Berent S, eds. Psychological Disturbances in Epilepsy. Boston: Butterworth Heinemann, 1996:45–97.

26. Horton AM Jr, Puente AE. Life-span neuropsychology: an overview. In: Horton AM Jr, ed. Neuropsychology Across the Life-Span: Assessment and Treatment. New York: Springer Publishing, 1990:1–15.

27. DeJong R. Adult age differences in goal activation and goal maintenance. Eur J Cogn Psychol 2001; 13:71–89.

28. Fuster JM. The Prefrontal Cortex. In: Anatomy, Physiology and Neuropsychology of the Frontal Lobe. 3d ed. Philadelphia: Lippincott-Raven, 1997.

29. Norman DA, Shallice T. Attention to action: willed and automatic control of behavior. In: Davidson JL, Schwartz GE, Shapiro D, eds. Consciousness and Self-regulation: Advances in Theory and Research. New York: Plenum, 1986: 1–18.

30. Mayr U, Liebscher T. Is there an age deficit in the selection of mental sets? Eur J Cogn Psychol 2001; 13(1–2):47–69.

31. Teasdale N, Bard C, LaRue J, Fleury M. On the cognitive penetrability of posture control. Exp Aging Res 1993; 19:1–13.

32. Teasdale N, Stelmach GE, Breunig A. Postural sway characteristics of the elderly under normal and altered visual and support surface conditions. J Gerontol 1991; 46(6):B238–B244.

33. Alexander NB, Guire KE, Thelen DG, Ashton-Miller JA, Schultz AB, Grunawalt JC et al. Self-reported walking ability predicts functional mobility performance in frail older adults. J Am Geriatr Soc 2000; 48(11):1408–1413.

34. Cress ME, Schectman KB, Mulrow CD, Fiatarone MA, Gerety MB, Buchner DM. Relationship between physical performance and self-perceived physical function. J Am Geriatr Soc1995(43):93–101.

35. Yardley L, Redfern MS. Psychological factors influencing recovery from balance disorders. Anxiety Disord 2001; (13):107–119.

36. Balaban CD, Thayer JF. Neurological bases for balance–anxiety links. Anxiety Disord2001(15):53–79.

37. Wada M, Sunaga N, Nagai M. Anxiety affects the postural sway of the anteroposterior axis in college students. Neurosci Lett 2001; 302(2–3):157–159.

38. Bolmont B, Gangloff P, Vouriot A, Perrin PP. Mood states and anxiety influence abilities to maintain balance control in healthy human subjects. Neurosci Lett 2002; 329(1):96–100.

39. Tinetti ME, Richman D, Powell L. Falls efficacy as a measure of fear of falling. J Gerontol Psychol Sci 1990; 45(6):P239–P243.

40. Tinetti ME, Mendes de Leon CF, Doucette JT, Baker DI. Fear of falling and fall-related efficacy in relationship to functioning among community-living elders. J Gerontol Med Sci 1994; 49(3):140–147.

41. Giordani B, Miller AC, Alexander NB, Guire KE, Ashton-Miller JA, Berent S, et al. Neuropsychological factors relate to self-report and performance-based measures of functional mobility. Annual Meeting of Tenth Gerontological Society of America, Los Angeles, CA, 1995. Ref Type: Abstract.

42. Giordani B, Persad CC, Miller AC, Alexander NB, Ashton-Miller JA, Guire KE, et al. Cognitive and personality measures as predictors of successful mobility performance. Annual Meeting of the American Psychological Association, Toronto, Ontario, Canada, 1996. Ref Type: Abstract.

43. Baddeley AD. Working Memory. Oxford, England: Oxford University Press, 1986.

44. Moscovitch M, Winocur G. The neuropsychology of memory and aging. In: Craik FIM, Salthouse TA, eds. The Handbook of Aging and Cognition. Hillsdale, NJ: Lawrence Erlbaum Associates, 1992:315–372.

45. Bjork RA. Retrieval inhibition as an adaptive mechanism in human memory. In: Roehrs T, Craik FIM, eds. Varieties of Memory and Consciousness. Essays in Honour of Endel Tulving. New Jersey: Lawrence Erlbaum Associates, 1989.

46. Tipper SP, Weaver B, Houghton G. Behavioural goals determine inhibitory mechanisms of selective attention. Quart J Exp Psychol 1994; 47A:809–840.

47. Neumann E, DeSchepper BG. An inhibition-based fan effect: evidence for an active suppression mechanism in selective attention. Canad J Psychol 1992; 46: 1–40.

48. Kahneman D. Attention and Effort. Englewood Cliffs, N J: Prentice-Hall, 1973.

49. Neumann O. A functional view of attention. In: Heuer H, Sanders AF, eds. Perspectives on Perception and Action. Hillsdale, NJ: Lawrence Erlbaum Associates, 1987:361–394.

50. Allport DA. Attention and performance. In: Claxton G, ed. New Directions in Cognitive Psychology. London: Routledge & Kegan Paul, 1980:112–153.

51. McDowd JM, Shaw RJ. Attention and aging: a functional perspective. In: Craik FIM, Salthouse TA, eds. The Handbook of Aging and Cognition. Mahwah, NJ: Lawrence Erlbaum Associates, 2000:221–292.

52. Adkin AL, Frank JS, Carpenter MG, Peysar GW. Postural control is scaled to level of postural threat. Gait Posture 2000; (12):87–93.

53. Brown LA, Gage WH, Polych MA, Sleik RJ, Winder TR. Central set influences on gait—age-dependent effects of postural threat. Exp Brain Res 2002; 145(3):286–296.

54. Bond JM, Morris M. Goal-directed secondary motor tasks: their effects on gait in subjects with Parkinson disease. Arch Phys Med Rehabil 2000; 81: 110–116.

55. Morris M, Iansek R, Smithson F, Huxham F. Postural instability in Parkinson's disease: a comparison with and without a concurrent task. Gait Posture 2000; 12(3):205–216.

56. Jahanshahi M, Frith CD. Willed action and its impairments. Cogn Neuropsychol 1998; 15(6/7/8):483–533.

57. Raz N, Gunning-Dixon FM, Head D, Dupuis JH, Acker JD. Neuroanatomical correlates of cognitive aging: evidence from structural magnetic resonance imaging. Neuropsychology 1998; 12(1):95–114.

58. Anderson PG, Nienhuis B, Mulder T, Hulstijn W. Are older adults more dependent on visual information in regulating self-motion than younger adults? J Motor Behav 1998; 30(2):104–113.

59. Patla AE, Vickers JN. Where and when do we look as we approach and step over an obstacle in the travel path? NeuroReport 1997; 8(17):3661–3665.

60. Shumway-Cook A, Woollacott M, Kerns KA, Baldwin M. The effects of two types of cognitive tasks on postural stability in older adults with and without a history of falls. J Gerontol 1997; 52A(4):M232–M240.

61. Albert M, Moss M. The assessment of memory disorders in patients with Alzheimer's disease. In: Squire LR, Butters N, eds. Neuropsychology of Memory. New York: Guilford, 1984.

62. Welford AT. Ageing and human skill. London: Oxford University Press, 1958.

63. Li YS, Meyer JS, Thornby J. Longitudinal follow-up of depressive symptoms among normal versus cognitively impaired elderly. Int J Geriatr Psychiatry 2001; 16(7):718–727.

64. Kemper S, Herman RE, Lian CHT. The costs of doing two things at once for young and older adults: talking while walking, finger tapping, and ignoring speech or noise. Psychol Aging 2003; 18(2):181–192.

65. Chen HC, Schultz AB, AshtonMiller JA, Giordani B, Alexander NB, Guire KE. Stepping over obstacles: dividing attention impairs performance of old more than young adults. J Gerontol Ser A—Biol Sci Med Sci 1996; 51(3): M116–M122.

66. Schrodt LA, Mercer VS, Giuliani CA, Hartman M. Characteristics of stepping over an obstacle in community dwelling older adults under dual-task conditions. Gait Posture 2004; 19(3):279–287.

67. Courtemanche R, Teasdale N, Boucher P, Fleury M, Lajoie Y, Bard C. Gait problems in diabetic neuropathic patients. Arch Phys Med Rehabil 1996; 77(9):849–855.

68. Turano KA, Geruschat DR, Stahl JT. Mental effort required for walking: effects of retinitis pigmentosa. Optom Vis Sci 1998; 75(12):879–886.

69. Bowen A, Wenman R, Mickelborouogh J. Dual-task effects while walking on velocity and balance following a stroke. Age Ageing 2001; 30:319–323.

70. Morris JC, Rubin EH, Morris EJ, Mandel SA. Senile dementia of the Alzheimer's type: an important risk factor for serious falls. J Gerontol 1987; 42(4):412–417.

70a. Walsh JS, Welch G, Larson EB. Survival of outpatients with Alzheimer-type dementia. Annals of Internal Medicine 1990; 113:429–434.

71. Finlay OE, Bayles TB, Rosen C, Milling J. Effects of chair design, age and cognitive status on mobility. Age Ageing 1983; 12:329–335.

72. Brody EM, Kleban MH, Moss MS, Kleban F. Predictors of falls among institutionalized women with Alzheimer's disease. J Am Geriatr Soc 1984; 32(12):877–882.

73. Van Kijk PTM, Meulenberg OGRM, Vandesande HJ, Habbema JDF. Falls in dementia patients. Gerontologist 1993; 33(2):200–204.

74. Baddeley A, Logie R, Bressi S, DellaSala S, Spinnler H. Dementia and working memory. Quart J Exp Psychol Sec A—Hum Exp Psychol 1986; 38(4): 603–618.

75. Rapp MA, Krampe RTH, Bondar A, Baltes PB. Resource competition between cognitive and sensorimotor functioning in old age: The role of a cognitive impairment. Annual Meeting of the Gerontological Society of America, Washington, D.C., Nov 19–23, 2000.

76. Alexander NB, Mollo JM, Giordani B, Ashton-Miller JA, Schultz AB, Grunawalt JA, et al. Maintenance of balance, gait patterns, and obstacle clearance in Alzheimer's disease. Neurology 1995; 45:908–914.

77. Camicioli R, Howieson D, Lehman S, Kaye J. Talking while walking: the effect of a dual task in aging and Alzheimer's disease. Neurology 1997; 48:955–958.

78. Chong RKY, Jones CL, Horak FB. Postural set for balance control is normal in Alzheimer's but not in Parkinson's disease. J Gerontol Ser A—Biol Sci Med Sci 1999; 54(3):M129–M135.

79. Morris ME, Iansek R, Matyas TA, Summers JJ. Stride length regulation in Parkinson's disease normalization strategies and underlying mechanisms. Brain 1996; 119:551–568.

80. Hausdorff JM, Balash Y, Giladi N. Effects of cognitive challenge on gait variability in patients with Parkinson's disease. J Geriatr Psychiatry Neurol 2003; 16:53–58.

81. Alapin I, Fichten CS, Libman E, Creti L, Bailes S, Wright J. How is good and poor sleep in older adults and college students related to daytime sleepiness, fatigue, and ability to concentrate? J Psychosom Res 2000; 49:381–390.

82. Saucier D, Bowman M, Elias L. Sex differences in the effect of articulatory or spatial dual-task interference during navigation. Brain Cogn 2003; 53(2): 346–350.

83. Lundin-Olsson L, Nyberg L, Gustafson Y. Attention, frailty, and falls: the effect of a manual task on basic mobility. J Am Geriatr Soc 1998; 46(6): 758–761.

84. Alexander NB, Ashton-Miller JA, Giordani B, Guire K, Schultz AB. Stepping accuracy with increasing cognitive and visual demand: a trails step test. Gerontologist 2000; 40:269.

85. Berg WP, Alessio HM, Mills EM, Tong C. Circumstances and consequences of falls in independent community-dwelling older adults. Age Ageing 1997; 26(4):261–268.

86. Richardson JK, Thies S, Demott T, Ashton-Miller JA. Interventions improve gait regularity in patients with peripheral neuropathy while walking on an irregular surface under low light. J Am Geriatr Soc 2004; 52:510–515.

87. Wright DL, Kemp TL. The dual-task methodology and assessing the attentional demands of ambulation with walking devices. Phys Ther 1992; 72(4): 306–312.

88. Sparrow WA, Bradshaw EJ, Lamoureux E, Tirosh O. Ageing effects on the attention demands of walking. Hum Mov Sci 2002; 21(5–6):961–972.

89. Patla AE, Prentice SD, Gobbi LT. Visual control of obstacle avoidance during locomotion: strategies in young children, young and older adults. In: Ferrandez AM, Teasdale N, eds. Changes in Sensory Motor Behavior in Aging. Elsevier Science, 1996:257–277.

90. Lindenberger U, Marsiske M, Baltes PB. Memorizing while walking: increase in dual-task costs from young adulthood to old age. Psychol Aging 2000; 15(3):417–436.

91. Melzer I, Oddsson LIE. The effect of a cognitive task on voluntary step execution in healthy elderly and young individuals. J Am Geriatr Soc 2004; 52: 1255–1262.

92. Brauer S, Woollacott M, Shumway-Cook A. The interacting effects of cognitive demand and recovery of postural stability in balance-impaired elderly persons. J Gerontol 2001; 56A(8):M489–M496.

93. Nevitt MC, Cummings SR, Hudes ES. Risk factors for injurious falls: a prospective study. J Gerontol Med Sci 1991; 46(5):164–170.

94. Nutt JG, Marsden CD, Thompson PD. Human walking and higher-level gait disorders, particularly in the elderly. Neurology 1993; 43:268–279.

95. Persad CC, Giordani B, Chen HC, Ashton-Miller JA, Alexander NB, Wilson CS, et al. Neuropsychological predictors of complex obstacle avoidance in healthy older adults. J Gerontol 1995; 50B(5):272–277.

96. Yogev G, Giladi N, Gruendlinger L, Baltadjieva R, Simon ES, Hausdorff JM. Executive function, mental loading and gait variability in Parkinson's disease. AGS Annual Meeting. Vol. 53. Abstract, 2004.

97. Sheridan PL, Solomont J, Kowall N, Hausdorff JM. Influence of executive function on locomotor function: divided attention increases gait variability in Alzheimer's disease. J Am Geriatr Soc 2003; 51(11):1633–1637.

98. Haggard P, Cockburn J, Cock J, Fordham C, Wade D. Interference between gait and cognitive tasks in a rehabilitating neurological population. J Neurol Neurosurg Psychiatry 2000; 69(4):479–486.

99. Camicioli R, Oken BS, Sexton G. Verbal fluency task affects gait in Pakinson's disease with motor freezing. J Geriatr Psychiatry Neurol 1998; 11:181–185.

100. Cockburn J, Haggard P, Cock J, Fordham C. Changing patterns of cognitive-motor interference (CMI) over time during recovery from stroke. Clin Rehabilitat 2003; 17(2):167–173.

101. Meinhart P, Kramer M, Ashton-Miller JA, Persad CC. Kinematic analyses of the 180° standing turn: effects of age on strategies adopted by healthy young and older woman. Gait Posture. In press.

102. Cumming RG, Klineberg RJ. Fall frequency and characteristics and the risk of hip-fractures. J Am Geriatr Soc 1994; 42(7):774–778.

103. Persad CC, Giordani B, Alexander N, Ashton-Miller JA, Guire K, Kemp TL. Cognition and motor performance in healthy old and cognitively impaired subjects. J Int Neuropsychol Soc 2003; 9(2):226.

104. Abernethy B. Dual-task methodology and motor-skills research—some applications and methodological constraints. J Hum Mov Stud 1988; 14(3): 101–132.

105. Lundin-Olsson L, Nyberg L, Gustafson Y. "Stops walking when talking" as a predictor of falls in elderly people. "Stops walking when talking" as a predictor of falls in elderly people. Lancet 1997; 349:617.
106. Shumway-Cook A, Woollacott M. Attentional demands and postural control: the effect of sensory context. J Gerontol Med Sci 2000; 55A(1):M10–M16.
107. Bootsma-van der Wiel A, Gussekloo J, de Craen AJM, van Exel E, Bloem BR, Westendorp RGJ. Walking and talking as predictors of falls in the general population: The Leiden 85-Plus Study. J Am Geriatr Soc 2003; 51(10): 1466–1471.

7

Gait Assessments and Interventions: A Glimpse into the Future

Jennifer Healey

Cambridge Research Laboratory, Hewlett–Packard, Cambridge, Massachusetts, U.S.A.

Jeffrey M. Hausdorff

Movement Disorders Unit, Tel Aviv Sourasky Medical Center, Sackler School of Medicine, Tel Aviv University, Tel Aviv, Israel and Division on Aging, Harvard Medical School, Boston, Massachusetts, U.S.A.

In the previous chapters of this book, current methods for monitoring gait and for optimizing treatment of balance and gait disorders were described (e.g., see Chapters 2 and 3). Here, we take a brief look at the future. It might take a few years or maybe a few decades, but there is little doubt. The practice of medicine, in general, and the methods for evaluating and treating balance and gait disorders, more specifically, are headed toward some dramatic changes that should, ultimately, improve diagnostic capabilities and functional outcomes. Here, we briefly describe some of the technologies, already on the horizon, that have a good chance of enhancing the gait and balance of many patients.

I. MONITORING EVERYWHERE

New models and methods of analysis are constantly being developed—but how will we obtain the signal for analysis? The future holds many possibilities as computers, cameras, and electronics become smaller, more ubiquitous, and require less power than ever before. Soon, methods for signal acquisition may be in our clothes, in our cars, and in our homes. These signals can either be processed by high-end personal digital assistants (PDAs) that can be carried in a pocket or sent to remote computers using radio frequency (RF) transmission or wireless Internet connections. In addition, cameras may be keeping an eye on us, watching our every move, and passing judgment. For example, the LifeShirt™ by VivoMetrics (http://www.vivometrics.com) is a comfortable, washable "shirt" containing numerous embedded sensors that continuously monitor multiple physiological signs including EKG, respiration, BP, PO_2, leg movements, and posture. The shirt can be worn at home, work, or play. Data from the sensors are captured on a small belt-worn recorder and sent to VivoMetrics Data Center by cellular telecommunication. Terrier et al. (1,2) at the University of Lausanne in Switzerland have recently begun to evaluate gait (e.g., stride length, gait speed) using high-precision global positioning satellite receivers. Biomechanical parameters can be captured throughout the day, in a totally unconstrained environment.

II. PRÊT À PORTER (READY TO WEAR)

Numerous studies have shown that patients with disturbances of balance and gait perform differently on measures of static balance. Collins and colleagues (3,4) sought to analyze the noisy center of pressure fluctuations using methods from statistical physics to predict a patient's response to a nudge or perturbation and, hence, the likelihood of falling. In recent pilot studies, they were able to show that quiet standing measures do indeed predict the response to a mechanical perturbation. Some have envisioned turning a force platform that measures center of pressure movements and sway into a fixture in older adults' homes in much the same way that a scale can be found in almost everyone's bathroom. A "super"-scale could give important new insights into mechanics of balance and gait. Every morning, people could monitor their balance from the comfort of their homes simply by stepping on a super-scale. This kind of daily monitoring could enable doctors to track changes in their patients' balance over time to see if their condition might be deteriorating due to aging or disease, or improving due to some new therapy.

However, why stop at just an intelligent bathroom scale? New advances in technology allow sensors and computers to follow us everywhere. A wearable computer that measures gait on an ongoing basis could warn of an increased risk of a fall before it happens, wherever the person is located. Several such devices are already in development and, in the future, they could become so inexpensive and unobtrusive that they could become part of everyday clothing or even be as disposable as bandages.

In Japan, Soichiro Matsushita of Tokyo University and researchers from Tokyo Saiseiki Central Hospital and Keio University have created a wearable "sense of balance" monitoring system that can be used any time, anywhere. The device, which could easily be mistaken for a set of headphones, tracks the patients' center of gravity (COG) in real time. Inside the headset, reside three accelerometers that measure changes in acceleration in three directions: forward and back, side to side, and up and down. A computer algorithm transforms these readings into a tracing of the wearer's COG that has been calibrated against standard force plate stabilometry tracings at Saiseiki Central Hospital. However, unlike the hospital apparatus, the headset COG device allows the wearer to perform a balance test on any solid surface just by standing still for a minute. A wearable computer or PDA can monitor the sensors and provide the wearer with a real-time assessment of their likeliness to fall. Certain changes in the COG tracing appear to be related to fatigue, dizziness, or illness. So before performing a difficult task such as climbing stairs or entering the shower, a person could do a "spot check" on their balance to help avoid injury. Such a balance check might also be useful for drivers before entering a vehicle.

In addition to static balance measurements, wearable sensors will also be able to tell us about the dynamics of our gait from measurements obtained via clothing and shoes and accessories. At the Veteran's Administration in Palo Alto, Eric Sabelman (5) has created a wearable system of accelerometers called "WAMAS" to identify patterns of human body movement that accompany loss of balance before a fall occurs, warn of pre-fall behavior, and if necessary, signal that the wearer has fallen. At Virginia Tech, Mark Jones of the Electrical Engineering Department is developing an e-textile approach to gait monitoring. He has developed a set of very colorful pants wired with sensors that detect the acceleration of the wearer's waist and upper and lower legs. Using these acceleration signals, researchers can extract the inter-stride variation and variations in walking patterns. These smart pants are different from the other strain gauge sensor clothing (6) because they are very loose fitting and easy to put on, making them ideal for elderly wearers for whom wriggling into tight-fitting spandex may not only be distasteful, but also sometimes physically impossible. Another appealing quality of these pants is that they have no buttons to push and no interface to master. The wires and sensors are all part of the fabric; so, all patients have to do is put them on and go about their normal daily routine.

At MIT's Media Lab, Professor Joseph Paradiso has been taking a different approach, developing an all in one sensor shoe that includes its own on board-signal processing and RF transmitter (7).

The shoe includes an insole with four force-sensitive resistors, used to measure stride timing and left to right weight distribution, two piezoelectric sensors made of polyvinylidine fluoride to measure heel strike and toe-off events, and two pairs of resistive bend sensors. An attached circuit board contains accelerometers and gyroscopes that provide motion three-dimensional information. The board weighs only 200 g and is powered by a 9 V battery. With a detection algorithm installed on the processing board, this system could be used to warn the wearer of an impending fall. The sneaker can also broadcast signals from all the sensors to a nearby PDA or embedded computer system for more complex real-time analysis. These shoes are already being assessed for clinical gait analysis in joint work with Massachusetts General Hospital's Biomotion Laboratory.

However, what if you just want something simple? T. Degen and colleagues at the Swiss Federal Institute of Technology in Zurich have been working on a fall detector that can be worn in a wristwatch. Nicknamed "SPEEDY," the "watch" can detect forwards, backwards, and sideways falls using two sensors that measure acceleration. SPEEDY uses signal processing and pattern recognition to identify a three phase "fall event" consisting of high velocity towards the ground followed by impact and inactivity. Once a fall is identified, the watch can send an alert via a wireless connection to the Internet to the patient's physician or a monitoring call center to quickly call for assistance. In the future, such fall detectors could be used to deploy a personal airbag such as James Bond's "inflatable skiwear" or Demolition Man's "safety foam," to minimize the impact, risk of fractures, and fear of falling. Other accelerometer- and footswitch-based systems are being used to measure walking speed and to identify freezing of gait in Parkinson's disease (8,9).

III. HOME SAFE HOME

Wearable sensors are likely to bring about a tremendous revolution in future monitoring fashion. In addition, these sensors will be able to interact with the wired home, office and car of the future to enable dynamic adaptation of these environments so that they can respond to people's needs. These environments may also be able to provide physicians with a more complete picture of a person's health. Dr. Vera Novak, Director of the Syncope and Falls in the Elderly (SAFE) resource, is exploring just such an interaction in her joint work with the House_n ("house of the future") project (http://architecture.mit.edu/house_n/) at MIT. Dr. Novak studies how the deterioration of sensorimotor feedback mechanisms with aging contributes to fall risk and has begun to identify differences in how elderly fallers and non-fallers adapt to the demands of everyday life such as standing, walking, and climbing the stairs. Dr. Novak's group has developed a set of wearable sensors to measure gait, muscle activity, and heart rate, and a group at MIT has developed a set of sensors that will record the use of light switches, appliance dials, furniture, cabinets, and other objects as well as sensors that will track peoples' location throughout the house. Dr. Novak anticipates that by studying physiological readings from the wearable sensors in conjunction with the activity signals from the home sensors, she can develop an understanding of how daily activities affect people's balance and the amount of effort they expend to maintain their gait. This broader perspective could also help in the design of custom homes of the future to accommodate people as they become more frail.

Another way the home can give feedback about activities is to have gait-tracking sensors built right into the floor. Researchers at the Medical Automation Research Center at the University of Virginia in Charlottesville are developing just such an approach, developing a floor mat of highly sensitive optic fiber vibration sensors that detect walking patterns. It has the ability to distinguish between normal walking and limping or shuffling, potential precursors of a fall. The floor can also detect if a fall has occurred (10). Such passive sensing eliminates the burden of having to wear special sensor clothing. Residents simply walk across the floor and embedded computer systems will assess their gait.

IV. SHAKING THINGS UP

Engineers often scratch their heads in order to get rid of "noise" in a signal, and thus, noise has a bad reputation. Recent work suggests that the addition of a small amount of non-detectable noise, in the form of small vibrations, may actually enhance balance and possibly gait (11,12). In a study of 27 young and elderly participants who stood quietly on vibrating gel-based insoles, application of noise resulted in a significant reduction in seven out of eight sway parameters in young participants and all of the sway variables in elderly participants.

Vibrating platforms are probably not the answer to every balance and gait disturbance, but research on the potential use of this modality has shown potential in a wide variety of patient populations. Standing on a vibrating platform for just a few a day may reduce osteoporosis, strengthen muscles, and enahnce balance (13–15). Imagine what could happen to couch potatoes if this technology is proven successful and made accessible.

For a long time, the healthy heart beat was believed to be perfectly regular. In the conventional approach, it was assumed that there is no meaningful information in what appears to be noisy fluctuations about the average heart rate, and, therefore, one does not expect to gain any understanding or clinical utility through the study of these fluctuations. Over the last few decades, however, numerous researchers have applied methods from statistical physics to heart-rate time series and demonstrated, time and again, that diagnostic and prognostic information is hidden in the beat-to-beat fluctuations in heart rate (16). Similarly, recent application of "fractal physiology" to the study of balance and gait has demonstrated that noise in these systems also contains and reflects important information that may be used to enhance diagnosis, prognosis, and basic understandings of gait and balance (17). For example, in a study of older adults with "cautious" gait of unexplained origin, about 50% reported falling. A fractal scaling index of gait based on the analysis of the stride-to-stride fluctuations in gait timing was successful in discriminating fallers from non-fallers while a long list of other measures were similar in those subjects who reported falls (or multiple falls) and those who did not (18). Application of such methods to the study of the fluctuations in balance and gait offers the potential of enhancing the analyses of balance and gait.

V. LOOK WHO'S WALKING

Cameras have become small, cheap, and ubiquitous. They may be found in public places, on computers, and in cell phones, creating a big brother-like atmosphere. Researchers at the University of Rochester's Center for Future Health are trying to turn this story around. They have proposed to create a video analysis and feedback environment that supports wellness in the privacy of one's home. Currently, they are developing a system that will monitor daily changes in health, including differences in gait patterns, using a set of cameras backed by advanced video analysis. The system's computers will make comparisons over time, checking for any tell-tale gait disturbances that might predict a stroke or a fall or for the trembling that may indicate Parkinson's disease. Animated video characters will also give residents feedback on their health status. By identifying these ailments relatively early on, the hope is that a disease's full effects can be prevented or ameliorated to a much greater extent.

The goal of identifying ailments from video alone is not unfounded. Algorithms are being developed to extract a wide variety of information from video analysis, which go beyond the traditional approach. These include processing algorithms for extracting low-level information such as gait velocity, stance width, stride length, arm swing, cadence, and stance times and recognition algorithms for determining certain aspects of their emotional state (19–21). Further work is being conducted by Professor Jim Davis at University of Ohio to detect atypical gait patterns (22) and to determine the amount of effort that a person is putting into walking or lifting (23). From the Davis' analysis, a system to quantify qualitative properties of movement such as the leisureliness of walking styles or the strain in lifting has been developed. By monitoring changes in these parameters, Davis hopes to be able to detect onset of fatigue or illness, the kind of information the home of the future will need to support wellness.

VI. THE INFORMATION WORLD

So, what will the future hold? Eventually, cheap wireless sensors will be embedded into the very fabric of our clothes (24), our heart rate and respiration will be sensed from our shirts (25), and our every movement may be tracked by accelerometers on our wrists, arms, and shoulders. Our homes and offices will be alive with sensors and cameras, which, thanks to wireless technologies, will be able to communicate with each other with our on-line health records to construct a very detailed picture of our every move. However, where will all this information go?

In the best case, all modes of data will come together to give the most complete picture of our health, warning us of disease in its earliest form (26) and allowing us to self-monitor our progress towards our health goals. Recordings will be made without requiring substantial effort, and at the touch of a button, we will be able to review changes in our health over periods of days, weeks, or even years. This wealth of information could be used by physicians to review our progress and recommend changes to our medications remotely, saving an unnecessary trip to the hospital, or could be used in conjunction with a hospital visit to investigate the history of a problem to determine if the situation has improved or declined since the last visit. These kinds of remote monitoring technologies have already proved useful in the management of other conditions such as congestive heart failure (27–29). Certain forms of monitoring, such as fall detection, also have real-time applications, alerting others to our situation and sending us the help we need (30,31). With an enriched array of data at hand, it seems likely that our ability to diagnose, monitor, and improve balance and gait will be radically improved, perhaps, in the not-so-distant future.

REFERENCES

1. Terrier P, Ladetto Q, Merminod B, Schutz Y. High-precision satellite positioning system as a new tool to study the biomechanics of human locomotion. J Biomech 2000; 33(12):1717–1722.
2. Terrier P, Ladetto Q, Merminod B, Schutz Y. Measurement of the mechanical power of walking by satellite positioning system (GPS). Med Sci Sports Exerc 2001; 33(11):1912–1918.
3. Chow CC, Lauk M, Collins JJ. The dynamics of quasi-static posture control. Human Mov Sci 1999; 18(5):725–740.
4. Lauk M, Chow CC, Pavlik AE, Collins JJ. Human balance out of equilibrium: nonequilibrium statistical mechanics in posture control. Phys Rev Lett 1998; 80(2):413–416.
5. Sabelman EE, Schwandt D, Jaffe DL. The WAMAS wearable accelerometric motion analysis system: combining technology developement and research in human mobility. Conf. Intellectual Property in the VA: Changes, Challenges and Collabrations, Arlington, VA, 2001.
6. Scilingo EP, Lorussi F, Mazzoldi A, De Rossi D. Strain sensing fabrics for wearable kinaesthetic systems. IEEE Sens J 2002; 3(4):460–467.
7. Morris SJ, Paradiso JA. A compact wearable sensor package for clinical gait monitoring. Offspring 2003; 1(1):7–15.

8. Hausdorff JM, Balash Y, Giladi N. Time series analysis of leg movements during freezing of gait in Parkinson's disease: akinesia, rhyme or reason? Physica A—Stat Mech Appl 2003; 321(3–4):565–570.

9. Tetrud JW, Sabelman EE, Yap R. Accelerometric identification of freezing-of-gait in Parkinson's syndrome. 7th Intl Congr Parkinson's Disease and Movement Disorders, Miami Beach, FL, Nov 10–14, 2002.

10. Alwan M, Dalal S, Kell S, Felder R. Derivation of basic human gait characteristics from floor vibrations. Proceedings of the 2003 Summer Bioengineering Conference, Key Biscayne, FL, USA, June 25–29, 2003.

11. Priplata A, Niemi J, Salen M, Harry J, Lipsitz LA, Collins JJ. Noise-enhanced human balance control. Phys Rev Lett 2002; 89(23):238101.

12. Priplata AA, Niemi JB, Harry JD, Lipsitz LA, Collins JJ. Vibrating insoles and balance control in elderly people. Lancet 2003; 362(9390):1123–1124.

13. Hannan MT, Cheng DM, Green E, Swift C, Rubin CT, Kiel DP. Establishing the compliance in elderly women for use of a low-level mechanical stress device in a clinical osteoporosis study. Osteoporosis Int 2004; 15:918–926.

14. Russo CR, Lauretani F, Bandinelli S, Bartali B, Cavazzini C, Guralnik JM, et al. High-frequency vibration training increases muscle power in postmenopausal women. Arch Phys Med Rehabil 2003; 84(12):1854–1857.

15. Torvinen S, Kannus P, Sievanen H, Jarvinen TA, Pasanen M, Kontulainen S, et al. Effect of four-month vertical whole body vibration on performance and balance. Med Sci Sports Exerc 2002; 34(9):1523–1528.

16. Goldberger AL, Amaral LA, Hausdorff JM, Ivanov PC, Peng CK, Stanley HE. Fractal dynamics in physiology: alterations with disease and aging. Proc Natl Acad Sci USA 2002; 99(suppl 1):2466–2472.

17. Hausdorff JM, Mitchell SL, Firtion R, Peng CK, Cudkowicz ME, Wei JY, et al. Altered fractal dynamics of gait: reduced stride–interval correlations with aging and Huntington's disease. J Appl Physiol 1997; 82(1):262–269.

18. Herman T, Giladi N, Gurevich T, Hausdorff JM. Gait instability and fractal dynamics of older adults with a "cautious" gait: why do certain older adults walk fearfully? Gait Posture 2005, Feb; 21(2):178–185.

19. Kozlowski L, Cutting J. Recognizing the sex of a walker from dynamic point-light display. Percept Psychophys 1977; 21(6):575–580.

20. Troje N. Decomposing biological motion: a framework for analysis and synthesis of human gait patterns. J Vis 2002; 2:371–387.

21. Lemke MR, Wendorff T, Mieth B, Buhl K, Linnemann M. Spatiotemporal gait patterns during over-ground locomotion in major depression compared with healthy controls. J Psychiatr Res 2000; 34(4–5):277–283. Actigraphy, cinematography and ground reaction forces.

22. Davis J, Taylor S. Analysis and recognition of walking movements. International Conference on Pattern Recognition, Quebec City, Canada, August 11–15, 2002: 315–318.

23. Davis J, Gao H, Kannappan V. A three-mode expressive feature model of action effort. IEEE workshop on Motion and Video Computing, Orlando, Florida, December 5–6, 2002: 139–144.

24. Healy T, Donnelly J, et al. Resistive fibre-meshed transducers. Proceedings of the 7th IEEE International Symposium on Wearable Computers, White Plains, New York, Oct 21–23, 2003: 200–209.
25. Marculescu D, Marculescu R, Park S, Jayaraman S. Ready to ware. IEEE Spectrum 2003; 10(40):28–32.
26. Verghese J, Lipton RB, Hall CB, Kuslansky G, Katz MJ, Buschke H. Abnormality of gait as a predictor of non-Alzheimer's dementia. N Engl J Med 2002; 347(22):1761–1768.
27. Maglaveras N, Gogou G, Chouvarda I, Koutkias V, Lekka I, Adamidis D, Karvounis C, Louridas G, Balas EA. Using contact centers in tele-management and home care of congestive heart failure patients: the CHS experience. Proc IEEE Comput Cardiol 2003; 29:281–284.
28. Shah NB, Der E, Ruggerio C, Heidenreich PA, Massie BM. Prevention of hospitalizations for heart failure with an interactive home monitoring program. Am Heart J 1998; 135:373–378.
29. http://www.healthhero.com/
30. http://lifealert.com/
31. http://www.adtcs.com/tl/

8

Common Gait Disturbances: A Clinical Overview

Neil B. Alexander

Mobility Research Center, Division of Geriatric Medicine, Department of Internal Medicine, Institute of Gerontology, University of Michigan and Ann Arbor VA Health Care System, Geriatric Research Education and Clinical Center, Ann Arbor, Michigan, U.S.A.

Allon Goldberg

Ann Arbor VA Health Care System, Geriatric Research Education and Clinical Center, Ann Arbor, Michigan, U.S.A.

Gait disorders are frequently associated with falls, disability, and institutionalization in older adults. This chapter will review the epidemiology of these gait disorders, diagnoses contributing to these disorders, approaches to clinical gait-disorder assessment, and interventions to reduce the impact of these disorders. Other chapters in this volume will review gait disorder and falls assessment and intervention, particularly with respect to certain key diseases, in greater detail.

I. EPIDEMIOLOGY

At least 20% of non-institutionalized older adults admit to walking difficulty or require the assistance of another person or special equipment to walk (1). Limitations in walking also increase with age. In some samples of non-institutionalized older adults aged ≥ 85 years, the incidence of limitation in walking can be over 54% (1). While age-related gait changes, such as in speed, are most apparent past age 75 or 80 years, the majority of gait disorders appear in connection with underlying diseases, particularly as disease severity increases. For example, advanced age (>85 years), three or more chronic conditions at baseline and the occurrence of stroke, hip fracture, or cancer predict "catastrophic" loss of walking ability (2).

Determining that a gait is "disordered" is difficult because there are no clearly accepted standards of "normal" gait for older adults. Yet, an aesthetically "abnormal" gait seems identifiable even by the casual, untrained observer. Slowed gait speed may suggest the presence of a disorder while deviations in smoothness, symmetry, and synchrony of movement patterns also may suggest a disorder. However, slow or abnormal gait may in fact be safer and allow the older adult to be independent.

Longitudinal studies suggest that progression of gait-related mobility disorders occurs with age and that this progression associates with morbidity and mortality. Gait/postural disorders, as measured by the Unified Parkinson's Disease Rating Scale (UPDRS) (including abnormalities in rising from a chair and turning), increased in most (79%) of a sample of non-demented Catholic clergy without clinical Parkinson's disease (mean age 75 years) followed for up to 7 years in a prospective cohort study (3). This increase was more common in the older-age groups and was associated with a higher mortality rate. While the UPDRS is usually used in rating known Parkinson's patients, the increased UPDRS score over time in this study may reflect changes with increasing age, such as increased parkinsonian signs and the increasing burden of associated disease and inactivity. In addition, subjects in this cohort could also have developed other overt neurological disease and/or dementia. For example, declining gait speed is one of the factors that can independently predict cognitive decline prospectively in healthy older adults (4). Regardless of the underlying mechanisms, gait disorders seem to become more prevalent with age.

Sub-clinical, as well as clinically evident, cerebrovascular disease is increasingly recognized as a major contributor to gait disorders (see Sec. III). Non-demented subjects with clinically abnormal gait (particularly unsteady, frontal, or hemiparetic gait) and followed for ~7 years are at higher risk of developing non-Alzheimer's, particularly vascular, dementia (5). Of note, at baseline, those with abnormal gait may not have met criteria for dementia but already had abnormalities in neuropsychological function, such as in visual–perceptual processing and language skills. Gait disorders with no apparent etiology (also termed "idiopathic" or "senile" gait disorder) are associated with a higher mortality rate, primarily from cardiovascular causes; these cardiovascular causes are likely linked to concomitant, previously undetected cerebrovascular disease (6).

II. DIAGNOSES CONTRIBUTING TO GAIT DISORDERS

A growing body of evidence suggests that disordered gait is not an inevitable consequence of aging but rather a reflection of the increased prevalence and severity of age-associated diseases (7). Similar gait abnormalities are common to many diseases (8), and thus attributing a gait disorder to one-disease etiology in older adults is particularly difficult. These underlying diseases, both neurological and non-neurological, are the major contributors to disordered gait in the older adult. In a primary care setting, complaints of pain, stiffness, dizziness, numbness, weakness, and sensations of abnormal movement are the most common contributors to walking difficulties (9). The most common diagnoses found in a primary care setting thought to contribute to gait disorders include degenerative joint disease, acquired musculoskeletal deformities, intermittent claudication, post-orthopedic surgery and post-stroke impairments, and postural hypotension (9). Usually, more than one contributing diagnosis is found. In a group of community-dwelling older adults >88 years of age, joint pain was by far the most common contributor, followed by multiple causes such as stroke and visual loss (7). Factors such as dementia and fear of falling also contribute to gait disorders. The diagnoses found in a neurological referral population are primarily neurologically oriented (10,11), and include frontal gait disorders [usually related to normal pressure hydrocephalus (NPH) and cerebrovascular processes], sensory disorders (also involving vestibular and visual function), myelopathy, previously undiagnosed Parkinson's disease or parkinsonian syndromes, and cerebellar disease. Known conditions causing severe gait impairment, such as hemiplegia and severe hip or knee disease, are frequently not mentioned in these neurological referral populations. Thus, many gait disorders, particularly those which are classical and discrete (such as related to stroke and osteoarthritis) and those which are mild and/or may relate to irreversible disease (such as vascular dementia), are presumably diagnosed in a primary care setting and treated without a referral to a neurologist. Other less common contributors to gait disorders include metabolic disorders (related to renal or hepatic disease), central nervous system (CNS) tumors or sub-dural hematoma, depression, and psychotropic medications. Case reports also document reversible gait disorders due to clinically overt hypo- or hyperthyroidism and B-12 and folate deficiency (for detailed review, see Ref. 8).

Factors that contribute to slowed gait speed are also considered contributors to gait disorders. These factors are frequently disease-associated (such as related to cardiopulmonary or musculoskeletal disease) and include reductions in leg strength, vision, aerobic function, standing balance and physical activity, as well as joint impairment, previous falls, and fear of falling (12–18). Combining these factors may result in an effect greater than the sum of the single impairments [such as when combining balance and strength impairments (17)]. Furthermore, the effect of reduced strength and aerobic capacity on gait speed may be curvilinear, i.e., for very impaired individuals, small improvements in strength or aerobic capacity yield relatively larger gains in gait speed, although these small improvements yield little gait speed change in healthy old (15,19).

Although many older adults maintain a relatively normal gait pattern well into their 80s, some slowing occurs, and decreased stride length thus becomes a common feature described in older adult gait disorders (see Ref. 8 for review). Some authors have proposed the emergence of an age-related gait disorder without accompanying clinical abnormalities, i.e., essential "senile" gait disorder (20). This gait pattern is described as broad-based with small steps, diminished arm swing, stooped posture, flexion of the hips and knees, uncertainty and stiffness in turning, occasional difficulty initiating steps, and a tendency toward falling. These and other non-specific findings (such as the inability to perform tandem gait) are similar to gait patterns found in a number of other diseases, and yet the clinical abnormalities are insufficient to make a specific diagnosis. This "disorder" may be a precursor to an as-yet-asymptomatic disease (e.g., related to subtle extrapyramidal signs) and often is concurrent with progressive cognitive impairment [e.g., Alzheimer's disease or vascular dementia (21)]. "Senile" gait disorder may potentially reflect a number of potential disease etiologies and is generally not useful in labeling gait disorders in older adults.

III. APPROACH TO ASSESSMENT

A potentially useful approach to assessing contributors to a gait disorder (Table 1) (based on Ref. 22) categorizes deficits according to sensorimotor level. Low sensorimotor level deficits are divided into peripheral sensory and peripheral motor dysfunction, including musculoskeletal (arthritic) and myopathic/neuropathic disorders that cause weakness. These disorders are generally distal to the CNS. With peripheral sensory impairment, unsteady and tentative gait is commonly caused by vestibular disorders, peripheral neuropathy, posterior column (proprioceptive) deficits, or visual impairment. With peripheral motor impairment, a number of classical gait patterns emerge, including compensatory strategies. Examples of these strategies include Trendelenburg gait (hip abductor weakness causing weight shift over the weak hip); antalgic gait (avoidance of excessive weight bearing and shortening of stance on one side due to pain); and steppage gait (exaggerated lifting of the lower extremity, often due to ankle dorsiflexor weakness and subsequent foot drop). These conditions involve extremity (both body segment and joint) deformities, painful weight-bearing, and focal myopathic and neuropathic weakness. Note that if the gait disorder is limited to this low sensorimotor level (i.e., the CNS is intact), successful

Table 1 Classification System and Associated Physical and Gait Findings in Gait Disorders of Older Adults

Level	Within-level classification	Condition	Physical findings	Gait findings
Low	Peripheral sensory	Sensory ataxia	Loss of position sense, touch	Possible "steppage gait" (exaggerated lower extremity lift)
		Vestibular ataxia		May weave, fall to one side
		Visual ataxia	Visual loss	Tentative, uncertain, unco-ordinated
	Peripheral motor	Arthritic (antalgic, joint deformity)	Pain-related avoidance of weight-bearing on affected side	Shortened stance phase on affected side "Trendelenburg" (trunk shift over affected side)
			Limited flexion in painful extremity (especially knee) and may lead to loss of joint range and contracture	Painful limb may buckle with weight bearing Unequal leg length can produce trunk and pelvic motion abnormalities (including "Trendelenburg")
			Decreased lumbar lordosis in painful lumbar spine	
			Stooped posture in kyphosis and ankylosing spondylosis	
		Myopathic and neuropathic (weakness)	Pelvic/hip girdle weakness	Pelvic girdle weakness can lead to exaggerated lumbar lordosis and lateral trunk flexion ("Trendelenburg" and "waddling" gait
			Proximal motor neuropathy produces proximal muscle weakness	Proximal weakness can produce "waddling" and "foot slap"
			Distal motor neuropathy produces distal muscle weakness	Weak ankle dorsiflexors result in "foot drop" or "slap" or "steppage gait"
Middle	Spasticity	Hemiplegia/paresis	Leg weakness and spasticity	Leg circumduction (swing out in semi-circle)
			Knee hyperextension (genu recurvatum)	Loss of arm swing
			Ankle excessively plantar flexed and inverted (equinovarus)	Foot drag or scrape
			Arm weakness and spasticity	

(Continued)

Table 1 Classification System and Associated Physical and Gait Findings in Gait Disorders of Older Adults (*Continued*)

Level	Within-level classification	Condition	Physical findings	Gait findings
		Paraplegia/paresis	Leg weakness and spasticity	Bilateral leg circumduction, scraping feet, can "scissor" (knees cross in front of each other)
	Parkinsonism		Rigidity Bradykinesia Trunk flexed	Small shuffling steps, hesitation, acceleration ("festination"), falling forward ("propulsion"), falling backward ("retropulsion"), moving the whole body while turning ("turning en bloc"), absent arm swing, may freeze (especially with attention diversion)
	Cerebellar ataxia		May have poor trunk control, incoordination or other cerebellar signs	Wide-based with increased trunk sway, irregular stepping, staggering, especially on turns.
High	Cautious gait		Fear of falling	Normal to widened base, shortened stride, decreased velocity, and en bloc turns
	Frontal-related gait disorders, other white matter lesions	Cerebrovascular, NPH	May have evidence of other atherosclerotic disease May also have cognitive impairment, weakness and spasticity, and urinary incontinence	Range of findings including cautious gait findings (above), difficulty initiating gait and shuffling gait, upright posture, preservation of arm swing, leg apraxia (can imitate gait movements in non-weight-bearing position), freezing (especially with attention diversion)

Source: From Ref. 66.

adaptation to the gait disorder is common, compensating with an assistive device or learning to negotiate the environment safely.

At the middle level, the execution of centrally selected postural and locomotor responses is faulty, and the sensory and motor modulation of gait is disrupted. Gait may be initiated normally, but stepping patterns are abnormal. Examples include diseases causing spasticity (such as related to myelopathy and stroke), parkinsonism (idiopathic as well as drug-induced), and cerebellar disease (such as alcohol-induced). Classical gait patterns appear when the spasticity is sufficient to cause leg circumduction and fixed deformities (such as equinovarus), when Parkinson's disease produces shuffling steps and reduced arm swing, and when the cerebellar ataxia increases trunk sway sufficiently to require a broad base of gait support.

At the high level, the gait characteristics become more non-specific and cognitive dysfunction become more prominent. Dementia and depression may be major contributors to, although not necessarily the sole causes of, the gait disorder. Behavioral aspects such as fear of falling are also important, particularly in cautious gait. Frontal-related gait disorders often have a cerebrovascular component and are not merely the result of frontal masses and NPH. The spectrum of frontal-related disorders ranges from gait-ignition failure, i.e., difficulty with initiation, to frontal dysequilibrium, where unsupported stance is not possible. Cerebrovascular insults to the cortex, as well as basal ganglia and their inter-connections, may relate to gait ignition failure and apraxia (23,24). In apraxia, gait movements can be imitated but only in non-weight-bearing positions. With increasing severity of the dementia, particularly in patients with Alzheimer's disease, frontal-related symptoms also increase (25). Cognitive, pyramidal, and urinary disturbances may also accompany the gait disorder. Gait disorders that might fall in this category have been given a number of overlapping descriptions, including gait apraxia, marche' a petits pas, and arteriosclerotic (vascular) parkinsonism.

Often, more than one disease/impairment contributes to a gait disorder, for example, a diabetic with peripheral neuropathy and a recent stroke who is now very fearful of falls. Certain disorders may actually involve multiple levels, such as Parkinson's disease affecting high (cortical) and middle (sub-cortical) structures. Drug-metabolic etiologies (such as from sedatives, tranquilizers, and anticonvulsants) may involve more than one level: phenothiazines, for example, can cause high (sedation) and middle (extrapyramidal) level effects.

A. History and Physical Examination

A careful medical history and a review of the factors given in Table 1 will help elucidate the multiple factors contributing to the gait disorder. A brief systemic evaluation for evidence of sub-acute metabolic disease (such as thyroid disorders), acute cardiopulmonary disorders (such as a myocardial infarction), or other acute illness (such as infection) is warranted because an acute gait disorder may be the presenting feature of acute systemic decompensation in an older adult. The physical examination should include an attempt to identify motion-related factors, such as by provoking both vestibular and orthostatic responses. In the Hallpike-Dix maneuver, while the patient is seated on an examination table, the examiner holds the patient's head, turns the head to one side, and lowers the head below the level of the table. The patient then sits up and the maneuver is repeated again to the other side. Patients with dizziness and a sensation of motion may also be considered for additional vestibular screening utilizing motion of the head to provoke eye-motion changes (e.g., head thrust or head shaking manuever, as reviewed in Ref. 26) or disrupted gait (as in Sec. II.B.1 of Chapter 2 on Functional Gait Assessment). Blood pressure should be measured with the patient both supine and standing to rule out orthostatic hypotension. Vision screening, at least for acuity, is essential. The neck, spine, extremities, and feet should be evaluated for pain, deformities, and limitations in range of motion, particularly regarding subtle hip and/or knee contractures. Leg-length discrepancies, such as may occur post-hip prosthesis and, either as an antecedent or subsequent to low back pain (27), can be measured simply as the distance from the anterior superior iliac spine to the medial malleolus. A formal neurological assessment is critical to include assessment of strength and tone, sensation (including proprioception), co-ordination (including cerebellar function), and station and gait. In regards to the latter, the Romberg test (feet side by side with eyes open) screens for simple postural control and whether the proprioceptive and vestibular systems are functional. Some investigators have proposed one-legged stance time <5 sec as a risk factor for injurious falls (28), although even relatively healthy older adults aged 70 years may have difficulty with one-legged stance (29). Given the importance of cognition as a risk factor, screening for mental status is also indicated.

B. Laboratory and Imaging Assessments

Depending upon the history and physical examination, laboratory and diagnostic imaging evaluation may be warranted. Complete blood count, chemistries, and other metabolic studies may be useful where systemic disease is suspected. Head or spine imaging, including x-ray, computed tomography, or magnetic resonance imaging (MRI), is of unclear use unless there are neurologic abnormalities by history and physical examination, either preceding or of recent onset related to the gait disorder. However, cerebral white matter changes, often considered to be vascular in nature (termed leukoaraiosis), have been increasingly associated with non-specific gait disorders. Periventricular high-signal measurements on MRI, as well as increased ventricular volume, even in apparently healthy older adults (30), are associated with gait slowing. White-matter hyperintensities on MRI correlate with longitudinal changes in balance and gait (31), and the periventricular frontal and occipitoparietal regions appear to be most affected (32). Age-specific guidelines, sensitivity, specificity, and cost-effectiveness of these work-ups remain to be determined.

C. Performance-Based Functional Assessment

Technologically oriented assessments involving formal kinematic and kinetic analyses have not been applied widely in clinical assessments of older adult balance and gait disorders. Comfortable gait speed and a related measure, distance walked, are powerful predictors of a number of important outcomes such as disability, institutionalization, and mortality. Perhaps, the simplest assessment in the clinical setting is the Timed Up and Go (TUG) (33), a timed sequence of rising from a chair, walking 3 m, turning, and returning to the chair. A recent expert panel recommended that in those patients who report a single fall, difficulty or unsteadiness in TUG performance should prompt a more extensive evaluation of fall risk factors, many of which overlap with gait-disorder risk factors (34). For a full discussion of functional gait assessments, see Chapter 2.

IV. INTERVENTIONS TO REDUCE GAIT DISORDERS

Even if a diagnosable condition is found on evaluation, many conditions causing a gait disorder are only, at best, partially treatable. For a more extensive review by certain diseases, see Sec. III Chapters 12 to 18, as well as a previous review (8). The patient is often left with at least some residual disability. However, other functional outcomes such as reduction in weight-bearing pain, improvement in walking distance, and reductions in walking limitation justify considering treatment. Achievement of pre-morbid gait patterns may be unrealistic, and improvement in measures such as gait speed is reasonable as long as gait remains safe. Comorbidity, disease severity, and overall health status tend to strongly influence treatment outcome.

Many of the older reports dealing with treatment and rehabilitation of gait disorders in older adults are retrospective chart reviews and case studies and not randomized, controlled studies. These studies of gait disorders presumably secondary to B-12 deficiency, folate deficiency, hypothyroidism, hyperthyroidism, knee osteoarthritis, Parkinson's disease, and inflammatory polyneuropathy show improvement as a result of medical therapy. A variety of modes of physical therapy for diseases such as knee osteoarthritis and stroke also result in modest improvements but continued residual disability. For example, a combined aerobic, strength, and functionally based group exercise program increased gait speed ~5% in knee osteoarthritics (35).

The focus is on strengthening the extensor groups (especially knee and hip) and stretching commonly shortened muscles [such as the hip flexors (36)]. A recent review suggests unclear effects of conventional physical therapy in the treatment of Parkinson's gait disorders (37), but that cueing, specifically audio and visual, can improve gait speed (38). Recent studies suggest an incremental reduction of gait impairment with the use of a body weight support and a treadmill to provide task-specific gait training post-total hip arthroplasty (39), in Parkinson's disease (40) and particularly in hemiparetics post-stroke (for review see Ref. 41). However, a Cochrane review found no statistically significant effect favoring treadmill training with or without body support over conventional training to improve gait speed or disability in post-stroke patients (42). Note that the Cochrane review found a small but clinically important trend (an improvement of 0.24 m/sec in the body weight support plus treadmill group) in those who could walk independently.

A few studies of group exercise have demonstrated improvements in gait parameters such as gait speed. Generally, the most consistent effects are with a variety of exercises provided in the same program. A 12-week combined program of leg resistance, standing balance, and flexibility exercises increased usual gait speed 8% in minimally impaired life care community residents (43). A similar varied 16-week format with more intensive individual support and prompting in select demented older adults (mean MMSE:15) resulted in 23% improvement in gait speed (44). A number of these studies note improvement in functional, gait-oriented measures (although not strictly gait "disorder" measures) such as the distance walked in 6 min (6-min walk test), such as in knee osteoarthritics undergoing either an aerobic or resistance training program (45).

Behavioral and environmental modifications that can be used to negotiate the environment more safely include improved lighting (particularly for those with vestibular or sensory impairment) and avoidance of pathway hazards (such as clutter, wires, and slippery floors). Note that light touch of any firm surface like walls or "furniture surfing" (46) provides feedback and enhances balance (47).

Use of orthoses and other mobility aids will help reduce the severity of the gait disorder. While there are few data supporting their use, lifts (either internal or external) to correct for limb-length inequality may be provided in a conservative, gradually progressive manner (48). Other ankle braces, shoe inserts, shoe body and sole modifications, and their subsequent adjustments are part of standard care for foot and ankle weakness, deformities, and pain but are beyond the scope of this review (for a recent case study, see Ref. 49). In general, well-fitting walking shoes with low heels, relatively thin firm soles, and if feasible, high, fixed heel collar support are recommended to maximize balance and improve gait (50). Mobility aids, such as canes reduce load on a painful joint and walkers, increase stability. Van Hook (51) recently reviewed the different types of canes and walkers and the appropriate candidates for their use.

Modest improvement and residual disability are also the results of surgical treatment for compressive cervical myelopathy, lumbar stenosis, and NPH. Few controlled prospective studies and virtually no randomized studies address the outcome of surgical versus non surgical treatment for compressive cervical myelopathy, lumbar stenosis, and NPH. A number of problems plague the available series: outcomes such as pain and walking disability are not reported separately; the source of the outcome rating is not clearly identified or blinded; the criteria for classifying outcomes differ; the outcomes may be subjective and subject to interpretation; the follow-up intervals are variable; the subjects who are reported in follow-up may be a highly select group; the selection factors for conservative vs. surgical treatment between studies differ or are unspecified, and there is publication bias (only positive results are published). Many of the surgical series include all ages, although the mean age is usually above 60 years. A few studies document equivalent surgical outcomes with conservative, non-surgical treatment.

Regarding lumbar stenosis, many older adults have reduction in pain and improvement in maximal walking distance following laminectomies and lumbar fusion surgery, although they have continued residual disability. In a somewhat younger cohort (mean age 69 years) and after an average of 8 years of follow-up after surgery for lumbar stenosis, approximately half reported that they were unable to walk two blocks and many of them attributed their decreased walking ability to their back problem (52). Part of the problem in determining long-term lumbar stenosis surgical outcomes are other mobility-influencing comorbidities such as cardiovascular or musculoskeletal disease (53). Nevertheless, some improvement can be found in select patients older than 75 years; a recent uncontrolled study found that 45% of patients (mean age 78 years) with preoperative "severe" limitation of ambulatory ability wound up with either "minimal" or "moderate" limitation post-operatively after an average of 1.5-year follow-up (54). Non-operative treatment (with a variety of interventions including oral anti-inflammatory medications, heating modalities, exercise, mobilizations, and epidural injections) may also result in modest improvements such as in walking tolerance (reviewed in Ref. 55). Recent studies involving cervical stenosis gait outcomes in older adults are limited (such as in Ref. 56, a case report), although significant improvement in walking speed post-cervical myelopathy decompression, in most patients, can be expected (57).

In a recent non-controlled study post-shunt for NPH (follow-up interval not specified), walking speed increased by over 10% in 75% of the patients and by >25% in over 57% of the patients (58). While there may be initial improvement following shunt placement, long-term results are often disappointing (e.g., 65% of post-shunt patients have initial improvement in their gait disorder, but only 26% maintain this improvement by 3-year follow-up, in Ref. 59). The poor long-term outcomes may be related to concurrent cerebro-vascular and cardiovascular disease, a frequent cause of mortality in these cohorts (60). Post-shunt gait outcomes may be better in those in whom the gait disturbance precedes cognitive impairment and in those who respond with gait speed improvement following a trial of cerebrospinal fluid removal (61) (for review, see Ref. 62).

Outcomes for hip and knee replacement surgery for osteoarthritis are better, although some of the same study methodological problems exist. Other than pain relief, sizable gains in gait speed and joint motion occur, although residual walking disability continues for a number of reasons including residual pathology on the operated side and symptoms on the non-operated side. For total knee replacements, despite rehabilitation post-operatively, some residual weakness, stiffness, and slowed/altered gait may remain (63,64). Simple function may be maintained post-knee replace-ment, such as maintaining the ability to safely clear an obstacle, but usually at the expense of additional compensation by the ipsilateral hip and foot (65).

V. CONCLUSIONS

Gait disorders are common in older adults and are a predictor of functional decline. The etiology of these disorders in older adults is frequently multifac-torial, and a full assessment must consider a number of different sensorimotor levels via standard medical (e.g., physical examination) and functional perfor-mance evaluations. Laboratory and imaging assessments may be warranted in the proper clinical setting. Interventions ranging from medical to surgical to exercise are effective and reduce the severity of the gait disorder, but residual impairment and disability may still remain. Orthoses and mobility aids are also important interventions to reduce the severity of the disorder. Appropriate evaluation of a gait disorder in older adults, with a careful con-sideration of a multifactorial etiology, should help in the identification of the most appropriate intervention.

REFERENCES

1. Ostchega Y, Harris TB, Hirsch R, et al. The prevalence of functional limitations and disability in older persons in the US: data from the National Health and Nutrition Examination Survey III. J Am Geriatr Soc 2000; 48:1132–1135.
2. Guralnik JM, Ferrucci L, Balfour JL, et al. Progressive versus catastrophic loss of the ability to walk: implications for the prevention of mobility loss. J Am Geriatr Soc 2001; 49:1463–1470.
3. Wilson RS, Schneider JA, Beckett LA, et al. Progression of gait disorder and rigidity and risk of death in older persons. Neurology 2002; 58:1815–1819.

4. Marquis S, Moore MM, Howieson DB, et al. Independent predictors of cognitive decline in healthy elderly persons. Arch Neurol 2002; 59:601–606.
5. Verghese J, Lipton RB, Hall CB, et al. Abnormality of gait as a predictor of non-Alzheimer's dementia. N Engl J Med 2002; 347:1761–1768.
6. Bloem BR, Gussekloo J, Lagaay AM, et al. Idiopathic senile gait disorders are signs of subclinical disease. J Am Geriatr Soc 2000; 48:1098–1101.
7. Bloem BR, Haan J, Lagaay AM, et al. Investigation of gait in elderly subjects over 88 years of age. J Geriatr Psychiatry Neurol 1992; 5:78–84.
8. Alexander NB. Gait disorders in older adults. J Am Geriatr Soc 1996a; 44: 434–451.
9. Hough JC, McHenry MP, Kammer LM. Gait disorders in the elderly. Am Fam Pract 1987; 30:191–196.
10. Sudarsky L, Rontal M. Gait disorders among elderly patients: a survey study of 50 patients. Arch Neurol 1983; 40:740–743.
11. Fuh JL, Lin KN, Wang SJ, et al. Neurologic diseases presenting with gait impairment in the elderly. J Geriatr Psychiatry Neurol 1994; 7:89–92.
12. Bendall MJ, Bassey EJ, Pearson MB. Factors affecting walking speed of elderly people. Age Ageing 1989; 18:327–332.
13. Tinetti ME, Mendes de Leon CF, Doucette JT, et al. Fear of falling and fall-related efficacy in relationship to functioning among community-living elders. J Gerontol 1994; 49:M140–M147.
14. Woo J, Ho SC, Lau J, et al. Age-associated gait changes in the elderly: pathological or physiological? Neuroepidemiology 1995; 14:65–71.
15. Buchner DM, Cress EM, Esselman PC, et al. Factors associated with changes in gait speed in older adults. J Gerontol 1996a; 51A:M297–M302.
16. Gibbs J, Hughes S, Dunlop D, et al. Predictors of walking velocity in older adults. J Am Geriatr Soc 1996; 44:126–132.
17. Rantanen T, Guralnik JM, Ferrucci L, et al. Coimpairments: strength and balance as predictors of severe walking disability. J Gerontol 1999; 54A: M172–M176.
18. De Rekeneire N, Visser M, Peila R, et al. Is a fall just a fall: correlates of falling in healthy older persons. The Health, Aging, and Body Composition Study. J Am Geriatr Soc 2003; 51:841–846.
19. Buchner DM, Larson EB, Wagner EH, et al. Evidence for a non-linear relationship between leg strength and gait speed. Age Ageing 1996b; 25:386–391.
20. Koller WC, Wilson RS, Glatt SL, et al. Senile gait: correlation with computed tomographic scans. Ann Neurol 1983; 13:343–344.
21. Elble RJ, Hughes L, Higgins C. The syndrome of senile gait. J Neurol 1992; 239:71–75.
22. Nutt JG. Classification of gait and balance disorders. In: Ruzicka E, Hallet M, Jankovic J, eds. Gait Disorders Advances in Neurology. Vol. 87. Philadelphia: Lippincott, Williams and Wilkins, 2001.
23. Liston R, Mickelborough J, Bene J, et al. A new classification of higher level gait disorders in patients with cerebral multi-infarct states. Age Ageing 2003; 32:252–258.

24. Jankovic J, Nutt JG, Sudarsky L. Classification, diagnosis, and etiology of gait disorders. In: Ruzicka E, Hallet M, Jankovic J, eds. Gait Disorders. Advances in Neurology. Vol. 87. Philadelphia: Lippincott, Williams and Wilkins, 2001.

25. O'Keefe ST, Kazeem H, Philpott RM, et al. Gait disturbance in Alzheimer's disease: a clinical study. Age Ageing 1996; 25:313–316.

26. Goebel JA. The ten-minute examination of the dizzy patient. Semin Neurol 2001; 4:391–398.

27. Gurney B. Leg length discrepancy. Gait Posture 2002; 15:195–206.

28. Vellas BJ, Wayne SJ, Romero L, et al. One-leg balance is an important predictor of injurious falls in older persons. J Am Geriatr Soc 1997; 45:735–738.

29. Rossiter-Fornoff JE, Wolf SL, Wolfson LI, et al. A cross-validation study of the FICSIT common data base static balance measures. J Gerontol 1995; 50A:M291–M297.

30. Camicioli R, Moore MM, Sexton G, et al. Age-related changes associated with motor function in healthy older people. J Am Geriatr Soc 1999; 47:330–334.

31. Baloh RW, Ying SH, Jacobson KM. A longitudinal study of gait and balance dysfunction in normal older people. Arch Neurol 2003; 60:835–839.

32. Benson RR, Guttmann CRG, Wei X, et al. Older people with impaired mobility have specific loci of periventricular abnormality on MRI. Neurology 2002; 58:48–55.

33. Posiadlo D, Richardson S. The timed "Up & Go": a test of basic functional mobility for frail elderly persons. J Am Geriatr Soc 1991; 39:142–148.

34. American Geriatrics Society. Guideline for prevention of falls in older persons. J Am Geriatr Soc 2001; 49:664–672.

35. Fransen M, Crosbie J, Edmonds J. Physical therapy is effective for patients with osteoarthritis of the knee: a randomized controlled clinical trial. J Rheumatol 2001; 28:156–164.

36. Kerrigan DC, Xenopoulos-Oddson A, Sullivan MJ, et al. Effect of a hip flexor stretching program on gait in the elderly. Arch Phys Med Rehabil 2003; 84:1–6.

37. Deane KHO, Jones D, Playford ED, et al. Physiotherapy versus placebo or no intervention in Parkinson's disease. In: Cochrane Library. Issue 1, Chechester, UK: John Wiley and Sons, Ltd, 2004.

38. Rubinstein TC, Giladi N, Hausdorff JM. The power of cueing to circumvent dopamine deficits: a review of physical therapy treatment of gait disturbances in Parkinson's disease. Mov Disord 2002; 17:1148–1160.

39. Hesse S, Werner C, Seibel H, et al. Treadmill training with partial body-weight support after total hip arthroplasty: a randomized clinical trial. Arch Phys Med Rehabil 2003a; 84:1767–1773.

40. Miyai I, Fujimoto Y, Yamamoto H, et al. Long-term effect of body weight-supported treadmill training in Parkinson's disease: a randomized controlled trial. Arch Phys Med Rehabil 2002; 83:1370–1373.

41. Hesse S, Werner C. Partial body weight supported treadmill training for gait recovery following stroke. In: Barnett HJM, Bogousslavsky J, Meldrum H, eds. Ischemic Stroke: Advances in Neurology. Vol. 92. Philadelphia: Lippincott, Williams and Wilkins, 2003b.

42. Moseley AM, Stark A, Cameron ID, et al. Treadmill training and bodyweight support for walking after a stroke (Cochrane Review). In: The Cochrane Library, Vol. 3. Oxford:Update Software, 2003.
43. Judge JO, Underwood M, Gennosa T. Exercise to improve gait velocity in older persons. Arch Phys Med Rehabil 1993; 74:400–406.
44. Toulotte C, Fabre C, Dangremont B, et al. Effects of physical training on the physical capacity of frail, demented patients with a history of falling: a randomized controlled trial. Age Ageing 2003; 32:67–73.
45. Ettinger WH, Burns R, Messier SP, et al. A randomized trial comparing aerobic exercise and resistance exercise with a health education program in older adults with knee osteoarthritis. JAMA 1997; 277:25–31.
46. Iezzonni LI. A 44-year-old woman with difficulty walking. JAMA 2000; 284: 2632–2639.
47. Jeka JJ. Light touch as a balance aid. Phys Ther 1997; 77:476–487.
48. Brady RJ, Dean JB, Skinner TM, et al. Limb length inequality: clinical implications for assessment and intervention. J Orthop Sport Phys Ther 2003; 33: 221–234.
49. Shrader JA, Siegel KL. Nonoperative management of functional hallux limitus in a patient with rheumatoid arthritis. Phys Ther 2003; 83:831–848.
50. Menz HB, Lord SR. Footwear and postural stability. J Am Pediatr Med Assoc 1999; 89:346–357.
51. VanHook FW, Demonbreun D, Weiss BD. Ambulatory devices for chronic gait disorders in the elderly. Am Fam Physician 2003; 67:1717–1724.
52. Katz JN, Lipson SJ, Chang LC et al. Seven- to 10-outcomes of decompressive surgery for degenerative lumbar spinal stenosis. Spine 1996; 21:92–98.
53. Katz JN, Stucki G, Lipson SJ, et al. Predictors of surgical outcome in degenerative lumbar spinal stenosis. Spine 1999; 42:2229–2233.
54. Vitaz TW, Raque GH, Shields CB et al. Surgical treatment of lumbar spinal stenosis in patients older than 75 years of age. J Neurosurg (Spine 2) 1999; 91:181–185.
55. Whitman JM, Flynn TW, Fritz JM. Nonsurgical management of patients with lumbar stenosis: a literature review and a case series of three patients managed with physical therapy. Phys Med Rehabil Clin N Am 2003; 14:77–101.
56. Engsberg JR, Lauryssen C, Ross SA, et al. Spasticity, strength, and gait changes after surgery for cervical spondylotic myelopathy. Spine 2003; 28:E136–E139.
57. Singh A, Crockard HA. Quantitative assessment of cervical spondylotic myelopathy by a simple walking test. Lancet 1999; 354:370–373.
58. Blomsterwall E, Svantesson U, Carlsson U, et al. Postural disturbance in patients with normal pressure hydrocephalus. Acta Neurol Scand 2000; 102:284–291.
59. Malm J, Kristensen B, Stegmayr B, et al. Three-year survival and functional outcome of patients with idiopathic adult hydrocephalus syndrome. Neurology 2000; 55:576–578.
60. Raftopoulos C, Massager N, Baleriaux D, et al. Prospective analysis by computed tomography and long term outcome of 23 adult patients with chronic idiopathic hydrocephalus. Neurosurgery 1996; 38:51–59.

61. Stolze H, Kuhtz-Buschbeck JP, Drucke H, et al. Gait analysis in idiopathic normal pressure hydrocephalus-which parameters respond to the CSF tap test. Clin Neurophys 2000; 111:1678–1686.

62. Krauss JK, Faist M, Schubert M, et al. Evaluation of gait in normal pressure hydrocephalus before and after shunting. In: Ruzicka E, Hallet M, Jankovic J, eds. Gait Disorders. Advances in Neurology. Vol 87. Philadelphia: Lippincott, Williams and Wilkins, 2001.

63. Ouellet D, Moffet H. Locomotor deficits before and two months after knee arthroplasty. Arthritis Rheum (Arthritis Care Res) 2002; 47:484–493.

64. Benedetti MG, Catani F, Bilotta TW, et al. Muscle activation pattern and gait biomechanics after total knee replacement. Clin Biomech 2003; 18:871–876.

65. Byrne JM, Prentice S. Swing phase kinetics and swing phase kinematics of knee replacement patients during obstacle avoidance. Gait Posture 2003; 18:95–104.

66. Alexander N. Gait disorders. In: Pompei P, Murphy JB, eds. Geriatrics Review Syllabus: A Core Curriculum in Geriatric Medicine. 6th ed. New York, NY: American Geriatrics Society, 2006. In Press.

9

Fall Risk Assessment: Step-by-Step

Laurence Z. Rubenstein

UCLA School of Medicine, Geriatric Research Education and Clinical Center (GRECC), VA Greater Los Angeles Healthcare System, Sepulveda, California, U.S.A.

Karen R. Josephson

Geriatric Research Education and Clinical Center (GRECC), VA Greater Los Angeles Healthcare System, Sepulveda, California, U.S.A.

I. INTRODUCTION

Falls are a common and complex geriatric syndrome causing considerable mortality, morbidity, reduced functioning, and pre-mature nursing home admission among older persons. Falls are a frequent and serious consequence of gait disorders. However, falls also have multiple precipitating causes and pre-disposing risk factors, which make their diagnosis, treatment, and particularly prevention a difficult clinical challenge. A fall may be the first indicator of an acute problem (infection, postural hypotension, and cardiac arrhythmia), or may stem from a chronic disease (parkinsonism, dementia, and diabetic neuropathy), or simply may be a marker for the progression of "normal" age-related changes in vision, gait, and strength. Moreover, most falls experienced by older persons have multifactorial and interacting pre-disposing and precipitating causes (e.g., a trip over an electrical cord contributed to by both a gait disorder and poor vision). Figure 1 provides a visual schematic of the complex relationship between selected risk factors, underlying causes, precipitating events and falls. Such multifactorial causality is typical of geriatric syndromes generally, which necessitates a systematic, multidimensional evaluation. This chapter will

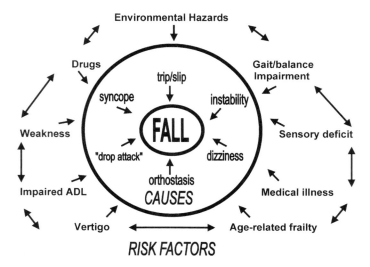

Figure 1   The multifactorial and interacting etiologies of falls.

review the risk factors for falls and discuss how their identification is the core of a multidimensional fall evaluation.

II.   EPIDEMIOLOGY

A.   Incidence of falls

Prospective studies have reported that 30–60% of community-dwelling older adults fall each year (1–6) with about half of fallers experiencing multiple falls. Fall incidence rates for community-dwelling older populations range from 0.2 to 1.6 falls per person per year, with a mean of about 0.7 falls per year (7). Incidence rises steadily after middle age and tends to be highest among individuals 80 years and older (8). These incidence rates are based on self-reported data, which may underestimate the true incidence of falls but may also over-represent the proportion of persons reporting multiple falls.

Incidence rates in institutionalized elderly populations are generally higher than in community-living elderly populations. This difference is due both to the frailer nature of institutionalized populations and to the more accurate reporting of falls in institutional settings. In surveys of nursing home populations the percentage of residents who fall each year ranges from 16% to 75%, with an overall mean of 43%.(9–12) Annual incidence of falls in long-term care facilities averages about 1.6 falls per occupied bed (range 0.2–3.6 falls) (7). Incidence rates from hospital-based surveys are somewhat lower with a mean of 1.4 falls per bed annually (range from 0.5 to 2.7 falls) (7). This variation in incidence rates between the institutionalized populations most likely reflects differences in case mix, ambulation levels, reporting practices, and institutional fall prevention policies and programs.

B. Fall-Related Mortality

Accidents are the fifth leading cause of death in older adults (after cardiovascular, cancer, stroke, and pulmonary causes), and falls constitute two-thirds of these accidental deaths. About three-fourths of deaths due to falls in the United States occur in the 13% of the population aged 65 and older (13). Fall-related mortality increases dramatically with advancing age, especially in populations after age 70. Older men have a higher mortality rate from falls than older women, and nursing home residents 85 years and older account for 1 out of 5 fatal falls (14). The estimated 1% of fallers who sustain a hip fracture has a 20–30% mortality rate within one year of the fracture (15).

C. Fall-Related Morbidity

A key issue of concern is not simply the high incidence of falls in elderly persons, since young children and athletes certainly have an even higher incidence of falls, but rather the combination of a high incidence and a high susceptibility to injury. This propensity for fall-related injury in elderly persons is due to a high prevalence of clinical diseases (e.g., osteoporosis) and age-related physiologic changes (e.g., slowed protective reflexes) that make even a relatively mild fall particularly dangerous. While most falls produce no serious injury, community surveys have reported that over half of falls result in at least minor injuries, and (16,17) between 5% and 10% of community-dwelling older persons who fall each year sustain a serious injury, such as a fracture, head injury, or serious laceration (16,17). The proportion of falls that result in serious injuries is similar in community-dwelling and institutionalized populations, but the range is wide (1–39%) because of differences in reporting practices. These injuries are often associated with considerable long-term morbidity. Among community-dwelling fallers with hip fractures, studies have shown that between 25% and 75% do not recover their pre-fracture level of function in ambulation or activities of daily living (15).

In addition to physical injuries, falls can produce other serious consequences for the elderly person. Repeated falls are a common reason for the admission of previously independent elderly persons to long-term care institutions (18). In one study, 50% of fall injuries that required hospital admission resulted in the elderly person being discharged to a nursing home (19). In a prospective study of a community-dwelling older population, the risk of nursing home placement for individuals who had sustained at least one fall with a serious injury was three times greater than for individuals with only one noninjurious fall (20).

Fear of falling has also been recognized as a negative consequence of falls. Surveys have reported that between 30% and 73% of older persons who have fallen acknowledge a fear of falling (21–23). This postfall anxiety syndrome can result in self-imposed activity restrictions among both home-living (22,24) and institutionalized elderly fallers (25). Loss of confidence in the ability to ambulate safely can result in further functional decline, depression, feelings of helplessness, and social isolation.

III. CAUSES OF FALLS

Table 1 lists the major causes of falls and their relative frequencies as reported by 6 studies (11,26–30) conducted among institutionalized populations and 6 studies conducted among community-living populations (31–36). The accuracy of these findings is limited by several factors including differences in classification methods, patient recall, and the multifactorial nature of many falls. However, these data provide useful general information about the reasons for falls among older adults. As shown in Table 1, so-called accidents, or falls stemming from environmental hazards, comprise the largest fall cause category, accounting for 25–45% in most series. Many of the falls in this category stem from interactions between environmental hazards or hazardous activities and increased individual susceptibility to hazards from accumulated effects of age and disease. These types of falls are more common in community-living populations than in institutions, probably because of the greater

Table 1 Causes of Falls in Older Persons: Summary of 12 Large Studies

Cause	Mean (%)[a]	Range[b]
Accident and environment-related	31	1–53
Gait and balance disorders or weakness	17	4–39
Dizziness and vertigo	13	0–30
Drop attack	9	0–52
Confusion	5	0–14
Postural hypotension	3	0–24
Visual disorder	2	0–5
Syncope	0.3	0–3
Other specified causes[c]	15	2–39
Unknown	5	0–21

Summary of 12 studies (Refs. 11, 26–36).
[a]Mean percent calculated from the 3628 reported falls.
[b]Ranges indicate the percentage reported in each of the 12 studies.
[c]This category includes: arthritis, acute illness, drugs, alcohol, pain, epilepsy, and falling from bed.

attention to creating hazard-free environments in institutions. The other major fall causes identified are related more directly to age-related changes or specific diseases. Overall, frail, high-risk populations tend to have more of these medically related falls, than do healthier populations.

IV. RISK FACTORS FOR FALLS

Because a single specific cause for falling often cannot be identified and because falls are usually multifactorial in their origin, many investigators have performed epidemiologic case–control studies to identify specific risk factors. A risk factor is defined as a characteristic found significantly more often in individuals who subsequently experience a certain adverse event than individuals not experiencing the event. While there are some differences in risk factors between community-living and institutionalized populations, most overlap. A review (7) of these fall risk factor studies analyzed the data from the 16 studies providing quantitative risk data, and summarized the relative risks of falls for persons with each risk factor. Eight of these studies were conducted in community-dwelling populations and eight in nursing home populations. The ranks and approximate mean relative risk data for the most commonly reported risk factors are listed in Table 2. It should be noted that some of these are directly involved in causing falls (e.g., weakness,

Table 2 Risk Factors for Falls Identified in 16 Studies[a] Examining Multiple Risk Factors: Results of Univariate Analysis

Risk factor	Significant/Total[b]	Mean RR-OR[c]	Range
Lower extremity weakness	10/11	4.4	1.5–10.3
History of falls	12/13	3.0	1.7–7.0
Gait deficit	10/12	2.9	1.3–5.6
Balance deficit	8/11	2.9	1.6–5.4
Use assistive device	8/8	2.6	1.2–4.6
Visual deficit	6/12	2.5	1.6–3.5
Arthritis	3/7	2.4	1.9–2.9
Impaired ADL	8/9	2.3	1.5–3.1
Depression	3/6	2.2	1.7–2.5
Cognitive impairment	4/11	1.8	1.0–2.3
Age >80 years	5/8	1.7	1.1–2.5

[a]From Ref. 7.
[b]Number of studies with significant odds ratio or relative risk ratio in univariate analysis/total number of studies that included each factor.
[c]Relative risk (RR) ratios calculated for prospective studies. OR calculated for retrospective studies.

gait, and balance disorder), while others are more markers of other underlying causes (e.g., prior falls, assistive device, age > 80).

Among these studies, lower extremity weakness (detected by either functional testing or manual muscle examination) was identified as the most potent risk factor associated with falls, increasing the odds of falling, on average, over four times (4.4, range 1.5–10.3). A recent meta-analysis looking at the relationship between muscle weakness and falls among purely prospective studies, reported that lower extremity weakness had a combined odds ratio of 1.76 for any fall and 3.06 for recurrent falls (37). In addition to having a strong association with falls, leg weakness is very common in older persons. As a whole healthy older people score 20–40% lower on strength tests than young adults (38), and the prevalence of detectable lower extremity weakness ranges from 57% among residents of an intermediate-care facility (12) to over 80% among residents of a skilled nursing facility (35). Weakness often stems from deconditioning due to limited physical activity or prolonged bed rest, together with chronic debilitating medical conditions, such as heart failure, stroke, or pulmonary disease.

Individuals who have already fallen have a three-fold risk of falling again. While recurrent falls in an individual are frequently due to the same underlying cause (e.g., gait disorder, orthostatic hypotension), they can also be an indication of disease progression (e.g., parkinsonism, dementia) or a new acute problem (e.g., infection, dehydration).

Gait and balance disorders are also common among older adults, affecting between 20% and 50% of people over the age of 65 years (39,40). Among nursing home populations, nearly three quarters of residents require assistance with ambulation or are completely unable to ambulate (41). Both gait and balance impairments were found to be a significant risk factor for falls, associated with about a three-fold increased risk of falling, and use of an assistive device for ambulation was associated with a 2.6 increased risk of falling.

Visual impairment has been found to increase the risk of falling about 2.5 times. At least 18% of noninstitutionalized persons 70 years and older have substantial visual impairment (42). The primary causes, most of which are treatable, include cataracts, glaucoma, and macular degeneration.

Arthritis, the most common chronic condition affecting persons 70 years and older in the United States (42), increases the risk of falling about 2.4 times. The relationship between arthritis and falls is most likely related to the gait impairment and weakness that are often associated with arthritis.

Functional impairment, usually indicated by inability to perform basic activities of daily living (ADLs) (e.g., dressing, bathing, and eating), has been shown to double the risk for falling. In the community, ADL impairment affects 20% of persons over age 70 (42). In the nursing home setting, the prevalence of functional impairment is higher with 96% of nursing home residents requiring assistance with bathing and 45% requiring assistance with eating (41).

Depression is associated with about a two-fold increased risk of falling. While the relationship between depression and falls is not well studied, depression may result in inattention to the environment, or cause more risk-taking behaviors. Conversely, it may be a reaction to previous fall-related morbidity and not be an actual causative risk at all. In addition, psychotropic medications have been shown to increase fall risk (43). Common risk factors have been identified for both depression and falls (i.e., poor self-rated health, cognitive impairment, functional impairment, and slow gait speed) (44). Mild depressive symptoms occur in close to a quarter of the older population, and about 5% of this population suffers major depression (45).

Cognitive impairment has been shown to almost double the risk of falling. A recent study confirmed this risk. Among residents of 59 nursing homes, the unadjusted fall rate for residents with dementia was 4.05 falls per year compared to 2.33 falls per year for residents without dementia ($p < 0.0001$) (adjusted relative risk = 1.74) (46). Confusion and cognitive impairment are frequently cited causes of falls and may reflect an underlying systemic or metabolic process (e.g., electrolyte imbalance, fever), as well as a dementing illness. Dementia can increase falls by impairing judgment, visuospatial perception, and orientation ability. Falls also occur when demented residents wander, attempt to get out of wheelchairs, or climb over bed siderails. Cognitive impairment affects between 5% and 15% of persons over age 65, and the prevalence rises with age and among institutionalized populations.

The risk of falls has also been shown to nearly double for individuals over the age of 80. This is probably due to the rising prevalence of multiple risk factors associated with age.

The relationship between medication use and falls has also been examined in many studies. A meta-analysis (43,47) found a significantly increased risk from psychotropic medication [odds ratio (OR) = 1.7], Class 1a antiarrhythmic medications (OR = 1.6), digoxin (OR = 1.2), and diuretics (OR = 1.1). Several studies also have shown strong relationships between use of three or more medications and risk of falls (8,26,35). While the size of these OR is not as large as the prior set of risk factors, they are nonetheless statistically and clinically significant.

Several of the studies shown in Table 2 used multivariate analysis to better understand possible interactions between the individual risk factors and to rank their relative importance. The risk factors and relative ranks emerging from these analyses were similar to the univariate factors, although the size of risk was altered for some of them. Muscle weakness remained the dominant risk factor with a four-fold increased risk of falls (range 3.0–5.9), and balance deficits and history of falls still were associated with about a three-fold increased risk of falls. However, cognitive impairment, age greater than 80 years and visual impairments increased in magnitude to about a three-fold increased risk, while gait deficits declined to a two-fold increased risk of falls in the multivariate analyses (7).

Many other case-control studies have examined the relationship between falls and single possible risk factors in isolation. For example, several studies examined the relationship of leg strength alone and fall status without exploring other possibly confounding risk factors. Gehlsen (48) reported that healthy older persons with a history of falling had significantly weaker leg strength than nonfallers. Whipple et al. (49) examined knee and ankle strength, and reported that weakness at both joints was found to be significantly more common among institutionalized fallers than nonfallers. They also performed gait analysis of 49 nursing home patients and found that fallers had significantly slower gait speed and shorter stride length than nonfallers (50). Studenski et al. (51) found that outpatients with impaired mobility had a significantly higher rate of recurrent falls over a 6-month period. Other studies have compared measures of dynamic balance in older fallers and nonfallers. Deficits in the ability to control lateral stability were associated with an increased risk of falling in a healthy ambulatory population (4). Other single-variable risk factor studies have documented significant relationships between falls and single leg stance (52), postprandial hypotension (53), impaired depth perception (54), musculoskeletal pain (55), and foot problems (56), to name only a few.

Possibly even more important than identifying risk factors for falling per se is identifying risk factors for injurious falls, since most falls do not result in injury. Risk factors associated with injurious falls have been identified by several research groups (16,17,50,57). Among community-living populations, risk factors identified as increasing the likelihood of an injurious fall include having a previous fall with a fracture, being Caucasian, having impaired cognitive function, and having impaired balance. A survey of elderly Medicaid enrollees revealed that the risk of hip fracture increased two-fold for both community-living elderly persons and nursing home residents who were taking psychotropic medications (58). Narcotic analgesics, anticonvulsants, and antidepressants were identified as independent risk factors for injurious falls among community living older adults receiving care in emergency departments (57). Among nursing home residents, lower extremity weakness, female sex, poor vision and hearing, disorientation, number of falls, impaired balance, dizziness, low body mass, and use of mechanical restraints have been identified as increasing the risk of an injurious fall (30,59–61). Surprisingly, patients who were functionally independent and not depressed also had a greater risk of injury (61)—probably because they were more active. Taken together, the risk factors for injurious falls are the same as for falls in general, with the addition of female sex and low body mass (both probably largely related to osteoporosis), and higher activity.

Once individual risk factors are identified, it is important to understand the interaction and probable synergism between multiple risk factors. Several studies have shown that the risk of falling increases dramatically as the number of risk factors increases (6,12,16,35). In their survey of community-living elderly persons, Tinetti et al. (6) reported that the percentage of persons falling increased from 27%, among those with none or one risk factor, to 78% among those with four or more risk factors. Their identified risk factors included sedative use, decreased cognition, leg and foot disabilities, gait and balance impairments, and the presence of a palmomental reflex. Similar results were found among an institutionalized population (12). In another study, Nevitt et al. (16) reported that the percentage of community-living persons with recurrent falls increased from 10% to 69% as the number of risk factors increased from one to four or more. Their identified risk factors included white race, a history of previous falls, arthritis, parkinsonism, difficulty rising, and poor tandem gait. In a study by Robbins et al. (35), involving an institutionalized and outpatient population, many risk factors were individually significantly related to falls. Multivariate analysis enabled simplification of the model so that maximum predictive accuracy could be obtained by using only three risk factors (i.e., hip weakness assessed manually, unstable balance, and taking four or more prescribed medications) in a branching logic, algorithmic fashion. With this model, the predicted one-year risk of falling ranged from 12% for persons with none of the three risk factors to 100% for persons with all three risk factors.

In summary, studies have shown that it is possible to identify persons at substantially increased risk of sustaining a fall or fall-related injury by detecting the presence of risk factors. Many, if not all, of these risk factors are amenable to treatment or rehabilitative approaches to ameliorate them. Consequently, risk factor identification appears to be a promising first step in developing effective fall-prevention programs targeted to high-risk patients. There are a large number of published fall-risk assessment tools available for assisting quantification of fall risk for older persons at home and residing in institutional settings. An analytic review of these fall-risk assessment tools recommended several that seem to be valid and potentially useful (62).

V. MULTIDIMENSIONAL FALL-RISK ASSESSMENT

Clinical practice guidelines on fall prevention and treatment have been published by the American and British Geriatrics Societies (63) after careful review of extensive published evidence. The purpose of these guidelines is to assist clinicians in the assessment of fall risk in older persons and the management of older patients found to be at increased risk of falling as well as those who have fallen. The guidelines recommend that a fall-risk assessment should be an integral part of primary healthcare for older persons. However, the intensity of the assessment will vary with the target population. For low-risk community-dwelling populations, the guidelines recommend that all older patients should be asked at least once a year about fall occurrence and circumstances. Older persons who report a single fall should be observed for mobility impairment and unsteadiness using a simple observational test. Those patients who demonstrate mobility problems or unsteadiness should be referred for further assessment. High-risk populations (e.g., older persons who report multiple falls in the past year, have abnormalities of gait and/or balance, seek medical attention because of a fall, or reside in a nursing home) should undergo a more comprehensive and detailed assessment.

The goals of the fall evaluation are two-fold: (1) to diagnose and treat patients after a fall and (2) to identify risk factors for future falls and implement appropriate interventions. Most of these risk factors can be easily assessed in the physician's office using basic examination techniques or standardized instruments. The fall evaluation should incorporate the basic principles of comprehensive geriatric assessment; namely, a multidimensional assessment to quantify medical, psychosocial, and functional capabilities and problems in order to develop a comprehensive plan for therapy.

The diagnostic approach should begin with a well-directed history aimed at uncovering any immediate precipitating cause as well as associated risk factors. A full report of the circumstances and symptoms surrounding a fall is crucial, including reports from witnesses. Certain historical factors can point to a specific cause or identify contributing risk factors, such as a fall associated with suddenly rising from a lying or sitting position (orthostatic hypotension), a trip or slip (gait, balance, or vision disturbance in addition to the apparent environmental hazard), antecedent cough or urination (reflex hypotension), a recent meal (postprandial hypotension), looking up or sideways (arterial or carotid sinus compression), and loss of consciousness (syncope or seizure). Symptoms experienced near the time of falling may also indicate a potential cause, such as dizziness or giddiness (e.g., orthostatic hypotension, vestibular problem, hypoglycemia, arrhythmia, and drug side effect), palpitations (e.g., arrhythmia), incontinence or tongue biting (e.g., seizure), asymmetric weakness (e.g., cerebrovascular disease), chest pain (e.g., myocardial infarction or coronary insufficiency), or loss of consciousness (any cause of syncope). Medications, especially those with hypotensive or psychoactive effects, and existence of concomitant medical problems may be important contributing factors.

Components of the physical examination often useful in identifying risk factors include postural pulse and blood pressure measurements, visual acuity testing, manual muscle testing of the lower extremities and neurologic assessment. A quantitative mental screening evaluation, such as the

Mini-Mental State Examination, is important to rule out cognitive impairment. The careful assessment of gait and balance is a particularly important component of the fall assessment, both to detect abnormalities and evaluate their impact on function. Gait and balance should be assessed by close observation of how the patient rises from a chair (which is also a functional test of lower extremity strength), stands with eyes open and closed, walks, turns, and sits down. Characteristics of gait to be noted include velocity and rhythm, stride length, symmetry, double support time (the time spent with both feet on the floor), height of stepping, and degree of trunk sway. The fit and use of any assistive device, as well as footwear, is also observed. Imbalance observed during head turning or flexion is an important finding associated with vestibular or vertebrobasilar pathology and an increased risk for falling. Simple scored screening scales for detecting and quantifying gait and balance problems have been developed and are reviewed in chapter 2. Useful examples include the Performance Oriented Mobility Index (12) and the Timed Up and Go test (64), both of which have been well validated for quantifying gait and balance impairment and assisting with diagnosis. The quantitative nature of these scales is useful for gauging severity of the problem and following progress over time.

In addition to identifying gait and balance deviations, it is important to assess functional mobility and physical activity. By determining the type of activities that a patient actually engages in, the clinician can make a more accurate appraisal of fall risk. Studies have suggested that patients with fall risk factors who are physically active are at somewhat greater risk of falling than similar patients who engage in little independent activity. However, activity has its own set of benefits that can often outweigh an increased fall risk. Inactivity can further accelerate muscle weakness and functional impairment, ultimately leading to more falls later (51,65). Optimally, it would be helpful to observe patients perform activities in their living environment, both to assess functional ability and to identify potential hazards. While this may be possible in the institutional setting, among community-living older adults the clinician must usually obtain this information indirectly through specific questioning. Numerous functional status scales have been developed for assessing different populations of older adults (66).

The fall evaluation should also include a careful review of the prescription and nonprescription medications that the patient is taking to identify those that have hypotensive or psychoactive effects. These types of medications should be altered or stopped as appropriate in light of the patient's risk for falls. Particular attention should be given to older people taking four or more medications.

Additional diagnostic evaluations should be directed by symptoms associated with the fall or a patient's medical history. For example, an assessment of vertigo should include the Dix–Hallpike maneuver to confirm benign positional vertigo (67). Ambulatory cardiac (Holter) monitoring may be advisable when a transient arrhythmia is suspected by history, in cases of syncope, or when the patient with unexplained falls has a history of cardiac disease and receives cardiac medication. In the presence of unexplained bradyarrhythmia or suspected carotid sinus hypersensitivity syndrome, carotid sinus massage (68) performed under monitored conditions may be indicated.

Laboratory evaluation is sometimes helpful in the falls evaluation, especially when the cause is not obvious: complete blood counts to search for anemia or infection; serum sodium, potassium, glucose, and creatinine levels; electrocardiography to document arrhythmia or ischemia and thyroid function tests. However, most of the important risk factors can be readily identified without use of laboratory testing.

Environmental hazards are frequently associated with falls, and are important to attend to, even though they do not generally appear on lists of intrinsic risk factors, largely because of methodological difficulties in quantifying them in case-control studies. Since most falls occur indoors at home, it is important for the clinician to include issues of home safety in the fall evaluation. Educational pamphlets and home safety assessment forms are widely available that the clinician can use to educate older persons about potential hazards (e.g., clutter, throw rugs, and poor lighting) and how to modify the environment to improve mobility and safety (e.g., installation of grab bars and handrails, raised toilet seat) (69).

Optimally, the multidimensional fall assessment will uncover direct causes and/or contributing risk factors amenable to medical therapy or other corrective interventions. Because of the multifactorial nature of falls, there is no standard approach to treatment or prevention. In cases where the cause of a fall is due to an obvious acute problem, treatment may be relatively simple, direct, and effective (e.g., discontinuing medication that causes postural hypotension). However, patients with multiple risk factors will often require a combination of medical, rehabilitative, environmental, and/or behavioral intervention strategies (e.g., treating syncope, removing environmental hazards, prescribing strengthening exercises, and supplying a properly fitted cane). The effectiveness of multifactorial interventions to prevent falls has been demonstrated in several randomized controlled trials, both among community-living (70–73) and nursing home (11,74) populations.

In conclusion, a large proportion of falls and fall injuries in older persons are probably preventable with careful medical and environmental evaluation and intervention, much of which involves identification and amelioration of risk factors. Therefore, as stated in the recent AGS/BGS guidelines, inquiry about recent falls and regular screening for fall risk factors is vitally important among older adults and forms the basis for effective falls prevention.

REFERENCES

1. Berg W, Alessio H, Mills E, Tong C. Circumstances and consequences of falls in independent community-dwelling older adults. Age Aging 1997; 26:261–268.
2. Campbell AJ, Borrie MJ, Spears GF, Jacson SL, Brown JS, Fitzgerald JL. Circumstances and consequences of falls experienced by a community population 70 years and over during a prospective study. Aging 1990; 19:136–141.
3. Luukinen H, Koski K, Hiltunen L, Kivela SL. Incidence rate of falls in an aged population in northern Finland. J Clin Epidemiol 1994; 47:843–850.
4. Maki BE, Holliday PJ, Topper AK. A prospective study of postural balance and risk of falling in an ambulatory and independent elderly population. J Gerontol 1994; 49:M72–M84.
5. Nevitt MC, Cummings SR, Kidd S, Black D. Risk factors for recurrent nonsyncopal falls. A prospective study. JAMA 1989; 261:2663–2668.
6. Tinetti ME, Speechley M, Ginter SF. Risk factors for falls among elderly persons living in the community. N Engl J Med 1988; 319:1701–1707.
7. Rubenstein LZ, Josephson KR. The epidemiology of falls and syncope. Clin Geriatr Med 2002; 18:141–158.
8. Campbell AJ, Borrie MJ, Spears GF. Risk factors for falls in a community-based prospective study of people 70 years and older. J Gerontol 1989; 44:M112–M117.
9. Gross YT, Shimamoto Y, Rose CL, Frank B. Monitoring risk factors in nursing homes. J Gerontol Nurs 1990; 16:20–25.
10. Gryfe CI, Amies A, Ashley MJ. A longitudinal study of falls in an elderly population: I. Incidence and morbidity. Aging 1977; 6:201–210.
11. Rubenstein LZ, Robbins AS, Josephson KR, Schulman BL, Osterweil D. The value of assessing falls in an elderly population: A randomized clinical trial. Ann Intern Med 1990; 113:308–316.
12. Tinetti ME, Williams TF, Mayewski R. Fall risk index for elderly patients based on number of chronic disabilities. Am J Med 1986; 80:429–434.
13. Hogue C. Injury in late life: I. Epidemiology, II. Prevention. J Am Geriatr Soc 1982; 30:183–190.
14. Baker S, Harvey A. Fall injuries in the elderly. Clin Geriatr Med 1985; 1:501–512.
15. Magaziner J, Simonsick EM, Kashner TM, Hebel JR, Kenzora JE. Predictors of functional recovery one year following hospital discharge for hip fracture: A prospective study. J Gerontol: Med Sci 1990; 45:M101–M107.
16. Nevitt MC, Cummings SR, Hudes ES. Risk factors for injurious falls: A prospective study. J Gerontol 1991; 46:M164–M170.
17. Tinetti M, Doucette J, Claus E, Marottoli R. Risk factors for serious injury during falls by older persons in the community. J Am Geriatr Soc 1995; 43:1214–1221.
18. Smallegan M. How families decide on nursing-home admission. Geriatr Consult 1983; 2:21–24.
19. Sattin RW, Huber DAL, DeVito CA, Rodriguez JG, Ros A, Bacchelli S. The incidence of fall injury events among the elderly in a defined population. Am J Epidemiol 1990; 131:1028–1037.

20. Tinetti ME, Williams CS. Falls, injuries due to falls, and the risk of admission to a nursing home. N Engl J Med 1997; 337:1279–1284.

21. King MB, Tinetti ME. Falls in community-dwelling older persons. J Am Geriatr Soc 1995; 43:1146–1154.

22. Tinetti ME, Mendes de Leon CF, Doucette JT, Baker DI. Fear of falling and fall-related efficacy in relationship to functioning among community-living elders. J Gerontol Med Sci 1994; 49:M140–M147.

23. Vellas BJ, Wayne SH, Romero LJ, Baumgartner RN, Garry PJ. Fear of falling and restriction of mobility in elderly fallers. Aging 1997; 26:189–193.

24. Walker JE, Howland J. Falls and fear of falling among elderly persons living in the community: Occupational therapy interventions. Am J Occup Ther 1991; 45:119–122.

25. Pawlson LF, Goodwin M, Keith K. Wheelchair use by ambulatory nursing home residents. J Am Geriatr Soc 1986; 34:860–864.

26. Lipsitz LA, Jonsson PV, Kelley MM, Koestner JS. Causes and correlates of recurrent falls in ambulatory frail elderly. J Gerontol 1991; 46:M114–M122.

27. Lucht U. A prospective study of accidental falls and injuries at home among elderly people. Acta Socio Med Scand 1971; 2:105–120.

28. Naylor R, Rosin AJ. Falling as a cause of admission to a geriatric unit. Practitioner 1970; 205:327–330.

29. Scott CJ. Accidents in hospital with special reference to old people. Health Bull (Edinb) 1976; 34:330–335.

30. Svensson ML, Rundgren A, Larsson M, Oden A, Sund V, Landahl S. Accidents in the institutionalized elderly: A risk analysis. Age Aging 1991; 3:181–192.

31. Brocklehurst JC, Exton-Smith An, Lempert-Barber SM, Hunt LP, Palmer MK. Fractures of the femur in old age: A two-centre study of associated clinical factors and the cause of the fall. Aging 1978; 7:7–15.

32. Clark ANG. Factors in fracture of the female femur. A clinical study of the environmental, physical, medical, and preventative aspects of this injury. Geront Clin 1968; 10:257–270.

33. Exton-Smith AN. Functional consequences of aging: clinical manifestations. In: Exton-Smith AN, Grimley Evans J, eds. Care of the Elderly: Meeting the Challenge of Dependency. London: Academic Press, 1977:41–53.

34. Morfitt JM. Falls in old people at home: Intrinsic versus environmental factors in causation. Public Health 1983; 97:115–120.

35. Robbins AS, Rubenstein LZ, Josephson KR, Schulman BL, Osterweil D, Fine G. Predictors of falls among elderly people. Results of two population-based studie. Arch Intern Med 1989; 149:1628–1633.

36. Sheldon JH. On the natural history of falls in old age. Br Med J 1960; 2:1685–1690.

37. Moreland JD, Richardson JA, Goldsmith CH, Clase CM. Muscle weakness and falls in older adults: a systematic review and meta-analysis. J Am Geriatr Soc 2004; 52:1121–1129.

38. Murray MP, Gardner GM, Mollinger LA, Sepic SB. Strength of isometric and isokinetic contractions: knee muscles of men aged 20 to 86. Phys Ther 1980; 60:412–419.

39. Alexander NB. Gait disorders in older adults. J Am Geriatr Soc 1996; 44(4):434–451.

40. Sudarsky L. Geriatrics: gait disorders in the elderly. N Engl J Med 1990; 322:1441–1446.

41. Sahyoun NR, et al. The changing profile of nursing home residents: 1985–1997. Aging Trends 4, Hyattsville, Maryland: National Center for Health Statistics, 2001.

42. Kramarow E, et al., 1999. Health and Aging Chartbook. Health, United States, 1999 Hyattsville, Maryland: National Center for Health Statistics.

43. Leipzig RM, Cumming RG, Tinetti ME. Drugs and falls in older people: A systematic review and meta-analysis: I. Psychotropic drugs. J Am Geriatr Soc 1999; 47:30–39.

44. Biderman A, Cwikel J, Fried, AV, Galinsky D. Depression and falls among community dwelling elderly people: a search for common risk factors. J Epidemiol Community Health 2002; 56:631–636.

45. Blazer D, Williams CD. Epidemiology of dysphoric and depression in an elderly population. Am J Psychiatry 1980; 137:413–417.

46. Van Doorn C, Gruber-Baldini AL, Zimmerman S, Hebel JR, Port CL, Baumgarten M, Quinn CC, Taler G, May C, Magaziner J. Dementia as a risk factor for falls and fall injuries among nursing home residents. J Am Geriatr Soc 2003; 51:1213–1218.

47. Leipzig RM, Cumming RG, Tinetti ME. Drugs and falls in older people: A systematic review and meta-analysis: II. Cardiac and analgesic drugs. J Am Geriatr Soc 1999; 47:40–50.

48. Gehlsen GM, Whaley MH. Falls in the elderly: Part II, balance, strength, and flexibility. Arch Phys Med Rehabil 1990; 71:739–741.

49. Whipple RH, Wolfson LI, Amerman PM. The relationship of knee and ankle weakness to falls in nursing home residents: an isokinetic study. J Am Geriatr Soc 1987; 35:13–20.

50. Wolfson L, Whipple R, Amerman P, Tobin JN. Gait assessment in the elderly: A gait abnormality rating scale and its relation to falls. J Gerontol 1990; 45:M12–M19.

51. Studenski S, Duncan PW, Chandler J, Samsa G, Prescott B, Hogue C, Bearon LB. Predicting falls: the role of mobility and nonphysical factors. J Am Geriatr Soc 1994; 42:297–302.

52. Vellas BJ, Wayne SH, Romero LJ, Baumgartner RN, Rubenstein LZ, Garry PJ. One-leg balance is an important predictor of injurious falls in older persons. J Am Geriatr Soc 1997; 45:735–738.

53. Ooi WL, Hossain M, Lipsitz LA. The association between orthostatic hypotension and recurrent falls in nursing home residents. Am J Med 2000; 108:106–111.

54. Lord R, Dayhew J. Visual risk factors for falls in older people. J Am Geriatr Soc 2001; 49(5):508–515.

55. Leveille SG, Bean J, Bandeen-Roche K, Jones R, Hochberg M, Guralnik JM. Musculoskeletal pain and risk for falls in older disabled women living in the community. J Am Geriatr Soc 2002; 50(4):671–678.

56. Menz HB, Pod B, Lord SR. The contribution of foot problems to mobility impairment and falls in community-dwelling older people. J Am Geriatr Soc 2001; 49(12):1651–1656.

57. Kelly KD, Pickett W, Yiannakoulias N, Rowe BH, Schopflocher DP, Svenson L, Voaklander DC. Medication use and falls in community-dwelling older persons. Aging 2003; 32:503–509.

58. Ray WA, Griffin MR, Schaffner W. Psychotropic drug use and the risk of hip fracture. N Engl J Med 1987; 316:363–369.

59. Thapa P, Brockman K, Gideon P, Fought RL, Ray WA. Injurious falls in nonambulatory nursing home residents: a comparative study of circumstances, incidence and risk factors. J Am Geriat Soc 1996; 44:273–276.

60. Tinetti ME, Liu WL, Ginter SF. Mechanical restraint use and fall-related injuries among residents of skilled nursing facilities. Ann Intern Med 1992; 116:369–374.

61. Tinetti ME. Factors associated with serious injury during falls by ambulatory nursing home residents. J Am Geriatr Soc 1987; 35:644–648.

62. Perell KL, Nelson A, Goldman RL, Luther SL, Prieto-Lewis N, Rubenstein LZ. Fall risk assessment measures: an analytic review. J Gerontol 2001; 56A:M761–M766.

63. American Geriatrics Society, British Geriatrics Society, American Academy of Orthopaedic Surgeons Panel on Falls Prevention. Guideline for the prevention of falls in older persons. J Am Geriatr Soc 2001; 49:664–672.

64. Podsiadlo D, Richardson S. The timed 'Up & Go': A test of basic functional mobility for frail elderly persons. J Am Geriatr Soc 1991; 39:142–148.

65. Stevens JA, Powell KE, Smith SM, Wingo PA, Sattin RW. Physical activity, functional limitations, and the risk of fall-related fractures in community-dwelling elderly. Ann Epidemiol 1997; 7:54–61.

66. Applegate WB, Blass JP, Williams TF. Instruments for the functional assessment of older patients. N Eng J Med 1990; 322:1207–1214.

67. Norre ME, Beckers A. Benign paroxysmal positional vertigo in the elderly. Treatment by habituation exercises. J Am Geriatr Soc 1988; 36:425–429.

68. Kenny RA. Neurally mediated syncope. Clin Geriatr Med 2002; 18:191–210.

69. Kercher BJ, Rubenstein LZ. Home-safety checklists for elders in print and on the Internet. Generations 2003; 26(4):69–74.

70. Hornbrook MC, Stevens VJ, Wingfield DF, Hollis JF, Greenlick MR, Ory MG. Preventing falls among community-dwelling older persons: results from a randomized trial. Gerontologist 1994; 34:16–23.

71. Tinetti ME, Baker DI, McAvay G, Claus EB, Garrett P, Gottschalk M, Koch ML, Trainor K, Morwitz RI. A multifactorial intervention to reduce the risk of falling among elderly people living in the community. N Engl J Med 1994; 331:821–827.

72. Wagner EH, LaCroix AZ, Grothaus L, Leveille SG, Hecht JA, Artz K, Odle K, Buchner DM. Preventing disability and falls in older adults: A population-based randomized trial. Am J Public Health 1994; 84:1800–1806.

73. Close J, Ellis M, Hooper R, Glucksman E, Jackson S, Swift C. Prevention of falls in the elderly trial (PROFET): a randomized controlled trial. Lancet 1999; 353:93–97.

74. Ray WA, Taylor JA, Meador KG, Thapa PB, Brown AK, Kajihara HK, Davis C, Gideon P, Griffin MR. A randomized trial of a consultation service to reduce falls in nursing homes. J Am Med Assoc 1997; 278:557–562.

10

Best Clinical Practice Models to Reduce Falls

Robert J. Przybelski

Section of Geriatrics and Gerontology, University of Wisconsin Medical School, Falls Prevention Clinic, Madison, Wisconsin, U.S.A.

Jane Mahoney

Section of Geriatrics and Gerontology, University of Wisconsin Medical School, Elder Care of Dane County, Madison, Wisconsin, U.S.A.

I. INTRODUCTION

Although falls among older adults occur commonly, many falls are preventable. The best clinical practice approach to prevent falls and associated injuries is to identify the person most likely to fall, isolate the factors causing, precipitating, or complicating the fall, and modify or eliminate as many of those factors as possible.

Individuals at high risk for falls and fall injuries are those with a history of two or more falls in 1 year, one fall with significant injury (more than a bruise), or one fall with balance or gait problems (1). The U.S. Preventive Services Task Force recommends that individuals of age 70–74 years with a risk factor for falls and all those ≥75 years be counseled on falls prevention (2). Conditions that have been shown in two or more observational studies to be associated with increased fall risk are use of four or more medications, cognitive impairment, orthostatic hypotension, balance or gait problems, muscle weakness, arthritis, vision problems, and depressive symptoms (3).

As the number of risk factors a patient manifests increases, the likelihood of falling increases precipitously. For example, in community-dwelling elders, the percentage of persons falling increased from 27% for those with no or one risk factor to 70% for those with four or more risk factors (4). Another study showed that maximum predictive accuracy could be obtained using only three risk factors: hip weakness, unstable balance, and taking more than four medications; this combination increased the predicted risk of falling from 12% in persons with none of these risk factors to 100% for people with all three (5).

The American Geriatrics Society, British Geriatrics Society, and American Academy of Orthopedic Surgeons Panel on Falls Prevention recommend that older patients undergoing a routine care assessment should be asked at least once a year about falls (1). A more aggressive approach is to ask each elderly, frail, or high-risk patient at each visit "When did you last fall?" This approach sends the message that falls are not unexpected and calls for more than one "yes" or "no" answer from the patient. Those who report even a single fall should be checked for gait and balance problems.

Older persons who present for medical attention because of a fall, report recurrent falls in the past year, or who report one fall with demonstrated abnormalities of gait and/or balance, should have a comprehensive fall evaluation (1). The primary care physician, nurse practitioner, or physician's assistant, with physical therapy and subspecialty consultative resources, can provide this assessment and the interventions directed toward prevention of subsequent falls.

This chapter reviews the evidence supporting a multifactorial intervention approach to preventing falls, examines the documented success of specific single interventions, and provides a set of recommendations for the most effective intervention strategies. These strategies are recommended on the basis of previous multifactorial intervention trials that have included such approaches in their interventions or on the basis of existing epidemiologic, clinical, or other research data suggesting the approaches are likely to be of benefit.

II. OVERVIEW OF EVIDENCE BASE FOR FALLS INTERVENTIONS

A. Multifactorial Interventions

The Panel on Falls Prevention has recommended that, for older adults living in their own homes, a falls evaluation be followed by a multifactorial intervention to address remediable factors (1). The multifactorial intervention should include gait training and advice on assistive devices; modification of medications, particularly psychotropic medications; provision of exercise including balance training; treatment of postural hypotension; modification of environmental hazards; and treatment of cardiovascular disorders/ arrhythmias (1).

Among high risk, community-dwelling older adults, a consistent reduction in rate of falls has been demonstrated from multifactorial interventions (6,7). A 2004 meta-analysis found a 40% reduction in fall rate with multifactorial intervention (8). Successful multifactorial intervention trials have utilized a targeted intervention approach, with specifics of the intervention based on the deficits identified in the falls evaluation. Typically, the intervention occurs over at least several months. Interventions have included physical therapy or group exercise, referrals for further medical care, decrease in psychotropic medications, behavior modification to decrease risky behavior, and modification of the environment (6,7,9,10).

Applying a multifactorial intervention to a general, non-high risk population of community-living older adults has resulted in lesser reduction in fall risk (9,10). A multifactorial strategy also may be less successful for older adults with cognitive impairment or dementia. A recent study found no reduction of falls in this patient group (11).

A multifactorial intervention approach may be more efficacious than a single intervention strategy. A recent study examined the efficacy of home hazard modification, vision improvement, or exercise as single interventions or combined as a multifactorial intervention. Neither home hazard modification nor vision improvement was efficacious as single interventions. Exercise as a single intervention was efficacious. However, the combined intervention of home hazard management, vision improvement, and exercise was almost twice as effective in reducing falls rates as exercise alone (12).

B. Single Interventions

1. Exercise

Exercise has shown efficacy as a single intervention to prevent falls. In older adults at high risk for falls, it is likely that to be effective, exercise needs to be individualized, progressive, of long duration (at least 10 weeks), and include balance exercises (1). A meta-analysis of exercise as an intervention has demonstrated that the type of exercise is important, with exercise incorporating balance training appearing to be the most efficacious (13). The Guideline for the Prevention of Falls in Older Persons has recommended that older adults with a history of falls receive long-term exercise and balance training (1).

The best method for delivery of exercise is unclear. Two positive randomized trials of exercise for high-risk older adults both utilized individualized, progressive home exercise programs delivered by a physical therapist or by a trained nurse (14,15). More recently, several studies have also shown benefit with group exercise. One study provided individualized high-intensity endurance, strength training, or both in a group setting (16). A second study found a 40% reduction in falls rate with weekly exercise classes designed to improve balance, co-ordination, aerobic capacity, and muscle strength (17). A third study of group exercise found a 22% reduction in falls (18). A fourth randomized trial of exercise in weekly classes supplemented by daily home exercise also showed a reduction in falls (12). It is unclear if individualized physical therapy and group exercise are equally efficacious in reducing falls. It is possible that the relative efficacy of individualized vs. group exercise may depend on the degree of risk of the target population, but this has not been well evaluated.

The efficacy of Tai Chi as an exercise intervention to reduce falls is unclear. An earlier study found a 47% reduction in risk of multiple falls for older adults receiving Tai Chi (19). A recent randomized trial examining Tai Chi in older adults with multiple fall risk factors found a 25% reduction in risk of falling, which was not significant (20). However, the study was not designed to detect a 25% reduction as significant. A recent meta-analysis showed an overall 14% reduction in risk of falling from exercise (8). It is likely that Tai Chi has modest benefit as a single intervention in reducing falls, but future studies with larger sample sizes or meta-analysis with existing studies will be required to provide definitive results. See Chapter 12 for further discussion of Tai Chi and other exercises.

2. Psychotropic Medication Withdrawal

A randomized, controlled trial evaluating the benefit of psychotropic medication withdrawal for older men and women on benzodiazepines, other hypnotics, antidepressants, or major tranquilizers demonstrated a marked reduction in falls with medication reduction. In the medication withdrawal group, after 44 weeks the relative hazard for falls was 0.34 compared with the group not reducing medication (21). Although many patients returned to the prior medication use after the study period, this study provides evidence that psychotropic medication reduction should be a key component of the falls intervention.

3. Vitamin D and Calcium Supplementation

Vitamin D deficiency is prevalent among frail older adults. Hypovitaminosis D was noted in 72% of patients attending a referral falls clinic (22). Vitamin D deficiency is characterized by muscle weakness, limb pain, and impaired physical function and has been associated with increased risk of falls (23). A randomized trial showed that vitamin D plus calcium decreased body sway and reduced falls (24). Another randomized trial evaluated the benefit of vitamin D 800 IU per day plus calcium 1200 mg per day for 12 weeks compared with calcium 1200 mg per day alone in decreasing falls among a population of older women with low vitamin D status (25-OH vitamin D level < 50 nmol/L). There was a 49% reduction in falls in the vitamin D plus calcium group, compared with the calcium alone group. This was associated with a significant improvement in musculoskeletal function (25).

In a meta-analysis of five randomized trials including 1237 participants, vitamin D therapy reduced the corrected odds ratio (OR) of falling by 22% (corrected OR = 0.78; 95% confidence ratio 0.64–0.02). The number needed to treat was 15 patients to prevent one patient from falling. The subgroup analyses suggested that the beneficial effect of vitamin D was independent of calcium supplementation, type of vitamin D used, duration of therapy, and sex of the participant (26).

4. Home Environment Modification and Home Safety Visits

In general, modification of the home environment is not beneficial as a single intervention. However, one randomized trial found a significant reduction in falls from one home safety visit for older adults after hospitalization. A single home visit by an occupational therapist after hospital discharge was associated with a 20% reduction in the risk of falls (27). A second study evaluated the benefit of a hospital-based comprehensive geriatric assessment followed by two home safety visits after hospital discharge, compared to the comprehensive assessment without home visits. The group that received the home safety visits in addition to the comprehensive assessment had 31% fewer falls than the group with no home visits (28). The Guideline for the Prevention of Falls in Older Persons recommends that an in-home safety assessment be considered for high-risk older adults who are recently discharged from the hospital (1).

Apart from the post-hospitalization period, home-safety intervention as a single intervention is not efficacious. Two randomized trials found no benefit from home environmental modification as a sole intervention (12,29). However, home environment modification is an important part of a multifactorial intervention. Day et al. (12) found that when home hazard modification was combined with exercise and vision improvement, it added to the efficacy of the latter two in reducing falls.

5. Vision Improvement

Visual factors associated with recurrent falls and hip fractures include poor visual acuity, visual acuity that differs between two eyes, reduced contrast sensitivity, decreased visual field, posterior subcapsular cataract, use of multifocal lenses, and non-miotic glaucoma medications (30–34). A prospective study of the rate of falls before and after cataract surgery found a significant reduction in falls 6 months postoperatively compared with 6 months prior to surgery (35). In a general population of older adults, however, recommendations and referrals for vision improvement were not effective in reducing falls as a single intervention. As noted previously, however, when vision improvement was added to an intervention of home hazard modification and exercise, the efficacy of the intervention was increased (12).

6. Pacemaker Placement for Select Patients

Some patients with recurrent, unexplained falls may have carotid sinus hypersensitivity as the etiology. A randomized trial evaluated the benefit of pacemaker placement for older adults with recurrent unexplained falls who had cardioinhibitory carotid sinus hypersensitivity on examination (36). Patients randomized to dual chamber pacemaker implant ($n = 87$) were significantly less likely to fall (OR $= 0.42$) in follow-up compared with usual care controls ($n = 88$). There were fewer syncopal episodes in the pacemaker group (28 vs. 47) as well as fewer injurious falls (61 vs. 202). It should be noted that cardioinhibitory carotid sinus syndrome was only infrequently seen as a cause of falls in this study. Of adults aged ≥ 50 years seen in the emergency room, only 13% had an unexplained fall. Of the group with unexplained falls who received carotid sinus massage for diagnosis, only 16% actually had cardioinhibitory or mixed carotid sinus hypersensitivity.

7. Hip Protector Pads

Early studies demonstrated a remarkable efficacy of hip protector pads in reducing hip fractures (37,38). Several recent studies, however, have found no significant benefit in intention-to-treat analysis (39,40). Post hoc analysis has suggested that the risk of hip fracture from a fall while wearing hip protectors is significantly decreased compared with a fall without a hip protector (RR $= 0.23$) (39). Negative findings in intention-to-treat analysis may be due to problems with compliance. A study in community-dwelling older adults found 53% compliance with use over the course of the study (39). A study in residential facilities found a compliance rate of 61% at 1 month, dropping to 45% at 6 months, and 37% at 1 year (40). Thus, although fractures may occur with hip protectors in place, these devices may play a role in fracture prevention, particularly in the long-term care setting where compliance may be easier to achieve.

C. Long-Term Care Setting Interventions

Data from randomized trials suggest that the approach to falls prevention is different for the long-term care setting. Although the individualized multifactorial intervention is efficacious in reducing falls in the community, it appears to be of no benefit in the long-term care setting. Rubenstein et al. (41) evaluated an individualized multifactorial intervention for nursing home residents with a recent fall. There was no significant reduction in falls in patients receiving the individualized intervention. Two studies have found no benefit from exercise as a single intervention to reduce falls in long-term care. One study evaluated the benefit of individually tailored physical therapy that included strength, endurance, and mobility exercises (42). A second study evaluated two different exercise groups (resistance/endurance or Tai Chi). There was no reduction in falls with either exercise group (43).

In contrast, an approach that provides a multifactorial intervention superimposed on staff and physician education has successfully decreased falls in nursing home and assisted living settings. In that study, an individualized multifactorial intervention was provided for high-risk patients. The intervention consisted of therapy to improve walking and transferring, psychotropic medication review, repair of wheelchairs, and environmental modifications. In addition to the individualized strategy, staff and physician education was provided. Facilities receiving the intervention showed a 19% reduction in the mean proportion of recurrent fallers, compared with control usual care facilities (44). A second randomized trial evaluated a multifaceted intervention consisting of staff and resident education on fall prevention, advice on environmental adaptation, progressive balance and resistance training, and hip protectors (45). The relative risk of falls was 0.55 in the intervention group compared with the control group. A cluster randomized trial of a multidisciplinary program that included both general and resident-specific, tailored strategies showed a risk ratio of 0.78 in the intervention facilities compared to control facilities (46). The strategies consisted of staff education, environmental modification, exercise programs, supply and repair of ambulation aids, medication review, hip protectors, post-fall problem-solving conferences, and staff consultation.

D. Hospital Setting Interventions

While there are few randomized trials evaluating falls prevention strategies among hospital inpatients, some data suggest that a multifactorial approach is likely to be efficacious (47,48). A recent randomized, controlled trial evaluated a targeted risk-factor reduction core care plan in reducing the risk of falls on intervention acute care wards compared with control wards receiving usual care. Introduction of the care plan resulted in a 21% reduction in relative risk of falls on intervention wards, significantly different from control wards (48). Other evaluations of multifaceted fall prevention programs using historical controls have also shown decreases in fall rates (49,50). Falls prevention programs have included staff education, identification of high-risk inpatients, increased toileting, medication review, and environmental modification.

Other controlled trials of interventions to prevent falls in the acute care setting have been negative (51–53). These trials evaluated bed alarms, use of risk identification bracelets, and a multifaceted nursing plan. However, these studies were small and potentially underpowered. At this time, data suggest that a multifaceted fall prevention program in acute care is likely to be successful. A recent randomized, controlled trial found a reduction in falls from a targeted multiple intervention program in the subacute care setting as well (54). The most effective components of a falls prevention strategy for the acute and post-acute care setting may vary depending on the inpatient population served; for example, neurologic, vs. medical, vs. psychiatric (55).

III. SPECIFIC COMPONENTS OF A MULTIFACTORIAL INTERVENTION

Table 1 lists specific interventions that have generally been included as part of a multifactorial intervention to reduce falls.

A. Medications

Medication adjustment based on the falls history is often the most effective and timely intervention the clinician can make, because falling is one of the most common adverse effects of drugs (56,57). Geriatric patients often accrue numerous and sometimes redundant medications as they visit various subspecialists. Furthermore, most medications have never been safety-tested in older patients, with or without the chronic renal and hepatic insufficiencies common in the geriatric patient. New or recent changes in prescriptions, additions of other medications that affect drug metabolism, and lack of adjustment for age, renal, and hepatic function should make one suspicious of a causal relationship between medications and falls.

Psychotropic medications are of particular concern because of their effect on the central nervous system. Neuroleptics, antidepressants (both tricyclic antidepressants and serotonin-reuptake inhibitors), and anticonvulsants have been linked with falls and fractures (58,59). Both short- and long-acting benzodiazepines and zolpidem have been associated with hip fracture in a dose-dependent manner (58,60). Cardiovascular medications such as digoxin, type I antiarrhythmics, and diuretics have also been associated with falls, although less strongly so than psychotropic medications (61).

Table 1 Eleven Interventions to Reduce Falls

1. Medication reduction or change
2. Vision improvement
3. Orthostatic hypotension treatment
4. Physical theraphy for exercise and balance and gait training
5. Chronic disease and pain management optimization
6. Better shoes and foot care
7. Vitamins D and B_{12} supplementation
8. Dementia and depression diagnosis and treatment
9. Assistive and protective devices
10. Home safety
11. Behavioral modifications

Although sedating antihistamines have not been strongly associated with falls in epidemiologic studies, they produce drowsiness and decrease attention. It is prudent to consider that sedating antihistamines may increase the risk of falls for individuals who are already at risk. Over-the-counter sleep aids often contain sedating antihistamines, most commonly diphenhydramine. Other antihistamines, such as scopolamine and second-generation antiallergy medications, can also cause drowsiness and dizziness. Ironically, meclizine, commonly used to treat vertigo, has ototoxicity as a serious adverse effect and commonly causes drowsiness due to its antihistaminic and anticholinergic properties. Thus, meclizine should be used with caution and only for a short duration.

As a "rule of thumb" any medication that has unsteadiness, incoordination, somnolence, dizziness, ataxia, blurred vision, confusion, disorientation, weakness, drowsiness, or fatigue as a side effect should be considered a risk factor for falls. A quick review of the patient's medications against the "adverse reaction" table for each drug will help the clinician select the drugs that may be contributing the most to gait or balance problems. Although a temporal relationship is helpful, the patient may have been on the offending drug for years before its side effects present in a fall, as the side effects may be exacerbated by infection, dehydration, the addition of another medication, concomitant alcohol use, or a change in renal or hepatic metabolism.

Medications that are requisite for patient health, such as an H_2 blocker for acid suppression in patients with peptic ulcer disease, can be replaced with an equally effective agent, such as a proton pump inhibitor, that carries less risk for central nervous system side effects. Regarding psychotropic medications, if the clinician can make even a minor reduction in the dose of such a medication, this may be all that is necessary to reduce or eliminate falls. It is important to remember that a drug may contribute to falls or balance problems even when the dosage falls within the usual adult dosage range or when the blood level is in the "normal range." An empiric trial of dosage reduction may be warranted to determine if there is a causal association with falls.

In the case of psychotropic medications, every attempt should be made to switch patients off of first generation tricyclic antidepressants (amitriptyline, imipramine, doxepin) to other agents with less sedation. Better alternatives exist for the indications of depression, neuropathic pain, and urinary incontinence. Alternatives may include the newer tricyclic antidepressants (nortriptyline or desipramine), serotonin-reuptake inhibitors, anticonvulsants for neuropathic pain, and oxybutinin or tolterodine for urinary incontinence. Dosages of any alternative agents should be kept to the lowest effective dose, as higher doses of these agents may contribute to falls due to anticholinergic properties and other side effects.

When initiating treatment with any psychotropic medication, in general, the dosage for older adults should be approximately half of the younger adult dosage. Patients with dementia may require even further dosage reduction. The risk of hip fracture increases as dose increases for multiple classes of psychotropic drugs, and for many psychotropic drug classes, risk has been elevated even at dosages considered moderate, rather than high (58,62).

Sleep agents, whether prescribed or over the counter, should be eliminated or at least reduced in the falling patient. Sleep strategies should be reviewed, with daytime naps and caffeinated beverages discouraged. Conservative, non-pharmacologic treatments should be tried, and a referral to sleep specialist is warranted if restless leg syndrome or sleep disordered breathing is suspected (63). Lastly, alcohol intake should be evaluated. Consumption of 14 or more drinks per week is associated with an increased risk of falls in prospective follow-up (64).

B. Vision Improvement

Visual factors associated with falls include poor visual acuity, reduced contrast sensitivity, decreased visual fields, cataracts, and the use of glaucoma medication (30–33). Iatrogenic visual impairment resulting from bifocal and other multifocal lens prescriptions might also contribute to balance problems and falls, especially when older patients with those lenses have to negotiate curbs or stairs (34). Single vision lenses for walking are preferred. In particular, older adults who wear multifocal lenses and have had a history of tripping falls, or falls associated with changes in depth, should be strongly encouraged to switch to single vision lenses.

Cataracts are a common cause of visual impairment in elderly patients. Fuzzy vision, halos around car lights at night, or merely a gradual decline in vision is a complaint that suggests cataracts. If a patient with falls or balance problems has vision that is affected by cataracts, corrective surgery is indicated. If only one eye is affected, corrective surgery should still ensue, as this could help with depth perception. In a pre–post-study design, cataract surgery was effective in decreasing the rate of falls (35).

C. Orthostatic Hypotension and Hypovolemia

Orthostatic hypotension can result from insufficient oral hydration, over-diuresis, as a medication side effect, or from autonomic dysregulation. Hypovolemia frequently results from poor fluid intake combined with increased urine output. The heavy use of caffeinated beverages can promote hypovolemia through diuresis while giving the patient a false sense of hydration. Diuretics prescribed for hypertension, congestive heart failure, and peripheral edema constitutes a potential iatrogenic cause of hypovolemia leading to falls. Treatment of orthostatic hypotension has been a component of most multifactorial intervention studies and is recommended as part of a multifactorial approach to falls (1,3,8).

Thus, if hypovolemia is considered to be a potential contributor to the risk of falls for an individual patient, it is desirable to reduce diuretics if possible, including caffeine. Nocturia and urgency, which may contribute to falls, may also decline with diuretic reduction. Water prescription, with electrolytes provided through a diluted sports rehydration beverage, if not contraindicated, may also improve orthostatic hypotension and hypovolemia and should promote renal and hepatic perfusion for better drug metabolism.

When hypovolemia is adequately treated, wrist and ankle pumps can enhance venous return and counter orthostatic blood pressure drops. These should be done while sitting at the edge of the bed or prior to rising from a chair. Compression stockings may be of benefit as well. For those with persistent orthostatic hypotension, especially with evidence of autonomic dysfunction or mineralocorticoid deficiency, treatment with midodrine or fludrocortisone, respectively, should be considered.

D. Exercise and Balance Training

Exercise is effective in preventing falls in both high- and low-risk older adults. Although the optimal type of exercise program for falls prevention is unknown, the Guidelines for Prevention of Falls in Older Persons recommends that older adults with recurrent falls be offered long-term exercise and balance training (1). Current studies suggest that balance training, as prescribed by a physical therapist, may be an important component.

The individualized course of physical therapy ideally should be of several months duration and should be followed by a long-term exercise program that incorporates exercises to maintain or improve balance. These may include group-based programs such as Tai Chi or other supervised exercise classes, supplemented by daily home exercises. To improve or maintain balance, exercises should be done in the standing position and should include weight shifts and head turns.

Although walking is beneficial in many regards, there is no evidence that it effectively reduces the risk of falls among high-risk older adults. In fact, a large randomized trial of brisk walking for women with previous upper limb fractures showed a significantly increased risk of falls in the brisk walking group compared with that in the control upper extremity exercise group (65). Walking should not be discouraged, but older adults should be instructed to pay attention to foot placement and to move slowly in certain environments, in particular, when on unfamiliar ground or in dim lighting. A cane or a walking stick may provide added stability.

E. Disease and Pain Management

Approximately 10% of falls is due to acute causes (4). Any acute or chronic medical condition that causes weakness or a significant decline in neurologic or cardiovascular function can contribute to falls. Infections such as pneumonia or urosepsis often present as falls in older patients.

Parkinson's disease, stroke, brain tumors, multiple sclerosis, lumbar or cervical spinal stenosis, amyotropic lateral sclerosis, progressive supranuclear palsy, and subdural hematoma can present as falls or increase the risk of falls of the patient. Along with optimal medical treatment, such patients need a multifaceted assessment and targeted interventions to reduce other factors contributing to balance problems and falls.

Muscle weakness has been associated with falls in numerous epidemiologic studies. The most common cause of muscle weakness in older adults is disuse. Proximal muscle weakness that makes rising from the chair especially difficult should suggest polymyalgia rheumatica, vitamin D deficiency, or statin-associated myopathy as possible causes.

Dementia and depression are associated with falls. Consideration should be given to potentially reversible causes of dementia, including normal pressure hydrocephalus, hypothyroidism, and vitamin B_{12} deficiency. Cholinesterase inhibitors or the NMDA receptor antagonist, memantine, may be considered to treat patients with dementia who fall. It is unknown, however, if treatment of dementia will decrease the risk of falls. Depression should be treated if present, as associated symptoms of decreased concentration and psychomotor impairment may contribute to the risk of falls. No particular antidepressant has been shown to be safest for older adults who have fall risk factors. Lower doses of selective serotonin-reuptake inhibitors are generally well tolerated in the elderly, but higher doses have been associated with hip fractures, similar to tricyclic antidepressants (59).

Cardiovascular dysfunction should be considered in patients falling with little or no warning. This can occur with or without palpitations. Patients may have amnesia for loss of consciousness; thus, in an unwitnessed fall, denial of syncope does not rule it out (66). Atrial fibrillation with rapid ventricular response and other conduction abnormalities causing abnormally rapid or slow heart rates are often underlying conditions. Treatment with a pacemaker for those selected patients with carotid sinus syndrome, as noted previously, can be of profound benefit to some patients.

Electrolyte abnormalities should be considered if the history and physical assessment do not suggest a clear cause for falls. Hyponatremia from diuretic use and elevated calcium levels from hyperparathyroidism or malignancy should be suspected in patients with other signs or symptoms of these diseases. Hypo- or hyperglycemia may also be a cause of falls.

Pain producing an antalgic gait should be treated aggressively. Underlying arthritic and anatomic problem should be referred to orthopedic, rheumatologic, or podiatric specialists for definitive care. Providing medications for chronic pain on a scheduled rather than "as needed" basis may provide greater efficacy and a constant level of pain control. Narcotics and neuroleptic medications used for pain should only be part of a complete regimen including such topical treatments as ice and capsaicin cream, along with physical therapy for stretching and strengthening. Narcotics and neuroleptics should be used cautiously, and in the lowest effective dose, because their use has been associated with falls and fractures (67).

F. Shoes and Foot Care

Poor footwear is an easily correctable risk factor for falls. Indoor and outdoor footwear should be examined as part of the comprehensive assessment of the falls patient. Particular attention should be paid to the fit, stability, arch support, thickness of sole and heel, and propensity for grabbing when the patient moves from rug to linoleum, for example. While indoors, patients should not walk barefoot or wear only stockings or socks. Functional reach and timed mobility tests have been improved when women wear walking shoes, compared with going barefoot (68). Foot position awareness and balance improve with use of firm, thin-soled shoes and low, rather than high, heels (69,70).

Patients who fall need to wear tie or Velcro shoes indoors with thin, smooth soles and good arch support, even at night during toileting activity. Outdoor walking shoes need enhanced traction but still should have thin soles and low heels as possible, along with good arch support. Foot and ankle deformities and leg-length discrepancies need to be corrected or accommodated with special footwear or orthotic devices. See Chapter 19 for further discussion.

G. Vitamin D, Calcium, and Vitamin B$_{12}$

As noted previously, vitamin D supplementation has been shown to reduce falls (24–26), and the combination of vitamin D (800 IU daily) and calcium (1200–1500 mg daily) supplementation is the cornerstone of osteoporosis prevention and treatment. Vitamin D (25-OH) level > 30 ng/mL should be the target. Ergocalciferol 50,000 IU tablets should be used for rapid treatment for values < 20 ng/mL, and sunlight exposure, even indirect or through windows, should be encouraged. Vitamin D levels need to be rechecked after treatment, as absorption is unpredictable. Daily supplementation with 800 IU vitamin D is recommended for older adults.

Vitamin B$_{12}$ deficiency should be considered if cognitive impairment or loss of proprioception or vibration is present. Vitamin B$_{12}$ levels should exceed 400 ng/mL in patients with falls, balance issues, or generalized weakness. Intramuscular injection of 1000 μg given at monthly intervals, or more often if necessary, may be used for replacement. High-dose oral supplementation of 1000–2000 μg daily may also be effective.

H. Assistive and Protective Devices

Assistive devices for support during walking may be of benefit. The selection of the best device should be made by a physical therapist. The wrong device, such as a providing wheeled walker when a standard walker would be more appropriate, can actually promote trips and falls. Canes and walking sticks provide proprioceptive input, as well as providing minimal support, and should be encouraged in diabetic patients and others with sensory losses, including peripheral neuropathies, vestibular impairment, or visual impairment. Physical therapy should measure and train the patient for proper use with all assistive devices. The individual should be assessed for outdoor and indoor mobility needs, as a different assistive device may be required for outdoor use.

   Hip protectors have been shown in some studies to reduce hip fractures and reduce fear of falling (37,38) and should be considered for patients at significant risk for falls or with prior hip fracture. They may be particularly helpful for patients in the long-term care setting.

I. Home Safety

This intervention, when provided to patients returning home from acute hospitalization, constitutes an effective single intervention to significantly reduce falls (27). Patients with a history of multiple falls in the home should have a home safety evaluation as part of a multifactorial falls intervention. Whenever possible, the evaluation should be provided by a trained occupational or physical therapist. Family members and care providers are instrumental in identifying problems and instituting changes.

   Lighting should be increased in bedrooms, halls, and bathrooms, and night-time safety can be enhanced with nightlights and lighted switches. Clutter and throw rugs should be removed to produce wide, clear walkways through the house. All stairs, even those with only one or two steps, need sturdy rails, and patients must be instructed to consistently use them. Marking step edges with brightly colored tape may improve stair safety for patients who have problems with depth perception. Raised toilet seats, grab rails and bars around the toilet and tub, and shower or tub benches may improve bathroom safety for patients with lower extremity muscle weakness or balance impairment due to central nervous system dysfunction or proprioceptive loss.

J. Behavioral Modification

As a single intervention to reduce falls, behavioral modification is not effective (71–74). However, it is an essential part of a multifactorial intervention. Patients should be informed of their specific fall risk factors and the particular types of maneuvers or activities that increase risk. In addition, patients

Table 2 Behavioral Interventions and Home Adaptations for Specific Deficits Related to Falls

Deficit	Behavioral intervention	Home adaptation
Vision <20/40 either eye	Extra caution in dark and outdoors Use cane or other assistive device	Good lighting Remove clutter, throw rugs, cords
Vision differs between 2 eyes	Caution on stairs, ramps, curbs, inclines, rough outdoor surfaces Consider cane or other assistive device for stairs, ramps, curbs, inclines, outdoors	Railings for stairs Bright-colored tape on step edges
Loss of vision or decreased vision in 1 or more quadrants of visual field	Caution with maneuvers, turns Caution regarding obstacles in that area of vision Turn head to compensate	Clear walking path in home
Proprioceptive loss	Educate patient regarding increased need for visual cues to maintain balance Avoid carrying things that could obstruct vision Extra caution in dark, in shower with eyes closed Extra caution on uneven surfaces Consider cane or assistive device Keep wide stance	Maximize lighting, decrease glare Railings on both sides of stairs Mark edges of steps with contrasting tape
Vestibular dysfunction	Consider cane or assistive device Extra caution in dark Extra caution with head turns	Maximize lighting Move kitchen, bedroom, and commonly -used closet items to shoulder level Remote clutter
Cognitive impairment, psychotropic medication use, evidence of gait slowing with cognitive task, or history of falls with divided attention	Instruct patient in paying attention to walking Avoid carrying objects while turning or walking Caution with talking while walking – stop to have conversations Avoid rushing to answer phone or door	

should be informed of the need for increased attention to mobility tasks. Recent data suggests that balance-impaired older adults may have more impairment in postural control in situations where their attention is divided. In one study, balance-impaired older adults had difficulty maintaining balance in response to a perturbation while simultaneously performing a cognitive task (75). Most fallers can identify attention factors that were involved in the falls (such as rushing, carrying objects, not paying attention, etc.). Table 2 identifies specific behavioral modifications and home adaptations appropriate for specific fall risk factors.

IV. CONCLUSION

All patients should be asked about falls, balance, and gait problems at their routine or periodic visits, and those with a history of recurrent falls or one fall with gait and balance problems should have a multifactorial assessment. Interventions targeting multiple risk areas for a given patient, such as medication adjustments, vision improvements, exercise and balance training, and footwear correction, constitute the best clinical practice to prevent falls.

REFERENCES

1. American Geriatrics Society, British Geriatrics Society, and American Academy of Orthopaedic Surgeons Panel on Falls Prevention. Guideline for the prevention of falls in older persons. J Am Geriatr Soc 2001; 49:179–187.
2. Preventive Services Task Force. Guide to Clinical Preventive Services: Report of the U.S. Preventive Services Task Force. 2nd ed. Baltimore: Williams and Wilkins, 1996:659–685.
3. Tinetti ME. Preventing falls in elderly persons. N Engl J Med 2003; 48:42–49.
4. Tinetti ME, Speechley M, Ginter SF. Risk factors for falls among elderly persons living in the community. N Engl J Med 1988; 319:1701–1707.
5. Robbins AS, Rubenstein LZ, Josephson KR, Schulman BL, Osterweil D. Predictors of falls among elderly people. Results of two population-based studies. Arch Intern Med 1989; 149:1628–1633.
6. Close J, Ellis M, Hooper R, Glucksman E, Jackson S, Swift C. Prevention of falls in the elderly trial (PROFET): a randomized controlled trial. Lancet 1999; 353:93–97.
7. Tinetti ME, Baker DI, McAvay G, Claus EB, Garrett P, Gottschalk M, Koch ML, Trainor K, Horwitz RI. A multifactorial intervention to reduce the risk of falling among elderly people living in the community. N Engl J Med 1994; 331:821–827.
8. Chang JT, Morton SC, Rubenstein LZ, Mojica WA, Maglione M, Suttorp MJ, et al. Interventions for the prevention of falls in older adults: systematic review and meta-analysis of randomized clinical trials. Br Med J 2004; 328:680–687.
9. Hornbrook MC, Stevens VJ, Wingfield DJ, Hollis JF, Greenlick MR, Ory MG. Preventing falls among community-dwelling older persons: results from a randomized trial. Gerontologist 1994; 34:16–23.

10. Wagner EH, LaCroix AZ, Grothaus L, Leveille SG, Hecht JA, Artz K, Odle K, Buchner DM. Preventing disability and falls in older adults: a population-based randomized trial. Am J Public Health 1994; 84:1800–1806.
11. Shaw FE, Bond J, Richardson DA, Dawson P, Steen IN, McKeith IG, Kenny RA. Multifactorial intervention after a fall in older people with cognitive impairment and dementia presenting to the accident and emergency department: randomized controlled trial. Br Med J 2003; 326:73–75.
12. Day L, Fildes B, Gordon I, Fitzharris M, Flamer H, Lord S. Randomised factorial trial of falls prevention among older people living in their own homes. Br Med J 2002; 325:128–132.
13. Province MA, Hadley EC, Honrbrook MC, Lipsitz LA, Miller JP, Mulrow CD, Ory MG, Sattin RW, Tinetti ME, Wolf SL. The effects of exercise on falls in elderly patients: a preplanned meta-analysis of the FICSIT trials. J Am Med Assoc 1995; 273:1341–1347.
14. Campbell AJ, Roberson MC, Gardner MM, Norton RN, Tilyard MW, Buchner DM. Randomised controlled trial of a general practice programme of home-based exercise to prevent falls in elderly women. Br Med J 1997; 315:1065–1069.
15. Robertson MC, Devlin N, Gardner MM, Campbell AJ. Effectiveness and economic evaluation of a nurse delivered home exercise programme to prevent falls. 1: randomised controlled trial. Br Med J 2001; 322:697–701.
16. Buchner DM, Cress ME, de Lateur BJ, Esselman PC, Margherita AJ, Price R, Wagner EH. The effect of strength and endurance training on gait, balance, fall risk, and health services use in community-living older adults. J Gerontol Med Sci 1997; 52:M218–M224.
17. Barnett A, Smith B, Lord SR, Williams M, Baumand A. Community-based group exercise improves balance and reduces falls in at-risk older people: a randomized controlled trial. Age Ageing 2003; 32:407–414.
18. Lord SR, Castell S, Corcoran J, Dayhew J, Matters B, Shan A, Williams P. The effect of group exercise on physical functioning and falls in frail older people living in retirement villages: a randomized, controlled trial. J Am Geriatr Soc 2003; 51:1685–1692.
19. Wolf SL, Barnhart HX, Kutner NG, McNeely E, Coogler C, Xu T, the Atlanta FICSIT Group. Reducing frailty and falls in older persons: an investigation of Tai Chi and computerized balance training. J Am Geriatr Soc 1996; 44:489–497.
20. Wolf SL, Sattin RW, Kutner M, O'Grady M, Greenspan AI, Gregor RJ. Intense Tai Chi exercise training and fall occurrences in older, transitionally frail adults: a randomized, controlled trial. J Am Geriatr Soc 2003; 51:1693–1701.
21. Campbell AJ, Robertson MC, Gardner MM, Norton RN, Buchner DM. Psychotropic medication withdrawal and a home-based exercise program to prevent falls: a randomized, controlled trial. J Am Geriatr Soc 1999; 47:850–853.
22. Dhesi JK, Moniz C, Close JCT, Jackson SHD, Allain TJ. A rationale for vitamin D prescribing in a falls clinic population. Age Ageing 2002; 31:267–271.

23. Stein MS, Wark JD, Scherer SC, Walton SL, Chick P, Di Carlantonio M, Zajac JD, Flicker L. Falls relate to vitamin D and parathyroid hormone in an Australian nursing home and hostel. J Am Geriatr Soc 1999; 47:1195–1201.

24. Bischoff HA, Stahelin HB, Dick W, Akos R, Knecht M, Salis C, Nebiker M, Thelier R, Pfeifer M, Begerow B, Lew RA, Conzelmann M. Effects of vitamin D and calcium supplementation of falls: a randomized controlled trial. J Bone Miner Res 2003; 18:343–351.

25. Pfeifer M, Begerow B, Minne HW, Abrams C, Nachtigall D, Hansen C. Effects of a short-term vitamin D and calcium supplementation on body sway and secondary hyperparathyroidism in elderly women. J Bone Miner Res 2000; 15:1113.

26. Bischoff-Ferrari HA, Dawson-Hughes B, Willett WC, Staehelin HB, Bazemore MG, Zee RY, Wong JB. Effect of vitamim D on falls: a meta-analysis. J Am Med Assoc 2004; 291:1999–2006.

27. Cumming RG, Thomas M, Gzonyi G, Salkeld G, O'Neill E, Westbury C, Frampton G. Home visits by an occupational therapist for assessment and modification of environmental hazards: a randomized trial of falls prevention. J Am Geriatr Soc 1999; 47:1397–1402.

28. Nikolaus T, Bach M. Preventing falls in community-dwelling frail older people using a home intervention team (HIT): results from the randomized falls-HIT trial. J Am Geriatr Soc 2003; 51:300–305.

29. Stevens M, Holman CDJ, Bennett N, deKlerk N. Preventing falls in older people: outcome evaluation of a randomized controlled trial. J Am Geriatr Soc 2001; 49:1448–1455.

30. Glynn RJ, Seddon JM, Krug JH, Sahagian CR, Chiavelli ME, Campion EW. Falls in elderly patients with glaucoma. Arch Ophthalmol 1991; 109:205–210.

31. Ivers RQ, Cumming RG, Mitchell P, Simpson JM, Peduto AJ. Visual risk factors for hip fracture in older people. J Am Geriatr Soc 2003; 51:356–363.

32. Lord SR, Dayhew J. Visual risk factors for falls in older people. J Am Geriatr Soc 2001; 49:508–515.

33. Felson DT, Anderson JJ, Hannan MT, Milton RC, Wilson PW, Kiel DP. Impaired vision and hip fracture, the Framingham study. J Am Geriatr Soc 1989; 37:495–500.

34. Lord SR, Dayhew J, Howland A. Multifocal glasses impair edge-contrast sensitivity and depth perception and increase the risk of falls in older people. J Am Geriatr Soc 2002; 50:1760–1766.

35. Brannan S, Dewar C, Sen J, Clarke D, Marshall T, Murray PI. A prospective study of the rate of falls before and after cataract surgery. Br J Opthalmol 2003; 87:560–563.

36. Kenny RA, Richardson DA, Steen N, Bexton RS, Shaw FE, Bond J. Carotid sinus syndrome: a modifiable risk factor for nonaccidental falls in older adults (SAFE PACE). J Am Coll Cardiol 2001; 38:1491.

37. Kannus P, Parkkari J, Niemi S, Pasanen M, Palvanen M, Jarvinen M, Vuori I. Prevention of hip fracture in elderly people with use of a hip protector. N Engl J Med 2000; 343:1506.

38. Parker MJ, Gillespie LD, Gillespie WJ. Hip protectors for preventing hip fractures in the elderly (Cochrane Review). Cochrane Database Syst Rev 2004; 2:CD001255.

39. Cameron ID, Cumming RG, Kurrle SE, Quine S, Lockwood K, Salkeld G, Finnegan T. A randomized trial of hip protector use by frail older women living in their own homes. Inj Prev 2003; 9:138–141.

40. Van Schoor NM, Smit JH, Twisk JWR, Bouter LM, Lips P. Prevention of hip fractures by external hip protectors: a randomized controlled trial. J Am Med Assoc 2003; 289:1957–1962.

41. Rubenstein LZ, Robbins AS, Josephson KR, Schulman BL, Osterweil D. The value of assessing falls in an elderly population: a randomized clinical trial. Ann Intern Med 1990; 113:308–316.

42. Ray WA, Taylor JA, Meador KG, Thapa PB, Brown AK, Kajihara HK, Davis C, Gideon P, Griffin MR. A randomized trial of a consultation service to reduce falls in nursing homes. J Am Med Assoc 1997; 278:557–562.

43. Becker C, Kron M, Lindemann U, Sturm E, Eichner B, Walter-Jung B, Nikolaus T. Effectiveness of a multifaceted intervention on falls in nursing home residents. J Am Geriatr Soc 2003; 51:306–313.

44. Jensen J, Lundin-Olsson L, Nyberg L, Gustafson Y. Fall and injury prevention in older people living in residential care facilities: a cluster randomized trial. Ann Intern Med 2002; 136:733–741.

45. Mulrow CD, Gerety MB, Kanten D, Cornell JE, De Nino LA, Chiodo L, Aguilar C, O'Neil MB, Rosenberg J, Solis RM. A randomized trial of physical rehabilitation for very frail nursing home residents. J Am Med Assoc 1994; 271: 519–524.

46. Nowalk MP, Prendergast JM, Bayles CM, D'Amico FJ, Colvin GC. A randomized trial of exercise programs among older individuals living in two long-term care facilities: the Falls FREE Program. J Am Geriatr Soc 2001; 49: 859–865.

47. Oliver D, Hopper A, Seed P. Do hospital fall prevention programs work? A systematic review. J Am Geriatr Soc 2000; 48:1679–1689.

48. Healey F, Monro A, Cockram A, Adams V, Heseltine D. Using targeted risk factor reduction to prevent falls in older in-patients: a randomized controlled trial. Age Ageing 2004; 33:390–395.

49. Barker SM, O'Brien CN, Carey D, Weisman GK. Quality improvement in action: a falls prevention and management program. Mt Sinai J Med 1993; 60: 387–390.

50. Mitchell A, Jones N. Striving to prevent falls in an acute care setting action to enhance quality. J Clin Nurse 1996; 5:213–220.

51. Mayo NE, Gloutney L, Levy AR. A randomised trial of identification bracelets to prevent falls among patients in a rehabilitation hospital. Arch Phys Med Rehabil 1994; 75:1302–1308.

52. Tideiksaar R, Feiner CF, Maby J. Falls prevention: the efficacy of a bed alarm system in an acute care setting. Mt Sinai J Med 1993; 60:522–527.

53. Fife D, Solomon P. A risk falls programme: code orange for success. Nurs Manage 1984; 15:50–53.

54. Haines TP, Bennell KL, Osborne RH, Hill KD. Effectiveness of targeted falls prevention program in subacute hospital setting: randomized controlled trial. Br Med J 2004; 328:676–682.

55. Mahoney JE. Immobility and falls. Clin Geriatr Med 1998; 14:699–726.

56. Field TS, Gurwitz JH, Avorn J, McCormick D, Jain S, Eckler M, Benser M, Bates DW. Risk factors for adverse drug events among nursing home residents. Arch Intern Med 2001; 161:1629–1634.

57. Hanlon JT, Schmader KB, Koronkowski MJ, Weinberger M, Landsman PB, Samsa GP, Lewis IK. Adverse drug events in high risk older outpatients. J Am Geriatr Soc 1997; 45:945–948.

58. Leipzig RM, Cumming RG, Tinetti ME. Drugs and falls in older people: a systematic review and meta-analysis. I. Psychotropic drugs. J Am Geriatr Soc 1999; 47:30–39.

59. Thapa PB, Gideon P, Cost TW, Milam AB, Ray WA. Antidepressants and the risk of falls among nursing home residents. N Engl J Med 1998; 339:875–882.

60. Glynn RJ, Wang PS, Bohn RL, Mogun H, Avorn J. Zolpidem use and hip fractures in older people. J Am Geriatr Soc 2001; 49:1685–1690.

61. Leipzig RM, Cumming RG, Tinetti ME. Drugs and falls in older people: a systematic review and meta-analysis. II. Cardiac and analgesic drugs. J Am Geriatr Soc 1999; 47:40–50.

62. Ray WA, Griffin MR, Schaffner W, Baugh DK, Melton LJ. Psychotropic drug use and the risk of hip fracture. N Engl J Med 1987; 316:363–369.

63. McDowell JA, Mion LC, Lydon TJ, Inoue SK. A nonpharmacologic sleep protocol for hospitalized older patients. J Am Geriatr Soc 1998; 46:700–705.

64. Mukamal KJ, Mittleman MA, Longstreth WT, Newman AB, Fried LP, Siscovick DS. Self-reported alcohol consumption and falls in older adults: cross-sectional and longitudinal analyses of the Cardiovascular Health Study. J Am Geriatr Soc 2004; 52:1174–1179.

65. Ebrahim S, Thompson PW, Baskaran V, Evans K. Randomized placebo-controlled trial of brisk walking in the prevention of postmenopausal osteoporosis. Age Ageing 1997; 26:253–260.

66. Kenny RA, Traynor G. Carotid sinus syndrome—clinical characteristics in elderly patients. Age Ageing 1991; 20:449–454.

67. Kelly KD, Pickett W, Yiannakoulias N, Rowe BH, Schopflocher DP, Svenson L, Voaklander DC. Medication use and falls in community-dwelling older persons. Age Ageing 2003; 32:503–509.

68. Arnadottir SA, Mercer VS. Effects of footwear on measurements of balance and gait in women between the ages of 65 and 93 years. Phys Ther 2000; 80:17–27.

69. Lord SR, Bashford GM. Shoe characteristics and balance in older women. J Am Geriatr Soc 1996; 44:429–433.

70. Robbins S, Waked E, Allard P, McClaran J, Krouglicof N. Foot position awareness in younger and older men: the influence of footwear sole properties. J Am Geriatr Soc 1997; 45:61–66.

71. Fabacher D, Josephson K, Pietruszka F, Linderborn K, Morley JE, Rubenstein LZ. An in-home preventive assessment program for independent older adults: a randomized controlled trial. J Am Geriatr Soc 1994; 42:630–638.

72. Carpenter GI, Demopoulos GR. Screening the elderly in the community: controlled trial of dependency surveillance using a questionnaire administered by volunteers. Br Med J 1990; 300:1253–1256.
73. Gallagher EM, Brunt H. Head over heels: impact of a health promotion program to reduce falls in the elderly. Can J Aging 1996; 15:84–96.
74. Vetter NJ, Lewis PA, Ford D. Can health visitors prevent fractures in elderly people? Br Med J 1992; 304:888–890.
75. Brauer SG, Woollacott M, Shumway-Cook A. The interacting effects of cognitive demand and recovery on postural stability in balance-impaired elderly persons. J Gerontol Med Sci 2001; 56A:M489–M496.

11

Fear of Falling

Sharon L. Tennstedt

New England Research Institutes, Watertown, Massachusetts, U.S.A.

I. INTRODUCTION

Falls are common among older adults and recognized as a serious health concern (see also Chapters 9 and 10). However, newly emerging as a health concern is the phenomenon of fear of falling. This fear can be a sequela of a fall (1–3, 9, 16) or independent of a history of falls. Falls can result in negative psychological outcomes and a loss of confidence in physical ability that was earlier referred to as "post-fall syndrome" (1) and now termed "fear of falling" (4,5). Fear of falling may also lead to a "cautious" gait that in turn produces its own negative sequelae. Persons with greater fear of falling tend to perform poorly on balance and lower extremity functional mobility tasks (6). As such, when considering the factors that contribute to gait and mobility changes, it is important to consider fear of falling.

Fear of falling is highly prevalent. Several studies (3,7–11) indicate that from 30% to 50% of independently living older adults are afraid of falling. In one of these studies (11), this fear ranked first when compared to the fear of being robbed in the street, forgetting an important appointment, losing a cherished item, or experiencing financial difficulties. The results of focus groups conducted to explore the etiology of fear of falling among the elderly suggested that many older adults do not discuss their fear of falling, or fall experiences, with support group members (family, friends, and health-care providers) because they perceive the falls as sentinel events in precipitating nursing home admissions (12).

II. CONSEQUENCES OF FEAR OF FALLING

It is now well recognized that fear of falling has a broad range of negative consequences for the health and well-being of older adults. It might be argued that a little fear is a good thing; for example, when a frail older person avoids activities beyond physical capability because of fear of falling. However, there is substantial evidence that fear of falling results in restriction of both physical and social activities that individuals are capable of performing (4,11,13–16). While this activity restriction often follows a fall (16), it also occurs independently of a history of falls.

Activity restriction is a concern with its own health consequences. Older persons often restrict their type or level of activity under the mistaken assumption that it will reduce their risk of falling. However, when fear of falling restricts activity to the point of causing physical deconditioning and associated muscle weakness (17), risk of falling has been found to increase (18). Similarly, fear of falling has been associated with decreased postural performance (19) and balance (6,10), also potential contributors to falls. Thus, fear of falling that restricts physical and social activity beyond a reasonable extent may increase rather than decrease falls risk.

The temporal relationship between fear of falling and falls was investigated by Friedman et al. (16) in a population-based, prospective study. While fear of falling increased after a fall as might be expected, they reported that fear of falling also increased the incidence of falls. Both falls and fear of falling shared predictors, resulting in a spiraling risk of falls, fear of falling and functional decline.

Fear of falling has been related to daily function in community-dwelling elderly (8). The degree of confidence in performing common daily activities without falling was related to the ability to carry out basic and instrumental activities of daily living as well as to higher order physical and social functioning. That is, persons who were afraid of falling or lacked confidence to perform activities without falling functioned at a lower level and were less active.

Results of longitudinal studies (16,20) are consistent with these findings. Older adults who reported greater fear of falling had an increased risk of falling and greater decline in ability to perform activities of daily living. In addition, nonfallers who said they were afraid of falling had an increased risk of nursing home admission.

There have been no investigations of the effect of fear of falling on one's mental health status. However, it is reasonable to assume that the negative effects on psychological well-being of a restricted social environment would hold true for those who have fear-related activity restrictions. Results of cross-sectional studies (9,10) support this conclusion.

III. FACTORS ASSOCIATED WITH FEAR OF FALLING

Little is known about the natural history of fear of falling (21). Growing evidence suggests that fear of falling has multiple causes (11,14,19) as has been reported for the etiology of falls (2,3,15). However, in most studies, the factors associated with falling and those related to fear of falling differ (11), reinforcing the need to understand and assess fear of falling as a distinct phenomenon. In one longitudinal study, risk factors for developing fear of falling included a history of multiple falls, dizziness, and poor self-rated health (22). While increasing age has been related to higher levels of fear of falling (7,16,22,23), another study (15) reported that among older adults expressing concerns about falling, this fear was more prevalent among the younger-old than among the older-old. This might be explained by efforts to reduce fear of falling through voluntary restrictions on mobility and physical activities. This study also reported more fear of falling among those with greater physical dysfunction, a lower sense of ability to manage a fall, and a sense of generalized fearfulness. The latter finding suggests that fear of falling, to some extent, might be a manifestation of a more generalized anxiety. However, the association with physical dysfunction and lower sense of ability to manage a fall remained significant even when controlling for generalized fearfulness.

IV. ASSESSMENT OF FEAR OF FALLING

With increasing recognition of fear of falling, attention has been directed to its assessment. Most of this work has been done in the research rather than clinical arena. The most straightforward approach has been to ask if an individual is afraid of falling (7,11,12,19). However, anecdotal evidence suggests that the term might be intimidating, especially to males. Use of the words "concerned" or "worried" has been found to increase likelihood of admission. A single question about fear of falling has the advantage of being straightforward and simple and lending itself easily to generating prevalence estimates. However, such direct measures have been questioned (8,24) because reports about global states, such as fear of falling, are often poor predictors of actual behavior and functioning. Tinetti et al. (24) have developed a measure that assesses fear of falling based on the impact that fear has on a sense of one's ability to perform routine activities without falling (self-efficacy). Their definition of fear of falling is based on Bandura's (25) theory of self-efficacy that posits that a person's beliefs about his/her capabilities affects how they behave in specific situations. This measure, the Falls Efficacy Scale, rates an individual's confidence to perform various activities of daily living without falling. The scale has been used in many studies and has been adapted for specific study populations. A similar measure, the Activities-Specific Balance Confidence (ABC) Scale (26), assesses the confidence that one can engage in a broader range of activities of daily living, including more difficult ones and ones that are performed outside the home than are included in the Falls Efficacy Scale. These measures ask persons to rate their confidence on a 10-point or 100-point scale.

Because fear of falling often results in activity restrictions, Lachman et al. (27) developed an instrument to assess the role of fear of falling in activity restriction. The survey of activities and fear of falling in the elderly (SAFE) consists of 11 activities, including activities of daily living (e.g., taking a tub bath, preparing simple meals), activities outside the home (e.g., going to a doctor or dentist, going to a place with crowds), and social activities (e.g., visiting a friend or relative). It gathers information about participation in each activity as well as the extent to which fear of falling is a source of activity restriction. One advantage of this measure is the potential for differentiating fear of falling that leads to activity restriction from fear of falling that accompanies activity restrictions. Subsequent validation testing by Li et al. (6) showed that the two-class (low fear and high fear) fear of falling profiles discriminated fallers from nonfallers. Their work supports the use of variation in response patterns to the SAFE instrument to identify individuals with differing levels of fear of falling for intervention.

Although developed for research purposes, these measures can also be used in clinical settings. Or, as proposed by Lach (21), clinicians can take a history of fear of falling, focusing on five key concepts:

- Presence of fear or concern about falling,
- Confidence in mobility and balance,
- Tasks and activities that generate concern,
- Excessive restriction of activities because of fear of falling,
- Concern about physical ability to navigate the environment, and
- Concerns about what would happen in case there is a fall.

A complete medical and physical assessment is indicated for the individual with fear of falling, including an assessment of mobility and balance. Formal testing options include the Tinetti (28) performance-oriented mobility assessment, the Berg Balance Test (29), or the "get up and go" tests (30,31) (see Chapter 2). Additional attention should also be paid to sensory impairments, medications, and other factors that often contribute to mobility and balance disorders and to falls risk (see Chapters 8 and 9).

V. INTERVENTIONS FOR FEAR OF FALLING

Intervention studies to reduce falls and falls risk were the first to report any treatment effect on fear of falling. Of the many fall prevention trials, including the FICSIT trials (32–45), only four included fear of falling among the outcomes of interest (34,40,41,43). Results of these studies were mixed. Both a multifactorial intervention to reduce risk of falling among community-dwelling elders (41) and a Tai Chi exercise intervention (42) found significant reductions in fear of falling in intervention subjects compared to control subjects. Two other fall-reduction interventions reported no change or increased fear of falling in intervention subjects (34,40).

A randomized trial of an intervention designed to reduce fear of falling and associated restrictions in activity levels among community-residing older adults (46) was conducted by the author and colleagues through the Boston University Roybal Center for the Enhancement of Late-Life Function. The intervention program (*A Matter of Balance*) consisted of eight group sessions designed to reduce fear of falling by increasing self-efficacy and the sense of control over falling. To accomplish this, the intervention was based on the principles of cognitive-behavioral therapy aiming to: (a) restructure misconceptions to promote a view of falls risk and fear of falls as controllable; (b) set realistic goals for increasing activity; (c) change the environment to reduce falls risk; and (d) promote physical exercise to increase strength and balance. The primary aim of the intervention was to reduce fear of falling. The secondary aim was to increase physical, social, and functional activity. At 12 months after the intervention, subjects in the intervention group reported decreased fear of falling and a greater perceived ability to manage a fall if it occurred when compared to the contact control subjects (Table 1). The results of the trial also showed enhanced activity, mobility, and social function (Sickness Impact Profile, SIP) at 12 months. Stronger and more extensive intervention effects were observed in participants who attended the majority (i.e., at least five) of the eight sessions. The intervention program was most beneficial for those persons who perceived that they could do something about the problem, had more concerns about falling, and whose participation was not hindered by disability (47). An important finding was that fear of falling increased over time in the control group not receiving the intervention. These findings support efficacy of this intervention, and the data support the hypothesis that physical and social activities can be enhanced by reducing fear of falling.

The findings from this study identified individuals who might derive more benefit from a different type of intervention. Participants who were more disabled, less active, and had lower self-efficacy about changing their falls concerns or risk reported less benefit from the intervention. Participants with these same characteristics were more likely to drop out of the trial. Interestingly, persons with greater fear of falling and restricted activity often declined enrollment in the trial, because it necessitated their leaving their apartment to attend the group sessions. The intervention was conducted in senior housing sites to facilitate participation by persons who, because of their fear of falling, might have restricted outside mobility. However, this

Table 1 Results of Intervention Trials to Reduce Fear of Falling: *A Matter of Balance* and *After a Fall*

	A Matter of Balance			After a Fall	
	12-Month follow-up			6-Month follow-up	
	Control	Intended	Compliant[a]	Control	Intended
	$N = 176$	$N = 170$	$N = 118$	$N = 113$	$N = 106$
Falls efficacy	−0.12	−0.04	0.09*	6.68	4.36
Falls management	0.02	0.15	0.26*	1.81	1.80
Control fear of falling	0.03	0.07	0.20	1.39	1.98
Intended activity	−0.07	−0.04	−0.02	2.35	1.55
SIP: total score	2.92	1.50	−0.43**	−4.30	−4.83

*$p < 0.01$.
**$p < 0.05$.
[a]Attended ≥5 sessions.

empirical and other anecdotal evidence indicates that proximal location of the intervention was not sufficient for inclusion of this more vulnerable population. The evidence suggested that perhaps an individually focused intervention provided in the home might be needed for a more vulnerable population.

Based on these findings, we conducted a second randomized clinical trial (*After a Fall*) targeted to a potentially more vulnerable population. Participants ($n = 259$) were recruited from the population of older patients who were admitted to emergency rooms for a fall-related injury. The intervention, consisting of three sessions conducted on a 1:1 basis, was delivered in the home to address the barrier to participation of limited outside mobility. The content of this intervention was also cognitive-behavioral and was based on the successful elements of the previous group intervention that could be conducted on a 1:1 basis in a home setting. Participants in the control group received limited printed materials about reducing falls risk.

The majority (66%) of study participants had no history of falls (prior to this event), but over half reported being somewhat or very afraid of falling. Similar to the participants in the group intervention, greater fear of falling was associated with a higher number of prior falls, more physical disability, and lower self-efficacy in terms of ability to manage a fall or do something to reduce fear of falling. However, unlike the group program, this intervention had no significant effect on reducing fear of falling or increasing activity levels (Table 1). In fact, reductions in fear of falling and/or increases in activity levels over the 6-month follow-up period in the control group sometimes exceeded changes in the intervention group.

There are a number of potential explanations for the lack of group differences, including the difference in study population and the difference in mode of administration.

While it was assumed that a fall-related injury might result in increased fear of falling, the sample included a large number of older adults for whom this fall was their first and not necessarily an indicator of heightened risk or vulnerability. An example is the man in his mid-60s who fell off a ladder while painting his house. For such participants, it would be reasonable to expect resolution in fear of falling and restricted activity level over time without the intervention. Whereas for the group intervention, an older adult had to report fear of falling and restricted activity level to be eligible for inclusion, this trial had no such inclusion criteria. This allowed persons with minimal or no fear of falling to enroll in the study.

While the change in mode of administration was informed by experience in the prior trial, the treatment exposure in this intervention was lower and less intense. In contrast to 8 two-hour group sessions, this intervention consisted of three sessions, each session of 60–90 min duration. Because the intervention was delivered on an individual basis, it also eliminated the group dynamics and the potential for mutual support inherent in the first intervention. This is a potentially critical difference in the two interventions. It is quite possible that the environment of a group with shared concerns (fear of falling) facilitated recognition of, and support to deal with, individual problems that was absent in the 1:1 sessions. The sharing with peers both of initial concerns and subsequent solutions may have been more effective than interactions with a professional interventionist. While the lack of treatment effects in this second intervention was discouraging, the experience yielded valuable information about the importance of specifying the content and mode of administration of an intervention to the needs of the targeted population as well as the importance of appropriately targeting a population for a specific intervention. This is particularly critical when considering a more resource intensive 1:1 intervention over a group intervention.

While falls reduction interventions have included balance and mobility as outcomes, the fear of falling interventions have not done so. In the two interventions described above, the outcomes were fear of falling and accompanying activity restriction. Neither of the interventions was designed to reduce falls or falls risk directly. While limited strength training exercises were included in most of the group sessions, there was no specific attempt to improve balance or gait. The results of the intervention studies by Tinetti et al. (41) and Wolf et al. (42) suggest that reduction in both falls/falls risk and fear of falling can be addressed in the same intervention. Such a combined intervention focus would likely include efforts to improve balance and gait, allowing the influence of such improvements on fear of falling and restricted activity to be investigated.

More recently, a randomized intervention trial (48) was conducted to determine and compare the relative effects of an exercise activity program and an education program on fear of falling, balance, strength, and general health status. Eight weekly group sessions were delivered to 17 older adults age in each intervention arm. The activity program consisted of low-resistance exercises and weight-shifting exercises. The education program focused on identifying and reducing risk factors for falls. At 6 weeks post-intervention, both groups showed a reduction in fear of falling ($p < 0.05$). The fact that the activity program, lacking the communication and social support in the education program, had a positive effect on fear of falling argues against the possibility that the results were due only to social contact or attention. However, the fact that both types of interventions were effective in reducing fear of falling provides support for a multifactorial intervention approach.

There is now general agreement that multifactorial interventions are the most effective in reducing falls, risk of falls, and fear of falling (see also Chapter 10). The Evidence-Based Guideline for Falls Prevention developed by the American Geriatrics Society, the British Geriatrics Society, and the American Academy of Orthopedic Surgeons (49) recommends that multifactorial interventions for community-residing older adults include gait training and advice on use of assistive devices; exercise programs with balance training; review and modification of medication; treatment of postural hypotension and cardiovascular disorders; and modification of environmental hazards. Multifactorial interventions for long-term care and assisted-living settings should also include staff education programs. Evidence to support fear of falling interventions lies outside the parameters of this guideline. However, inclusion of cognitive-behavioral techniques to address fear of falling (46,50) is consistent with a multifactorial approach to intervening on the related phenomena of falls and fear of falling.

VI. COMMUNICATION ABOUT THE PROBLEM

Falls and fear of falling are often referred to as dangerous secrets. Older persons view a fall as a sentinel event that signals functional decline and loss of independence. Psychologically, it is difficult to disclose information that may threaten one's independence. As discussed by Dugan and Bonds (51), effective communication between patient and health-care provider is critical to good medical care. Yet many factors impede good communication, including personal, relationship, and organizational issues. The time constraints and the problem-focused nature of most heath care visits do not provide opportunities for an older person to raise concerns about falling, particularly in the absence of a history of falls. Providers, in turn, are trained to address patient complaints, and given the time limits of the visit are less inclined to inquire about potential problems not identified by the patient. Problems with communication about fear of falling extend to family members as well. An older adult may be reluctant to reveal information that implies weakness or can be perceived as impending frailty, concerned that family members might over-react and place undesired, and likely inappropriate, limits on their independence. In turn, family members might not want to hear about an older relative's concerns about falling because it is perceived as loss in role and function.

Intervention with all concerned is indicated. Providers should be educated regarding the prevalence of fear of falling and its untoward consequences. Screening for fear of falling can be incorporated into the screening for risk of falls recommended by the binational panel (49). Awareness of interventions available in the community will facilitate referral. Family members should strive to open lines of communication about fear of falling, as well as other sensitive health topics, and to support older relatives in their efforts to maintain independence while controlling risk of falls. Older adults must learn that falls and fear of falling are not an inevitable part of growing older, and that proactive steps can be taken to reduce risk of falls without losing independence or curtailing physical and social activities. This realization will go a long way toward reducing their fear of falling and avoiding excess disability.

REFERENCES

1. Murphy J, Isaacs B. The post-fall syndrome. A study of 36 elderly patients. Gerontology 1982; 28:265–270.
2. Nevitt MC, Cummings SR, Kidd S, Black D. Risk factors for falls among elderly persons living in the community. N Engl J Med 1989; 319:1701–1706.
3. Tinetti ME, Speechley M, Ginter SF. Risk factors for falls among elderly persons living in the community. N Engl J Med 1988; 319:1701–1707.
4. Vellas B, Cayla F, Bocquet H, de Pemille F, Albarede JL. Prospective study of restriction of activity in old people after falls. Age Ageing 1987; 16:189–193.
5. Tinetti ME, Speechley M. Prevention of falls among the elderly. N Engl J Med 1989; 320:1055–1059.
6. Li F, Fisher KJ, Harmer P, McAuley E, Wilson NL. Fear of falling in elderly persons: association with falls, functional ability, and quality of life. J Gerontol B Psychol Sci 2003; 58B(5):P283–P290.
7. Arfken CL, Lach HW, Birge SJ, Miller JP. The prevalence and correlates of fear of falling in elderly persons living in the community. Am J Public Health 1994; 84:565–570.
8. Tinetti ME, Mendes de Leon CF, Doucette JT, Baker DI. Fear of falling and fall-related efficacy in relationship to functioning among community-living elders. J Gerontol 1994; 49:M140–M147.
9. Murphy SL, Williams CS, Gill TM. Characteristics associated with fear of falling and activity restriction in community-living older persons. J Am Geriatr Soc 2002; 50:516–520.

10. Kressig RW, Wolf SL, Sattin RW, O'Grady M, Greenspan A, Curns A, Kutner M. Associations of demographic, functional, and behavioral characteristics with activity-related fear of falling among older adults transitioning to frailty. J Am Geriatr Soc 2001; 49:1456–1462.
11. Howland J, Peterson EW, Levin WC, Fried L, Pordon D, Bak S. Fear of falling among the community-dwelling elderly. J Aging Health 1993; 5:229–243.
12. Walker JE, Howland J. Falls and fear of falling among elderly persons living in the community: occupational therapy interventions. Am J Occup Ther 1991; 45:119–122.
13. The prevention of falls in later life. A report of the Kellogg International Work Group on the prevention of falls by the elderly. Dan Med Bull 1987; 34(suppl 4): 1–24.
14. Nevitt MC, Cummings SR, Hudes ES. Risk factors for injurious falls: a prospective study. J Gerontol 1991; 46:M164–M170.
15. Lawrence RH, Tennstedt SL, Kasten LE, Shih J, Howland J, Jette AM. Intensity and correlates of fear of falling and hurting oneself in the next year: baseline findings from a Roybal Center fear of falling intervention. J Aging Health 1998; 10:267–286.
16. Friedman SM, Munoz B, West SK, Rubin GS, Fried LP. Falls and fear of falling: which comes first? A longitudinal prediction model suggests strategies for primary and secondary prevention. J Am Geriatr Soc 2002; 50:1329–1335.
17. Hindmarsh JJ, Estes EH Jr. Falls in older persons. Causes and interventions. Arch Intern Med 1989; 149:2217–2222.
18. Campbell AJ, Borrie MJ, Spears GF. Risk factors for falls in a community-based prospective study of people 70 years and older. J Gerontol 1989; 44: M112–M117.
19. Maki BE, Holliday PJ, Topper AK. Fear of falling and postural performance in the elderly. J Gerontol 1991; 46:M123–M131.
20. Cumming RG, Salkeld G, Thomas M, Szonyi G. Prospective study of the impact of fear of falling on activities of daily living, SF-36 scores, and nursing home admission. J Gerontol A Biol Sci Med Sci 2000; 55(5):M299–M305.
21. Lach HW. Fear of falling: an emerging public health problem. Generations 2002–2003; 26(Winter):33–37.
22. Lach HW. Incidence and risk factors for developing fear of falling. Public Health Nursing 2005; 22(1):45–52.
23. Murphy SL, Dubin JA, Gill TM. The development of fear of falling among community-living older women: predisposing factors and subsequent falls events. J Gerontol A Med Sci 2003; 58A(10):943–947.
24. Tinetti ME, Richman D, Powell L. Falls efficacy as a measure of fear of falling. J Gerontol 1990; 45:239–243.
25. Bandura A. Self-efficacy: the exercise of control. New York: W. H. Freeman, 1997.
26. Powell LE, Myers AM. The Activities-Specific Balance Confidence (ABC) Scale. J Gerontol A Biol Sci Med Sci 1995; 50A:M28–M34.
27. Lachman ME, Howland J, Tennstedt S, Jette A, Assmann S, Peterson EW. Fear of falling and activity restriction: the survey of activities and fear of falling in the elderly (SAFE). J Gerontol B Psychol Sci Soc Sci 1998; 53:43–50.

28. Tinetti ME. Performance-oriented assessment of mobility problems in elderly patients. J Am Geriatr Soc 1986; 34:119–126.
29. Berg K, et al. Measuring balance in the elderly: preliminary development of an instrument. Physiother Can 1998; 41:304–311.
30. Rose DJ, Jones CJ, Lucchese N. Predicting the probability of falls in community-residing older adults using the 8-foot up-and-go: a new measure of functional mobility. J Aging Phys Act 2002; 10:466–475.
31. Shumway-Cook A, Brauer S, Woollacott M. Predicting the probability for falls in community-dwelling older adults using the timed up & go test. Phys Ther 2000; 80:896–903.
32. Buchner DM, Cress ME, Wagner EH, de Lateur BJ, Price R, Abrass IB. The Seattle FICSIT/Move It Study: the effect of exercise on gait and balance in older adults. J Am Geriatr Soc 1993; 41:321–325.
33. Fiatarone MA, O'Neill EF, Ryan ND, Clements KM, Solares GR, Nelson ME, Roberts SB, Kehayias JJ, Lipsitz LA, Evans WJ. Exercise training and nutritional supplementation for physical frailty in very elderly people. N Engl J Med 1994; 330:1769–1775.
34. Hornbrook MC, Stevens VJ, Wingfield DJ. Seniors' program for injury control and education. J Am Geriatr Soc 1993; 41:309–314.
35. Hornbrook MC, Stevens VJ, Wingfield DJ, Hollis JF, Greenlick MR, Ory MG. Preventing falls among community-dwelling older persons: results from a randomized trial. Gerontologist 1994; 34:16–23.
36. Lord SR, Ward JA, Williams P, Strudwick M. The effect of a 12-month exercise trial on balance, strength, and falls in older women: a randomized controlled trial. J Am Geriatr Soc 1995; 43:1198–1206.
37. Mulrow CD, Gerety MB, Kanten D, Cornell JE, DeNino LA, Chiodo L, Aguilar C, O'Neil MB, Rosenberg J, Solis RM. A randomized trial of physical rehabilitation for very frail nursing home residents. J Am Med Assoc 1994; 271:519–524.
38. Obonyo T, Drummond M, Isaacs B. Domiciliary physiotherapy for old people who have fallen. Int Rehabil Med 1983; 5:157–160.
39. Province MA, Hadley EC, Hornbrook MC, Lipsitz LA, Miller JP, Mulrow CD, Ory MG, Sattin RW, Tinetti ME, Wolf SL. The effects of exercise on falls in elderly patients. A preplanned meta-analysis of the FICSIT Trials. Frailty and Injuries: Cooperative Studies of Intervention Techniques. J Am Med Assoc 1995; 273:1341–1347.
40. Reinsch S, MacRae P, Lachenbruch PA, Tobis JS. Attempts to prevent falls and injury: a prospective community study. Gerontologist 1992; 32:450–456.
41. Tinetti ME, Baker DI, McAvay G, Claus E, Garrett P, Gottschalk M, Koch M, Tramork K, Horowitz R. A multifactorial intervention to reduce the risk of falling among elderly people living in the community. N Engl J Med 1994; 331:821–827.
42. Wolf SL, Barnhart HX, Kutner NG, McNeely E, Coogler C, Xu T. Reducing frailty and falls in older persons: an investigation of Tai Chi and computerized balance training. Atlanta FICSIT Group. Frailty and Injuries: Cooperative Studies of Intervention Techniques. J Am Geriatr Soc 1996; 44:489–497.

43. Wolf-Klein GP, Silverstone FA, Basavaraju N, Foley CJ, Pascaru A, Ma PH. Prevention of falls in the elderly population. Arch Phys Med Rehabil 1988; 69:689–691.

44. Wolfson L, Whipple R, Judge J, Amerman P, Derby C, King M. Training balance and strength in the elderly to improve function. J Am Geriatr Soc 1993; 41:341–343.

45. Alkalay L, Alcalay J, Sherry C. Reducing falls among the elderly in a small community. Practitioner 1984; 228:698.

46. Tennstedt S, Howland J, Lachman M, Peterson E, Kasten L, Jette A. A randomized, controlled trial of a group intervention to reduce fear of falling and associated activity restriction in older adults. J Gerontol B Psychol Sci Soc Sci 1998; 53:384–392.

47. Tennstedt SL, Lawrence RH, Kasten L. An intervention to reduce fear of falling and enhance activity: who is most likely to benefit? Educ Gerontol 2001; 27:227–240.

48. Brouwer BJ, Walker C, Rydahl SJ, Culham, EG. Reducing fear of falling in seniors through education and activity programs: a randomized trial. J Am Geriatr Soc 2003; 51:829–834.

49. Guideline for the prevention of falls in older persons. American Geriatrics Society, British Geriatrics Society, and American Academy of Orthopaedic Surgeons Panel on Falls Prevention. J Am Geriatr Soc 2001; 49:664–672.

50. Peterson EW. Using cognitive behavioral strategies to reduce fear of falling: a matter of balance. Generations 2002–2003; 26(Winter):53–59.

51. Dugan E, Bonds D. Explaining the lack of communication about falls and the fear of falling. Generations 2002–2003; 26(Winter):48–52.

12

Therapeutic Exercise to Improve Balance and Gait and Prevent Falls

Tanya A. Miszko

Department of Physical Education and Sports Studies, The University of Georgia, Prescriptive Health, Inc., Snellville, Georgia, and Veterans Affairs Medical Center, Decatur, Georgia, U.S.A.

Steven L. Wolf

Departments of Rehabilitation Medicine, Medicine (Division of Geriatrics), and Cell Biology, Emory University School of Medicine, and Nell Hodgson Woodruff School of Nursing, Emory University, Atlanta, Georgia, U.S.A.

I. INTRODUCTION

Gait and balance are so intricately inter-related that being able to distinguish the independent contributions of each to the performance of daily tasks is difficult. Even the simple task of walking demonstrates a most fundamental form of dynamic balance movement. Integrating the multiple components that interface balance and gait, ambulation (gait) without falling is dependent on the successful shift of bodyweight between single- and double-limb support phases, while successfully moving the body orward (dynamic balance). Completion of most daily activities often demands a minimum effort at independent ambulation. Because this effort requires balance, both balance and gait can be considered important for most aspects of independent living.

The aging process includes physiological changes that predispose an individual to balance and gait difficulties. Documented deficits in the neurological, vestibular, visual, and musculoskeletal systems are critical to postural control (1,2). These control parameters, in turn, are highly related to performance in gait (3). Such physiological changes are manifest in reduced gait velocity, decreased stride length, increased stride width, and reduced single stance time (4–6). Slowed gait velocity is significantly related to fall risk (7,8), which impacts an older adult's independence.

Changes in balance and gait can negatively affect an older adult's activity level, thus adversely influencing functional level while promoting morbidity. Balance and gait abnormalities, such as poor postural control and gait instability, are associated with fear of falling and falls (9,10), which can also restrict an older adult's activities. Declines in muscle strength, flexibility, or the presence of neurological changes are other important factors that foster a reduced activity level in older adults. The resulting diminution in physical activity potentially increases the risk for heart disease, osteoporosis, obesity, hypertension, and diabetes and reduces independence (11). If an exercise intervention is applied; however, balance and gait abnormalities may be overcome or improved, physical activity increased, and functional decline and morbidity attenuated.

Equivocal evidence suggests that regular participation in exercise may improve balance (i.e., postural sway, single-limb support) and certain parameters of gait (i.e., gait velocity, step length, step frequency). Studies emphasizing strength, endurance, or balance training, as well as flexibility have independently, and in combination, examined the effects on balance and gait. Because poor gait and balance are associated with increased risk for falls, a reduction in fall rate and risk is ultimately the goal of exercise programs designed to improve gait and balance, and consequently improving physical function and independence. Against this background, the purpose of this chapter is to review the extent to which flexibility, strength, endurance, and balance components of exercise programs impact balance and gait among older adults and secondarily to ascertain if there are components that preferentially contribute to improvements in balance and gait for a select primary diagnosis. While we recognize the importance of factors other than balance and gait required for independent living (see, for example, Chapters 4–6), they are beyond the scope of this chapter.

II. FACTORS ASSOCIATED WITH ABNORMAL BALANCE AND GAIT

A. Muscular Strength and Power

Age-associated neuromuscular changes influence gait and balance performance. Both leg extension power and muscle strength are reduced with age (12,13); leg extension power being more sensitive to aging than strength in adults over the age of 65 years (3.5%/year vs. 1%/year) (13). Leg extension power, strength, and gait velocity are significantly related (14,15), such that the effects of aging are evident in a slowed gait speed and reduced swing phase (16). Riley et al. (5) suggest that gait velocity is reduced due to a shorter stride length, which may be due to loss in maximal hip extension power. Consequently, slower gait velocity may increase postural instability and the risk for falls (8).

B. Biomechanics and Falls Risk

Gait and balance abnormalities in older adults are typically associated with increased risk of falling and fear of falling (9,10). In a two-year prospective study, older adults who reported being fearful of falling at baseline experienced a greater increase in balance, gait, and cognitive disorders over time than those not fearful of falling at baseline (10). Reductions in peak hip extension, increased anterior pelvic tilt, and reduced ankle plantar flexion range of motion and power are physiological abnormalities relating gait and balance deficits to increased risk of falls (1). Consequently, older adults who fall tend to walk slower, have a shorter stride length, wider base of support, and spend more time in double support stance during gait (17). However, faster gait speed, longer step length relative to body height, and more rapid steps have also been associated with increased risk for falls after a trip (18). These conflicting statements would suggest that a range of safe walking speeds exist for which an older adult is not at increased risk for falls.

III. EXERCISE PROGRAMS TO IMPROVE BALANCE

Several exercise interventions have been designed and tested for their efficacy to improve balance (Table 1). Interventions have ranged from home-based exercise programs to more traditional, supervised programs (i.e., resistance and endurance training) and recently, to alternative interventions, such as Tai Chi. While a majority of the research indicates positive improvements in balance, results from some studies have yielded conflicting findings.

A. Endurance Training

Endurance-training programs have primarily involved weight-bearing activities (walking, running, aerobic dance) and require maintained postural control. The effect of such programs on improving balance is promising. Sedentary older adults (65–85 years old) with mild balance impairments who participated in a walking, cycling, or aerobic exercise program (3 days/week for 12 weeks; 35–40 min/day at 50–75% heart rate reserve) significantly improved the distance walked on a narrow (8.5 cm) 6-m balance beam, but no change was observed in any static balance measure (20). A dose–response improvement in balance was evident for the three types of endurance training; cycling elicited a 3% improvement, walking elicited a 7% improvement, and aerobic exercise elicited an 18% improvement. Thus

Table 1 Summary of Exercise Programs to Improve Balance

Author (reference)	Year	Intervention	Sample	Age	Physiological outcomes	Performance outcomes
Endurance training						
Brown and Holloszy (19)	1993	3 days/week for 12 weeks; low intensity ST and flexibility progressing to 12-month END (brisk walking, cycling, jogging; 30–50 min/day at 60–85% HRmax)	Men and women	60–72	Increased knee extension and flexion torque after the initial 12 weeks, then no additional increase after the END training program; reduced time to peak knee extension torque and total work performed significantly improved after the END training program; reduced forward trunk bending range of motion after END training	Increased single-limb stance time with eyes closed and open after the initial 12-week program and further improved after the END training program
Buchner et al. (20)	1997	3 days/week for 12 weeks with 6-month follow-up; walking, cycling, or aerobic exercise; 35–40 min/day at 50–75% HRreserve	Physically unfit, sedentary men and women	68–85	Walking increased VO_{2max} by 18%, aerobics increased VO_{2max} by 10%, cycling increased VO_{2max} by 8%; lower body isokinetic strength increased in all groups	Increase speed walked on narrow balance beam; increased distance walked on narrow balance beam; no change in static balance

Resistance training

Reference	Year	Age	Population	Protocol	Aim	Outcome
Vanderhoek et al. (21)	2000	Mean =67	Women with low bone mineral density	3 days/week for 32 weeks; lower extremity ST program (3×8–10 repetitions at 80% 1RM)	Increase dynamic muscular strength (41–96%); no change in isokinetic knee extension/flexion strength	Improved tandem stance time
Carter et al. (22)	2002	65–75	Women with osteoporosis	2 days/week for 20 weeks; community-based ST	Increase knee extension strength	Reduced time to walk figure eight course
Yates and Dunnagan (23)	2001			3 days/week for 10 weeks; home-based ST program (19 chair exercises with 5-lb adjustable weights) as part of multidimensional fall prevention program	Increased lower extremity power	Improved balance using the Tinetti balance assessment; reduced fear of falling; no change in Timed Up and Go score
Topp et al. (24)	1993	>65	Community-dwelling men and women	3 days/week for 12 weeks; home-based ST program (2–3×10 repetitions) using elastic tubing	Increased isokinetic eccentric knee flexor and extensor strength	No change in eyes-closed static or dynamic balance (backwards toe to heel walking on a narrow line)

Multidimensional training

Reference	Year	Age	Population	Protocol	Aim	Outcome
Hauer et al. (25)	2001	75–90	Women with a	3 days/week for 12 weeks; ST (2×10	Increase lower extremity dynamic muscular	Increased functional reach and static

(Continued)

Table 1 Summary of Exercise Programs to Improve Balance (*Continued*)

Author (reference)	Year	Intervention	Sample	Age	Physiological outcomes	Performance outcomes
		repetitions at 70–90% 1RM), balance training (45 min/day, dance, functional exercises, Tai Chi)	history of injurious falls		strength	balance; 25% reduction in secondary falls (not statistically significant) and fear of falling; reduced use of assistive devices; improved motor performance (walking, standing up, and stepping)
Judge et al. (26)	1993	24 weeks; flexibility training (incorporating Tai Chi movements) or combined strength, endurance, and balance training	Older women	62–75	Increased knee extension 1RM in exercise group	Improved single-limb stance (17%) in combined group (not statistically significant); no change in double-limb support for either group
Campbell et al. (27)	1997	3 days/week for 24 weeks; home-based ST and balance training; 1-year fall follow-up	Community-dwelling older women	>80		Improved chair stand, tandem stance, semitandem stance, single-leg stance, functional reach in exercise group; reduced rate of falls/year; no change in IADL scale

Study	Year	Subjects	Age	Protocol		Results
Messier et al. (28)	2000	Men and women with knee osteoarthritis	Mean = 60	3 days/week for 18 months (3 months supervised and 15 months at home); ST (2 × 10–12 repetitions using ankle weights and dumbbells) and walking (40 min/day at 50–85% HRreserve) program		Decreased center of pressure sway velocity; increased single-leg stance time
Tai Chi						
Wolfson et al. (29)	1996	Community-dwelling older adults	>75	3 days/week for 12 weeks; 45 min/session; balance, strength, or balance+ST (1×13 repetitions at 75% 1RM) followed by a 26-week Tai Chi maintenance phase	Improved peak joint moments in strength and balance+strength groups; improvements in strength were maintained only in the ST group after Tai Chi maintenance	Improved functional base of support in the balance group; reduced loss of balance in balance+strength and strength groups; improved single-limb stance in all groups, but only maintained in balance+ST group after Tai Chi
Hartman et al. (30)	2000	Older adults with osteoarthritis	49–81	2 days/week for 12 weeks; 60 min/session		No change in single-limb stance

ST, strength training; END, endurance training; HRmax, heart rate max; HRreserve, heart rate reserve.

an endurance-training program that includes challenging balance tasks may improve dynamic balance.

B. Resistance Training

More traditional facility-based resistance-training programs have also demonstrated benefits on balance. Older women (mean age $= 67 \pm 1.3$ years) with low bone density who participated in a thrice-weekly strengthening program for 32 weeks significantly improved static balance measures (36–54%) as well as dynamic muscular strength (mean increase of 57%) (21). Older women (65–75 years old) with osteoporosis participating in a community-based strength program (2 days/week for 20 weeks) significantly improved dynamic balance (7.7% increase in time to walk a figure eight course) and knee extension strength (3.2%), which are both significant predictors of fall risk (22).

C. Multidimensional Training

Similar to the results from one-dimensional exercise programs, multidimensional exercise programs incorporating strength, endurance, and/or balance components demonstrate consistent benefits to balance. After 12 weeks of strength (3 days/week; 2 sets of 10 repetitions at 70–90% maximal strength) and balance training (3 days/week; 45 min/day; Tai Chi, dance, and functional exercises), older adults (mean age $= 82 \pm 4.8$ years) with a history of injurious falls significantly improved lower extremity muscle strength (23–40%) and balance as measured by functional reach (23%) and a series of static balance postures (10%) (25). This program also produced a 25% reduction in secondary falls; however, due to a small group size, this finding was not significant. This randomized-controlled trial supports the efficacy of a multidimensional exercise-training program to improve measures of balance.

Home-based exercise programs, typically multidimensional in scope, have proven effective for improving balance in individuals with and without chronic conditions. Campbell et al. (27) found significant improvements in measures of balance (chair stand, tandem stance, semitandem stance, single-leg stance, and functional reach) after six months of a home-based strengthening and balance exercise program in community-dwelling, ambulatory women over the age of 80 years. Postmenopausal women (mean age $= 71.6 \pm 7.3$ years) diagnosed with osteoporosis and a vertebral fracture significantly improved their quality of life, center of pressure sway velocity, and center of pressure range of displacement during a static balance test after participating in a 12-month home-based exercise program (31). Similarly, older adults (> 60 years of age) with knee osteoarthritis improved postural stability by reducing center of pressure sway velocity (6%) after an 18-month walking and strengthening program (28). Yates and Dunnagan (23) incorporated an at-home strength-training program into their multifaceted fall prevention program (fall risk education, nutritional counseling, and environmental hazards education). After 10 weeks, independent, community-dwelling older adults over the age of 65 years demonstrated a significant improvement in balance, fear of falling, and lower extremity power, but no change in mobility. Contrary to these results, Topp et al. (24) found no significant effect of a home-based strength-training program (3 days/week for 12 weeks; 2 to 3 sets of 10 repetitions with elastic tubing) on the ability of community-dwelling older adults over the age of 65 years to improve static or dynamic balance (8.5 sec increase) greater than the no-exercise control group. Although results from some of these studies are conflicting, in general, they suggest that even "low-tech," home-based exercise programs may improve balance.

Few research studies have directly compared the effects of different training programs on balance to determine which is more efficacious. The Seattle FICSIT (Frailty and Injuries: Cooperative Studies of Intervention Techniques) study directly compared the effects of strength training, endurance training, and endurance + strength training on gait and balance measures, as well as other outcomes, in a group of older adults with mild deficits in strength and balance (32). Participants in the FICSIT study were between the ages of 68 and 85 years old, unable to do an eight-step tandem gait without errors, and knee extensor strength less than the 50th percentile for their height and weight. Interestingly, after six months of exercise, there was no significant change in any gait (33% reduction to 0% improvement) or balance measure (20% reduction to 3% improvement) for any intervention group, yet there was a significant reduction in time to first fall for the three exercise groups combined (relative hazard = 0.53). Improvements in lower body strength (13–40%) were observed for both the strength- and strength and endurance-training groups, but not the endurance-training group. This would suggest that strengthening exercises to overcome muscle weakness, not necessarily endurance training alone, contribute to reductions in fall rates, but changes are not necessarily manifest in the performance measures of gait and balance used in this study. When comparing six months of flexibility training to combined strength, endurance, and balance training, Judge et al. (26) found a significant improvement in single-limb support (18%) after the combined training program, but not the flexibility training group; however, this difference was not statistically significant. The less challenging, double-limb support measure remained unchanged after the intervention in the community-dwelling older women. A 10-month self-paced resistance-training program proved to be more efficacious than a self-paced walking endurance program and a no-exercise control for improving strength (+65% vs. –6% and –7%, respectively) and single-limb support (+9% vs. –23% and –39%, respectively) in somewhat active, community-dwelling older men and women (33). Both exercise groups improved their tandem stance time and stair climb ability from baseline, but they were not statistically different from each other. This evidence suggests that although each separate intervention has merit, the additive effects of the combined training are more efficacious.

D. Tai Chi

An alternative form of exercise, Tai Chi, an ancient Chinese exercise, has demonstrated promise as an intervention to improve balance in older adults. Healthy, independent older adults significantly improved single stance time after three months of balance training and balance + strength training (27% and 64%, respectively), yet this improvement was sustained through the addition of Tai Chi only in the balance + strength-training group (29). Thus, the Tai Chi maintenance program complimented the balance + strength-training program. Contrary to the results of others, a group of older adults diagnosed with lower extremity osteoarthritis did not improve balance (single-leg stance time; 10%) after twice-weekly Tai Chi classes for 12 weeks (30). Possibly the intensity of the Tai Chi classes was not sufficient to induce an improvement in balance in this population. Tai Chi's effect on balance may also help explain its effect on reduced fall rates. Recent evidence from our group supports this notion since older fallers with multiple comorbidities were able to significantly improve chair stand performance and the time necessary to bend down to pick up objects compared to non-exercise control participants (34). Both these tasks require strength and balance. There is some discrepancy regarding the actual changes that occur in control parameters. While specific studies examining kinetic and kinematic parameters are underway (35) [see Ref. 52 study cited later], we found that more robust older adults respond to dynamic "toes up" perturbations by increasing their anterior–posterior center of pressure, as though they have learned to move with the perturbation (36). This perspective of dynamic postural control following Tai Chi training in older adults differs from other studies (26) that found reduced center of pressure following Tai Chi training. This and other points requiring clarification on the benefits Tai Chi bestows upon older adults have been highlighted recently (37,38).

   While several types of interventions have demonstrated improvements in balance, some studies have provided results to the contrary. The review of literature suggests that specific components of an exercise program be incorporated for the best improvement in balance. Exercise programs that include strength, endurance, and some form of balance training appear to be the most beneficial for improving balance measures.

IV. EXERCISE PROGRAMS TO IMPROVE GAIT

Older adults can show kinetic and kinematic patterns during gait that differ from younger individuals, such as reduced stride length, increased double support stance time, decreased push-off power, a more flat footed landing, and decreased gait velocity (6). There are at least four major attributes of a normal gait pattern that can change profoundly as a function of aging and, consequently adversely affect walking. These factors include: (1) joint range of motion (16); (2) temporal patterns of muscle activation across the entire gait cycle (39); (3) muscle strength (12); and (4) sensory inputs from the visual, vestibular, and somatosensory systems (40,41). Given the overwhelming data to support the veracity of this contention, exercise interventions designed to overcome deficits in one or more of these factors should improve gait patterns in older adults (Table 2).

A. Flexibility Training

Knowing that muscle flexibility can affect joint range of motion and that joint range of motion and gait parameters are related, one would assume that a stretching/flexibility program should be one intervention to improve gait parameters. However, results from stretching programs designed to increase flexibility have provided little evidence for improved gait.

Improvements in flexibility have been observed, but a concomitant improvement in gait has not always been revealed. Kerrigan et al. (42) examined the effect of a 10-week hip flexor-stretching vs. shoulder-stretching program in healthy older adults. Although not statistically significant, an increase in gait velocity, peak ankle plantar flexor power (4%), peak hip extension range of motion (28%), and a reduction in anterior pelvic tilt (8%) were evident after the hip flexor-stretching program. These improvements were specific to the type of training performed: flexibility training.

B. Endurance Training

One-dimensional endurance-training programs are commonly used to improve gait parameters. Because of the weight-bearing nature of endurance training, which requires adequate postural control, balance should also be improved after such an intervention. In older patients with a right or left cortical stroke, six weeks of body weight supported or non-body weight supported treadmill walking (4 days/week for 20 minutes) resulted in significant improvements in balance (approximately 36%), motor recovery (approximately 35%), walking endurance (approximately 66%), and gait velocity (approximately 48%) (48). Because gait is a measure of physical function and can be improved after endurance training, one might conclude that endurance training can improve physical function, thus facilitating greater independence in older adults.

Table 2 Summary of Exercise Programs to Improve Gait

Author (reference)	Year	Intervention	Sample	Age	Physiological outcomes	Performance outcomes
Flexibility training						
Kerrigan et al. (42)	2003	Twice daily for 10 weeks; hip flexor stretching vs. shoulder stretching	Healthy men and women	>65	Increased peak ankle plantar flexor power, peak hip extension range of motion, reduced anterior pelvic tilt after hip stretching program (not statistically significant)	Increased gait velocity in hip stretching program (not statistically significant)
Endurance training						
Brown and Holloszy (19)		3 days/week for 12 weeks; low intensity ST and flexibility progressing to 12-month END (brisk walking, cycling, jogging; 30–50 min/day at 60–85% HRmax)			Increased knee extension and flexion torque after the initial 12 weeks, then no additional increase after the END training program; reduced time to peak knee extension torque and total work performed significantly improved	No change in gait after the 12-week ST and flexibility program; increased step length, stride length, gait velocity

Buchner et al. (20)	1997	3 days/week for 12 weeks with 6-month follow-up; walking, cycling, or aerobic exercise; 35–40 min/day at 50–75% HR reserve	Physically unfit, sedentary older adults	68–85	Walking increased VO_{2max} by 18%, aerobics increased VO_{2max} by 10%, cycling increased VO_{2max} by 8%; lower body isokinetic strength increased in all groups	after the END training program; reduced forward trunk bending range of motion after END training	Increased usual gait speed (5%) in walking group
Resistance training					
Krebs et al. (43)	1998	3 days/week for 24 weeks; home-based ST program using elastic tubing	Functionally limited men and women	62–89	Increase lower extremity isometric strength (17.6%)	No change in anteroposterior gait velocity; improved whole body center of gravity mediolateral stability; reduced center of gravity excursion and velocity

(Continued)

Table 2 Summary of Exercise Programs to Improve Gait (*Continued*)

Author (reference)	Year	Intervention	Sample	Age	Physiological outcomes	Performance outcomes
Topp et al. (24)	1993	3 days/week for 12 weeks; home-based ST program (2–3×10 repetitions) using elastic tubing	Community-dwelling men and women	>65	Increased isokinetic eccentric knee flexor and extensor strength	Decreased gait velocity
Judge et al. (44)	1993	3 days/week for 12 weeks; ST (3 sets to volitional fatigue at 75–80% 1RM)+ balance exercises (anterior–posterior and lateral movements)	Life-care community residents	>75	Increased knee extension strength (17–32%)	Increased usual gait velocity (8%), tend for improved maximal gait velocity (4%)
Judge et al. (45)	1994	3 days/week for 15 weeks; ST (3 sets to volitional fatigue at 60–75% 1RM) and ST+balance training or balance training only	Community-dwelling men and women	>75	Increase muscle strength (62–73%) and summed joint moments in strength groups	Increase gait velocity in strength groups only; No change in chair rise time
Multidimensional training						
Rubenstein et al. (49)	2000	3 days/week for 12 weeks; combined ST, balance, and END training	Community-dwelling fall-prone older men		No significant change in muscular endurance or strength	Greater distance walked in 6 min (10%), reduced fall rate relative to physical activity level

Tai Chi

Wolf et al. (47)	1996	2 days/week for 15 weeks; Tai Chi vs. computerized balance vs. no-exercise control	Community-dwelling men and women	Mean = 76	Tai Chi reduced systolic blood pressure; grip strength was reduced in balance and control groups	Tai Chi reduced gait velocity and rate of falls (47.5%); reduced fear of falling
Hartman et al. (30)	2000	2 days/week for 12 weeks; 60 min/session	Older adults with osteoarthritis	49–81		No change in gait velocity; improved arthritis self-efficacy and quality of life indicators
Wolfson et al. (29)	1996	3 days/week for 12 weeks; 45 min/session; balance, strength, or balance + ST (1×13 repetitions at 75% 1RM) followed by a 26-week Tai Chi maintenance phase	Community-dwelling older adults	>75	Improved peak joint moments in strength and balance + strength groups; improvements in strength were maintained only in the ST group after Tai Chi maintenance	Balance and balance + ST reduced gait velocity, but Tai Chi increased gait velocity after 24 weeks in the balance + ST group only

ST, strength training; END, endurance training; HRmax, heart rate max; HRreserve, heart rate reserve.

C. Resistance Training

Muscular strength and gait are curvilinearly related (14). This curvilinear relationship suggests that a significant increase in strength does not always lead to a significant increase in gait velocity. Thus, gains in strength above a certain threshold will not elicit significant improvements in gait velocity. Below the threshold, however, gains or losses in strength will be reflected in gains or losses in gait velocity. This observation was supported by results from a six-month home-based strength-training program performed by functionally limited older adults (62–89 years old) who improved lower extremity strength (17.6%), but not gait velocity (3–5%) (43). Although gait velocity did not increase, there was a significant improvement in the center of gravity mediolateral stability and a reduction in center of gravity excursion and velocity. This improvement in gait stability may be protective against falls in a population of functionally limited older adults. Community-dwelling older adults participating in a home-based strength-training program (3 days/week for 12 weeks; 2 to 3 sets of 10 repetitions with elastic tubing) significantly improved isokinetic eccentric knee flexor and extensor strength, but walked slower after the intervention (4.2%). In this study, gait velocity showed a non-significant inverse relationship with strength ($r = -0.08$ to -0.23) (24). The curvilinear relationship between strength and gait velocity is not always supported. Thus, improvements in strength can lead to improvements in gait velocity. Twelve weeks of strength training including some balance exercises, significantly improved maximal knee extension strength (17–32%) at several isokinetic speeds, self-selected gait velocity (8%), and resulted in a trend for improved maximal gait velocity (4%) in life-care community residents (44). Results from another study showed a significant increase in gait velocity (2.6%) and muscle strength (62%) after 15 weeks of resistance training in men and women over 75 years (45). Because of the conflicting results, these studies collectively demonstrate that physiological factors other than muscle strength must be responsible for improvements in gait.

D. Multidimensional Training

Multidimensional training programs may be more appropriate for improvements in gait parameters because they incorporate different training modalities, which may have additive benefits for improvement in gait. A 12-week multidimensional exercise program (combined strength training, balance training, and endurance training) resulted in improved strength (8–14%), global health (23%), greater distance walked in 6 minutes (10%), and reduced fall rate relative to physical activity level in community-dwelling, fall-prone older men (49). These older men presented with at least one of the following fall risk factors: lower extremity weakness; impaired gait; impaired balance; or >1 fall in the previous 6 months. A 16-week home-based exercise intervention designed to improve strength, proprioception, balance, and flexibility in frail, demented older adults with a history of falls resulted in a significant increase in flexibility (69%), gait velocity (23%), gait velocity during the Timed Up and Go test (41%), and improved static balance (40%) (50). The number of falls was reduced during the exercise-training intervention period; however, participants began to fall after the conclusion of the exercise program. When comparing a multidimensional restorative program (strength and balance exercises) to usual care for older adults after a hip fracture, Tinetti et al. (51) found no significant difference in measures of social activity levels, mobility tasks, balance, or lower extremity strength; however, intervention subjects had slightly higher upper body strength and improved gait compared to the usual care participants. Multidimensional exercise programs appear to be effective interventions to improve gait performance; however, because of the non-randomized design employed in some studies, these results must be interpreted with caution and within the scope of the study population.

E. Tai Chi

Tai Chi has proven to be no more effective or consistent at improving gait performance compared to traditional exercise. Interestingly, after 15 weeks of Tai Chi practice, community-dwelling adults over the age of 70 years reduced their walking speed compared to a balance training and no-exercise control group; however, the Tai Chi group also reported a 47.5% reduction in rate of falls (47). Even though time to complete a 6-min walk was increased among the Tai Chi participants, Tai Chi was still effective at reducing falls, suggesting that after Tai Chi training, these individuals may have increased their awareness and walked more deliberately. Contrary to these findings, older adults with osteoarthritis who participated in Tai Chi twice weekly for 12 weeks did not significantly improve gait velocity (13%) (30). When gait speed was assessed in younger individuals who learned a "Tai Chi gait" over the course of a week, they too demonstrated longer cycle duration and single-leg stance time (52). Wolfson et al. (29) examined changes in usual gait velocity after three months of balance training and balance + strength training and again after six months of Tai Chi maintenance. Balance training and balance + strength training significantly reduced gait velocity (3%) after the three-month interventions, but gait velocity was then increased (8%) after six months of Tai Chi maintenance in the balance + strength-training group. Thus, evidence suggests that Tai Chi provides mixed results on gait parameters. Further research is needed to determine if Tai Chi training instills in its students an ability to walk more deliberately (and by extension, more slowly), more quickly, or in a manner dependent upon the intent and orientation of the instructor.

V. AN EXAMPLE OF INTERFACING EXERCISE DESIGN PRINCIPLES TO THE PATIENT: CEREBROVASCULAR ACCIDENT (STROKE)

Having previously discussed design principles governing improvements in balance and gait and reducing falls, it would appear that a multidimensional program is appropriate. An effective multidimensional exercise program is one that combines resistance exercises, endurance training, and challenging balance tasks. Applying exercise design principles to patients following stroke is potentially valuable because these individuals often present with muscle weakness, reduced cardiovascular capacity, and problems with balance.

For several decades, clinicians believed that patients who had sustained strokes should be rehabilitated with considerable care, lest profound cardiorespiratory taxation, fatigue, or induced exaggerations of spasticity yield adverse effects (see, for example, Ref. 53). More recently, evidence seems to suggest that patients with stroke can assume more active roles early in their rehabilitation and that strengthening programs designed to overcome muscle weakness can be enacted without the fear of concomitantly exacerbating spasticity (54). For example, Teixeira-Salmela et al. (55) found that a 10-week aerobic exercise program applied to community-dwelling older adults, designed to target lower extremity musculature and included warm up and cool down intervals, yielded significant improvements in peak isokinetic torque in quadriceps and ankle plantar flexor muscle groups and gait speed without adversely affecting spasticity. Comparable results were obtained by Sharp and Brouwer (56). The sequence employed in these studies suggests an algorithm that might be applicable to many patients with stroke, if the goal is to improve muscle strength, balance, and gait speed. After assuring reasonable postural stability, with or without use of assistive devices, objective and subjective measures of fatigue should be acquired. Exercise programs should then include a general warm up period to promote circulation and then a very gradual increasing resistance program. The rate of progression needs to be tailored to the endurance of the patient without overstressing repetition, lest spastic muscles become overtaxed. Task specificity should be incorporated so that ambulation and monitoring of gait speed are undertaken and periodic feedback on performance offered to the patient. A cool down period should be considered. Pacing of an exercise program for patients with stroke, either as an individual prescription or, preferably, in a group setting should be instituted, so that the training does not exceed alternating days in intensity. Collectively, this construct suggests that a more aggressive approach to improving gait and balance than has typically been undertaken in this population should be pursued.

In this chapter, evidence has been provided to suggest that Tai Chi is an exercise form that can enhance balance and improve ambulation among older adults. Since many individuals who sustain strokes are older, the application of Tai Chi to improve posture and strength should be considered. Surprisingly, while reference has been made to the use of this exercise form as a therapeutic intervention for diagnosis-specific entities, little information has been published (57,58). Recently, we (59) suggested guidelines for the implementation of Tai Chi exercise among patients with stroke. The approach excludes patients with lower extremity dyskinesis, compromised mental competence that adversely impacts procedural memory, hemianopsia or other profound visual field deficits, or imbalance that requires constant guarding even if the back of a four-legged chair is available.

The training consists of progressive weight shifting leading toward the institution of a commencement form (Yang style). Eventually, patients make slow and deliberate "box steps" leading first to their better, less affected side. Backward ambulation to heighten somatosensation in the absence of visual guidance is encouraged, as is the monitoring of progressive "exercise" time. Many forms, including "grasp bird's tail" emphasize diagonal patterns of movement and continuous weight shifting. Movement forms progress toward single-limb support (compromised center of pressure to center of mass relationships), which emphasizes postural control capabilities. As yet, falls have not been experienced and patients report awareness of movement accomplishments with reduced feelings of fatigue. Patients also begin using fewer assistive devices and walking faster. However to date, there has been no systematic study of this intervention for patients with stroke and, much like the application to improve balance and gait with transitionally frail older adults, there is concern that the effectiveness of the intervention to improve gait and balance will only persist as long as Tai Chi is practiced safely and under supervision.

VI. EXERCISE TO REDUCE FALLS

With the increase in the aging population, the incidence of falls and fall-related injuries also increases, thus threatening an older adult's independence. Of utmost importance for older adults at increased risk for falls is fall prevention. Intuitively, one would assume that effective exercise interventions that improve factors associated with falls, such as gait and balance, would also impact fall risk. Although one-dimensional exercise interventions (i.e., strength training or endurance training) have demonstrated improvements in factors associated with falls, few have been successful at reducing the incidence of falls in older adults.

A meta-analysis of the seven FICSIT studies examined the efficacy of short-term exercise on fall rates and injuries in older adults (60). The sample of older adults was predominantly cognitively intact, yet some studies required further inclusion criteria such as functional impairments, high fall risk, or balance deficits. One-dimensional and multidimensional exercise programs that included strength, endurance, balance, flexibility, and/or Tai Chi performed for 10 to 36 weeks were examined. With respect to risk of falling, the Tai Chi training was the most effective (incident ratio =0.63). Recently, we demonstrated that older adult fallers, meeting the Speechley and Tinetti (61) criteria for transitioning to frailty, who underwent an intense Tai Chi training program experienced a 25% reduction in falls over the course of a 48-week program compared to a Wellness Education control group. This difference was 40% after the first four months of training (62). Although not as effective as Tai Chi, multidimensional programs that included a balance component were also effective for reducing fall risk (incident ratio = 0.76). Steadman et al. (63) also demonstrated that balance training (2 days/week for 8 weeks) could significantly improve balance, gait velocity, quality of life, and reduce the number of falls in balance-impaired older adults. Thus, providing further support for the efficacy of balance training to reduce falls.

Because many factors influence fall risk (waist to hip ratio, low bone density, poor balance, muscle weakness, impaired gait), a multifactorial intervention is needed to reduce fall risk (9,64). Thus far, multidimensional exercise interventions show more promise than one-dimensional exercise interventions as effective strategies to reduce the number of falls. An individually tailored home-based strength-training (2 sets of 10 repetitions; moderate intensity; 3 days/week for 1 year), balance-training (progressively challenging tasks; 3 days/week for 1 year), and walking program (30 min/day at usual pace; 2 days/week for 1 year) with 1 year of follow-up revealed a significant reduction in the rate of falls (range = 30–46%) in men and women over the age of 75 years (27,65). A meta-analysis of the four studies conducted by the New Zealand group concluded that their multidimensional fall prevention program consistently demonstrated an average 35% reduction in the number of falls and fall-related injuries in adults over the age of 80 years (66). From an economic standpoint, they also found this fall prevention program was more cost-effective per fall prevented when compared to a no-exercise control group (67,68). Fear of falling, time to first fall, and number of falls and injurious falls were reduced after a multidimensional home-based exercise program designed to improve balance and strength, and included behavioral instruction and medication adjustment for community-dwelling, ambulatory older men and women (69). Additionally, a smaller percentage of those participants in the intervention group continued to have balance or gait impairments and overall had less fall risk factors after 1 year of follow-up. As described in more detail in Chapters 9 and 10, other multidimensional programs have also been successful at reducing the rate of falls (25,70).

Multidimensional exercise programs do not always yield significant improvements in both falls and fall-related factors. While Rubenstein et al.'s (49) group exercise program (3 days/week for 12 weeks; strength training and endurance training) significantly improved factors that influence fall risk (i.e., strength, muscle and aerobic endurance, gait parameters), a significant reduction in rate of falls in fall-prone older men was not observed. Contrary to these findings, Buchner et al. (32) demonstrated a significant reduction in time to first fall, but no significant effect of exercise (3 days/week for 24-26 weeks; strength training, endurance training, or a combination of strength and endurance training) on factors influencing falls (gait, balance, strength, health status). These seemingly conflicting data on multidimensional programs highlight the importance of identifying those factors that most contribute to inducing falls through more systematic and specific inclusion criteria.

VII. ISSUES TO CONSIDER WHEN INTERPRETING THE LITERATURE

As demonstrated in the previous sections, profound variability in the design of research studies affecting the interpretation of results is present. This variability is evident because investigations have not adequately controlled for: participant selection, cultural differences, variability in exercise prescription between and within exercise modalities, and lack of standardization in measurement of dependent variables or outcomes. Thus choosing the "best" intervention to improve gait and balance becomes difficult.

Much variability is present in the inclusion criteria used to select participants. Participants range from robust and healthy community-dwelling older adults to frail institutionalized demented older adults. Thus, the results of each study are specific to the population studied. The age of participants covers a broad range from 60 to greater than 85 years. Because of the variability in function and physiological processes due to the aging process in this age range, results grouped in age categories might enhance interpretation of the results.

Also, cultural differences affect interpretation of the results. Older adults in many other countries tend to be more physically active than older adults living in the United States. Thus, results from exercise interventions may not be representative of *all* older adults, but rather the older adults in that specific country. Economical diversity is also different between cultures such that all older adults in the United States may not be eligible for the same type of exercise regimen prescribed by clinicians in another country and other countries, such as New Zealand, might have special programs for older adults where their health care (including exercise training) is paid from other resources (governmental, social insurance programs, etc.) and cultural diversity, which may expand perspectives on the role and value of exercise in aging, may be less profound.

Variability in exercise prescription also confounds interpretation of the results and makes implementation by clinicians difficult. Differences in the prescribed intensity, duration, and frequency of exercise exist between and within exercise modalities. For example, between exercise modalities, flexibility training is prescribed daily while strength and endurance training are prescribed 3 days per week. Within exercise modalities, strength training intensity can vary from 50% of maximal strength to 80% of maximal strength and the volume of exercise varies from one to three sets of 8 to 12 repetitions to volitional fatigue. The length of training programs also varies widely from a few weeks to as long as a year. Not controlling for these differences or making efforts to standardize exercise prescription widens the gap between research and clinical application.

The lack of standardization of test measures also makes interpretation difficult. Balance can be measured as static or dynamic, yet there are many ways to measure both. Standardized laboratory-based (SMART Balance Master, force platform) and clinical-based measures (Timed Up and Go, Berg Balance test) are widely used; however, there is not a single gold standard measure of balance. Gait parameters such as gait velocity, stride length, and step width are typically evaluated; however, the methods used to determine these outcomes vary. For example, the distance walked to calculate gait velocity can vary from 6 to 30 m. Collection of fall data also varies widely. Self-reported fall rates are typically used to evaluate the effect of an exercise intervention on falls, yet this method is not as accurate as directly measuring falls. Furthermore, the accuracy of self-reported falls is influenced by the age and recollection of participants, and the time between the actual event and falls ascertainment.

To reduce variability between research studies and improve interpretation of the results for the general population, the following recommendations are offered (Table 3). The population to be studied should be clearly defined, i.e., older adults at risk for falls if fall prevention is a main outcome, should be targeted. Within that population, grouping results by age categories or functional impairments should be considered. Based on past research findings, those exercise interventions and/or testing protocols that

Table 3 Recommendations to Reduce Variability in Research Findings

Target the population to be studied
Categorize participants by age and/or functional status
Standardize testing methodology of dependent variables
Review literature and determine which exercise program is "best" and implement that program
Design an exercise program with less variability in intensity, frequency, and duration
Directly measure falls
Consider cultural differences

are "best" or optimal should be determined and the appropriate protocols implement. Exercise programs with less variability in intensity, frequency, and duration should be designed. When possible, direct measurement of falls is preferred over self-report. Cultural differences should be considered when designing studies and implementing research findings so that the results can be interpreted accordingly. Reducing the variability between research studies can yield focused results and clarify interpretation and implementation of the data.

VIII. SUMMARY

An older adult's ability to successfully move within his/her environment is a function of balance and gait parameters, which are affected by aging. Age-associated changes in the sensory and neuromuscular systems are manifested in a slowed gait velocity, reduced step length, reduced single stance time, increased double support phase, etc. Because balance and gait are highly related, impairments in one will negatively affect the other; thus, poor balance can increase gait instability. Balance and gait affect one's ability to perform daily tasks and function independently.

Exercise interventions have demonstrated promise to improve balance and gait. Based on findings in the literature, the optimal exercise regimen to improve balance is one that incorporates strength, endurance, and challenging balance tasks. Given the relationship between balance and gait, an exercise program that improves balance should also impact gait parameters. Evidence suggests that a multidimensional exercise program is also best for improving gait. Multidimensional exercise programs have resulted in increased single stance time, gait velocity, and stride length, and reduced double support phase during gait, fear of falling, and fall rate. Not all exercise programs result in these improvements; however, this fact may be related to variability between studies rather than to a direct effect of the intervention.

Equivocal results from the literature influence their interpretation and application. Variability between exercise programs results from an inability to control for participant selection, cultural differences, variability in exercise modalities, and lack of standardization in measurement of outcomes. To reduce variability between studies, we recommend future research studies: (1) target the population, standardize outcome methodology; (2) consider cultural differences by making necessary adjustments to the study protocol; and (3) select exercise programs with reduced variability in intensity, duration, and frequency by seeking criteria (for example, the number and type of comorbidities, gender differences, diagnoses, level of independence, etc.) that enhance sample targeting and exercise specificity. This approach will improve the interpretation of results and implementation to the community.

In summary, multidimensional exercise programs are recommended to improve balance and gait in older adults. Since poor balance and impaired gait are factors related to falls, the effect of exercise on these factors should transfer to a reduction in fall rate. As evidenced by the existing literature, multidimensional exercise programs have been the most successful at reducing fall risk. Further research is still needed to determine the optimal dosage of exercise and specific modality utilized while considering the above-mentioned factors to reduce variability between studies.

ACKNOWLEDGMENTS

Portions of this work are funded by the Veterans Administration Associate Investigator Award E3133H and by NIH grant AG 14767.

REFERENCES

1. Kerrigan DC, Todd MK, Croce UD, Lipsitz LA, Collins JJ. Biomechanical gait alterations independent of speed in the healthy elderly: evidence for specific limiting impairments. Arch Phys Med Rehabil 1998; 79:317–322.
2. Woollacott M, Shumway-Cook A. Attention and the control of posture and gait: a review of an emerging area of research. Gait Posture 2002; 16:1–14.
3. Roma AA, Chiarella LA, Barker SP, Brenneman SK. Examination and comparison of the relationships between strength, balance, fall history, and ambulatory function in older adults. Issues Aging 2001; 24(2):21–30.
4. Judge JO, Davis RB, Ounpuu S. Step length reductions in advanced age: The role of ankle and hip kinetics. J Gerontol A Biol Sci Med Sci 1996; 51(6):M303–M312.
5. Riley PO, DellaCroce U, Kerrigan DC. Effect of age on lower extremity joint moment contributions to gait speed. Gait Posture 2001; 14(3):264–270.
6. Winter DA, Patla AE, Frank JS, Walt SE. Biomechanical walking pattern changes in the fit and healthy elderly. Phys Ther 1990; 70:340–347.
7. Imms FJ, Edholm OG. Studies of gait and mobility in the elderly. Age Ageing 1981; 10:147–156.
8. Tinetti ME, Speechley M, Ginter SF. Risk factors for falls among elderly persons living in the community. N Engl J Med 1988; 319:1701–1707.
9. Tinetti ME, Doucette J, Claus E, Marottoli R. Risk factors for serious injury during falls by older persons in the community. J Am Geriatr Soc 1995; 43:1214–1221.
10. Vellas BJ, Wayne SJ, Romero LJ, Baumgartner RN, Garry PJ. Fear of falling and restriction of mobility in elderly fallers. Age Ageing 1997; 26:189–193.
11. Hirvensalo M, Rantanen T, Heikkinen E. Mobility difficulties and physical activity as predictors of mortality and loss of independence in the community-living older population. J Am Geriatr Soc 2000; 48:493–498.
12. Larsson L, Grimby G, Karlsson J. Muscle strength and speed of movement in relation to age and muscle morphology. J Appl Physiol 1979; 46(3):451–456.

13. Skelton DA, Greig CA, Davies JM, Young A. Strength, power and related functional ability of healthy people aged 65–89 years. Age Ageing 1994; 23:371–377.
14. Buchner DM, Larson EB, Wagner EH, Koepsell TD, deLateur BJ. Evidence for a non-linear relationship between leg strength and gait speed. Age Ageing 1996; 25:386–391.
15. Rantanen T, Avela J. Leg extension power and walking speed in very old people living independently. J Gerontol A Biol Sci Med Sci 1997; 52(4):M225–M231.
16. Judge JO, Ounpuu S, Davis RB. Effects of age on the biomechanics and physiology of gait. Clin Geriatr Med 1996; 12(4):659–678.
17. Maki BE. Gait changes in older adults: Predictors of falls or indicators of fear? J Am Geriatr Soc 1997; 45(3):313–320
18. Pavol MJ, Owings TM, Foley KT, Grabiner MD. Gait characteristics as risk factors for falling from trips induced in older adults. J Gerontol A Biol Sci Med Sci 1999; 54(11):M583–M590.
19. Brown M, Holloszy JO. Effects of walking, jogging and cycling on strength, flexibility, speed and balance in 60- to 72-year olds. Aging Clin Exp Res 1993; 5:427–434.
20. Buchner DM, Cress ME, de Lateur BJ, Esselman PC, Margherita AJ, Price R, Wagner EH. A comparison of the effects of three types of endurance training on balance and other fall risk factors in older adults. Aging Clin Exp Res 1997; 9:112–119.
21. Vanderhoek KJ, Coupland DC, Parkhouse WS. Effects of 32 weeks of resistance training on strength and balance in older osteopenic/osteoporotic women. Clin Exerc Physiol 2000; 2(2):77–83.
22. Carter ND, Kham KM, McKay HA, Petit MA, Waterman C, Heinonen A, Janssen PA, Donaldson MG, Mallinson A, Riddell L, Kruse K, Prior JC, Flicker L. Community-based exercise program reduces risk factors for falls in 65- to 75-year-old women with osteoporosis: randomized controlled trial. CMAJ 2002; 167(9):997–1004.
23. Yates SM, Dunnagan TA. Evaluating the effectiveness of a home-based fall risk reduction program for rural community-dwelling older adults. J Gerontol A Biol Sci Med Sci 2001; 56(4):M226–M230.
24. Topp R, Mikesky A, Wigglesworth J, Holt W, Edwards JE. The effect of a 12-week dynamic resistance strength training program on gait velocity and balance of older adults. Gerontologist 1993; 33(4):501–506.
25. Hauer K, Rost B, Rutschle K, Opitz H, Specht N, Bartsch P, Oster P, Schlierf G. Exercise training for rehabilitation and secondary prevention of falls in geriatric patients with a history of injurious falls. J Am Geriatr Soc 2001; 49:10–20.
26. Judge J, Lindsey C, Underwood M, Winsemius D. Balance improvements in older women: Effects of exercise training. Phys Ther 1993; 73(4):254–262.
27. Campbell AJ, Robertson MC, Gardner MM, Norton RN, Tilyard MW, Buchner DM. Randomised controlled trial of a general practice programme of home based exercise to prevent falls in elderly women. BMJ 1997; 315:1065–1069.
28. Messier SP, Royer TD, Craven TE, O'Toole ML, Burns R, Ettinger WH. Long-term exercise and its effect on balance in older, osteoarthritic adults: results

from the Fitness, Arthritis, and Seniors Trial (FAST). J Am Geriatr Soc 2000; 48:131–138.

29. Wolfson L, Whipple R, Derby C, Judge J, King M, Amerman P, Schmidt J, Smyers D. Balance and strength training in older adults: intervention gains and tai chi maintenance. J Am Geriatr Soc 1996; 44:498–506.

30. Hartman CA, Manos TM, Winter C, Hartman DM, Li B, Smith JC. Effects of T'ai Chi training on function and quality of life indicators in older adults with osteoarthritis. J Am Geriatr Soc 2000; 48:1553–1559.

31. Papaioannou A, Adachi JD, Winegard K, Ferko N, Parkinson W, Cook RJ, Webber C, McCartney N. Efficacy of home-based exercise for improving quality of life among elderly women with symptomatic osteoporosis-related vertebral fractures. Osteoporosis Int 2003; 14(8):677–682.

32. Buchner DM, Cress ME, de Lateur BJ, Esselman PC, Margherita AJ, Price R, Wagner EH. The effect of strength and endurance training on gait, balance, fall risk, and health services use in community-living older adults. J Gerontol A Biol Sci Med Sci 1997; 52(4):M218–M224.

33. Rooks DS, Kiel DP, Parsons C, Hayes WC. Self-paced resistance training and walking exercise in community-dwelling older adults: Effects on neuromotor performance. J Gerontol A Biol Sci Med Sci 1997; 52(3):M161–M168.

34. Wolf SE, O'Grady M, Easley KA, Guo Y, Kressig RW, Kutner M. The influence of Tai Chi training of functional performance and hemodynamic outcomes in transitionally frail older adults. J Gerontol 2005; (In Review).

35. Wolf SL, Gregor RJ. Exploring unique applications of kinetic analyses to movement in older adults. J Appl Biomech 1999; 15:75–83.

36. Wolf SL, Barnhart HX, Ellison GL, Coogler CE. The effect of Tai Chi Quan and computerized balance training on postural stability in older subjects. Atlanta FICSIT Group. Frailty and Injuries: Cooperative Studies on Intervention Techniques. Phys Ther 1997; 77(4):371–381.

37. Wang C, Collet JP, Lau J. The effect of Tai Chi on health outcomes in patients with chronic conditions. Arch Intern Med 2004; 164:493–501.

38. Wu G. Evaluation of the effectiveness of Tai Chi for improving balance and preventing falls in the older population—a review. J Am Geriatr Soc 2002; 50:746–754.

39. Woollacott MH, Shumway-Cook A. Changes in posture control across the life span—a systems approach. Phys Ther 1990; 70:799–807.

40. Horak FB, Shupert CL, Mirka A. Components of postural dyscontrol in the elderly: a review. Neurobiol Aging 1989; 10(6):727–738.

41. Lord SR, Clark RD, Webster IW. Physiological factors associated with falls in an elderly population. J Am Geriatr Soc 1991; 39:1194–1200.

42. Kerrigan DC, Xenopoulos-Oddsson A, Sullivan MJ, Lelas JJ, Riley PO. Effect of a high flexor-stretching program on gait in the elderly. Arch Phys Med Rehabil 2003; 84:1–6.

43. Krebs DE, Jette AM, Assmann SF. Moderate exercise improves gait stability in disabled elders. Arch Phys Med Rehabil 1998; 79:1489–1495.

44. Judge JO, Underwood M, Gennosa T. Exercise to improve gait velocity in older persons. Arch Phys Med Rehabil 1993; 74(4):400–406.

45. Judge JO, Whipple RH, Wolfson LI. Effects of resistance and balance exercises on isokinetic strength in older persons. J Am Geriatr Soc 1994; 42(9):937–946.

46. Alexander NB, Guire KE, Thelen DG, Ashton-Miller JA, Schultz AB, Grunawalt JC, Giordani B. Self-reported walking ability predicts functional mobility performance in frail older adults. J Am Geriatr Soc 2000; 48: 1408–1413.

47. Wolf SL, Banrnhart HX, Kutner NG, McNeeley E, Coogler E, Xu C. Reducing frailty and falls in older persons: an investigation of Tai Chi and computerized balance training. Atlanta FICSIT Group. Frailty and Injuries: Cooperative Studies of Intervention Techniques. J Am Geriatr Soc 1996; 44:489–497.

48. Visintin M, Barbeau H, Korner-Bitensky N, Mayo NE. A new approach to retrain gait in stroke patients through body weight support and treadmill stimulation. Stroke 1998; 29:1122–1128.

49. Rubenstein LZ, Josephson KR, Trueblood PR, Loy S, Harker JO, Pietruszka FM, Robbins AS. Effects of a group exercise program on strength, mobility, and falls among fall prone elderly men. J Gerontol A Biol Sci Med Sci 2000; 55(6):M317–M321.

50. Toulotte C, Fabre C, Dangremont B, Lensel G, Thevenon A. Effects of physical training on the physical capacity of frail, demented patients with a history of falling: a randomised controlled trial. Age Ageing 2003; 32:67–73.

51. Tinetti M, Baker D, Gottschalk M, Williams C, Pollack D, Garrett P, Gill T, Marottoli R, Acampora D. Home-based multicomponent rehabilitation program for older persons after hip fracture: a randomized trial. Arch Phys Med Rehabil 1999; 80(8):916–922.

52. Wu G, Liu W, Hitt J, Milton D. Spatial, temporal and muscle action patterns of Tai Chi gait. J Electromyogr Kinesiol 2004; 14:343–354.

53. Riolo L, Fisher K. Evidence in practice: is there evidence that strength training could help improve muscle function and other outcomes without reinforcing abnormal movement patterns or increasing reflex activity in a man who has had a stroke? Phys Ther 2003; 83:844–851

54. Brandstater ME. Important practical issues in rehabilitation of the stroke patient. In: Branstater ME, Basmajian JV, eds. Stroke Rehabilitation. Rehabilitation Medicine Library Series. Baltimore: Williams & Wilkins, 1987:330–368.

55. Teixeira-Salmela LF, Olney SJNS, Brouwer B. Muscle strengthening and physical conditioning to reduce impairments and disability in chronic stroke survivors. Arch Phys Med Rehabil 1999; 80:1211–1218.

56. Sharp SA, Brouwer BJ. Isokinetic strength training of the hemiparetic knee: effects on function and spasticity. Arch Phys Med Rehabil 1997; 78:1231–1236.

57. Bottomley JM. T'ai Chi: choreography of body and mind. In: Davis CM, ed. Complementary Therapies in Rehabilitation. Thorofare, NJ: Slack, 1997: 133–156.

58. Hain TC, Kotsias J, Pai C. Tai Chi: Applications in neurology. In: Weintraub ME, ed. Alternative and Complementary Treatment in Neurologic Illness. New York: Churchill Livingstone, 2001:248–254.

59. Kressig RW, Wolf SL. Exploring guidelines for the application of T'ai Chi to patients with stroke. Neurol Rep 2001; 25:50–54.

60. Province MA, Hadley EC, Hornbrook MC, Lipsitz LA, Miller JP, Mulrow CD, Ory MG, Sattin RW, Tinetti ME, Wolf SL. The effects of exercise on falls in elderly patients. A preplanned meta-analysis of the FICSIT trials. JAMA 1995; 273(17):1341–1347.
61. Speechley M, Tinetti ME. Falls and injuries in frail and vigorous community elderly persons. J Am Geriatr Soc 1991; 39:46–52.
62. Wolf SL, Sattin RW, Kutner M, O'Grady M, Greenspan AI, Gregor RJ. Intense Tai Chi exercise training and fall occurrences in older, transitionally frail adults: a randomized, controlled trial. J Am Geriatr Soc 2003; 51: 1693–1701.
63. Steadman J, Donaldson N, Kalra L. A randomized controlled trial of an enhanced balance training program to improve mobility and reduce falls in elderly patients. J Am Geriatr Soc 2003; 51:847–852.
64. Lord SR, McLean D, Stathers G. Physiological factors associated with injurious falls in older people living in the community. Gerontology 1992; 38: 338–346.
65. Campbell AJ, Robertson MC, Gardner MM, Norton RN, Buchner DM. Falls prevention over 2 years: a randomized controlled trial in women 80 years and older. Age Ageing 1999; 28:513–518.
66. Robertson MC, Campbell AJ, Gardner MM, Devlin N. Preventing injuries in older people by preventing falls: a meta-analysis of individual-level data. J Am Geriatr Soc 2002; 50:905–911.
67. Robertson MC, Devlin N, Gardner MM, Campbell AJ. Effectiveness and economic evaluation of a nurse delivered home exercise programme to prevent falls. 1: Randomised controlled trial. BMJ 2001; 322:697–701.
68. Robertson MC, Gardner MM, Devlin N, McGee R, Campbell AJ. Effectiveness and economic evaluation of a nurse delivered home exercise programme to prevent falls. 2: Controlled trial in multiple centers. BMJ 2001; 322:701–4.
69. Tinetti ME, Baker DI, McAvay G, Claus EB, Garrett P, Gottschalk M, Koch ML, Trainor K, Horwitz RI. A multifactorial intervention to reduce the risk of falling among elderly people living in the community. N Engl J Med 1994; 331(13):821–827.
70. Barnett A, Smith B, Lord SR, Williams M, Baumand A. Community-based group exercise improves balance and reduces falls in at-risk older people: a randomised controlled trial. Age Ageing 2003; 32:407–414.

13

Clinical Gait Analysis in Neurology

Meg Morris, Belinda Bilney, Karen Dodd, and Sonia Denisenko
BPT, School of Physiotherapy, La Trobe University, Victoria, Australia

Richard Baker, Fiona Dobson, and Jennifer McGinley
School of Physiotherapy, La Trobe University and Hugh Williamson Gait Laboratory, Royal Children's Hospital, Victoria, Australia

Clinical gait analysis is central to the evaluation of medical and therapy outcomes in people with neurological conditions. Despite the rapid evolution and availability of laboratory-based technologies to evaluate the kinematics and kinetics of gait (see Chapter 3), visual observation remains the most frequently used method of gait analysis in the clinical setting (1). To illustrate the utility of visual observation, in this chapter, we explore common forms of locomotor disturbance in people with neurological conditions. We focus on four common representative examples: cerebral palsy (CP), Parkinson's disease (PD), Huntington's disease (HD), and stroke, as well as the major factors taken into account during clinical gait analysis. Consideration is given to the pathogenesis of locomotor disorders and to the way in which their clinical presentation varies according to constraints afforded by the environment, task, attention, age, medication, and rehabilitation therapies. Some of the ways in which the accuracy of clinical gait analysis can be enhanced are presented, and the major gait deviations to target are discussed.

I. GAIT ANALYSIS IN PEOPLE WITH CP

Cerebral palsy (CP) (2) describes a variety of motor impairments caused by non-progressive lesions in the immature brain. Although walking is only one aspect of the impaired gross motor function, it is a well-defined, more or less cyclic activity that is well suited to standardized methods of analysis. Gait analysis thus provides a useful assessment tool that is becoming a more widely accepted component of the clinical management of children with this condition (3). In the current chapter, the term "clinical gait analysis" refers to the overall process of assessing walking patterns in clinical settings, either by using observational gait analysis (OGA) (also referred to as "visual analysis") or computer-based three-dimensional gait analysis (3-DGA).

The lesion in CP leads directly to spasticity, hyper-reflexia, and co-contraction, as well as weakness and loss of selective motor control, balance, or co-ordination. Abnormalities in movement patterns that occur as a result of these are termed "primary" gait deviations. While the lesion itself is non-progressive, the musculoskeletal pathology progressively deteriorates over time. Because children with CP put abnormal loads through the muscles, bones and joints can develop abnormally. Abnormalities that eventually occur are termed "secondary" gait deviations. People with such primary and secondary problems will not, generally, be able to walk at all unless they adopt some abnormal compensatory mechanisms and these are termed "tertiary" gait deviations.

A wide range of gait deviations are observed across the CP syndromes, depending on the main type of movement disorder (spastic, dyskinetic, ataxic, hypokinetic, or mixed) and the topographical classification (monoplegia, hemiplegia, diplegia, triplegia, or quadriplegia). Because spastic type CP is the most common, representing ~87% of CP cases in developed countries such as Australia (2), typical gait deviations in this population will be the focus of this chapter. Unless complicated by severe epilepsy or cognitive disturbances, most children with spastic hemiplegia achieve independent walking (4,5). Likewise, the majority of children with spastic diplegia achieve walking either in the community or in the home, although many require assistive devices such as walking frames or crutches (6). Children with spastic quadriplegia rarely have functional walking (4,5).

The most obvious gait deviation seen in spastic hemiplegia is asymmetry between involved and uninvolved sides of the spatio-temporal, kinematic, and kinetic characteristics of gait. Typical gait deviations mainly affect distal regions and occur in the sagittal plane, although deviations more proximally and in the coronal and transverse planes, are also recognized (7–11). The most common and clinically relevant sagittal plane kinematic deviations in spastic hemiplegia are excessive ankle plantar-flexion in swing and/or stance (equinus), excessive knee flexion at initial contact and in stance, knee hyper-extension in stance, reduced and/or delayed peak knee flexion in swing, reduced hip range of motion, and a single-bump pelvic-tilt pattern (11,12). Typical kinematic deviations in the transverse plane include excessive internal foot progression and internal hip rotation and external pelvic rotation (4,12,13). The most common coronal plane kinematic deviation is pelvic obliquity with the involved side down, although this is usually secondary to limb-length discrepancy (12). The typical equinovarus foot deviation includes hind-foot varus and fore-foot supination in terminal swing (12,14).

Despite the wide range of gait disorders in spastic diplegia, the more common kinematic deviations have been described according to the sagittal patterns of knee involvement (10,15,16). These essentially include (i) true equinus, where the ankle is in plantar-flexion, the knee extends fully or is slightly hyper-extended, the hip extends fully, and the pelvis is in normal range or tilted anteriorly; (ii) jump gait, where the ankle is in plantar-flexion, the knee and hip are in excess flexion, and the pelvis is in normal range or tilted anteriorly; (iii) apparent equinus, where the ankle is within normal range, the hip and knee are in excess flexion, and the pelvis is in normal range or tilted anteriorly; and (iv) crouch gait, where the ankle is in excess dorsiflexion throughout stance, the knee and hip are in excess flexion, and the pelvis is in normal range or tilted anteriorly. Typical transverse plane kinematic deviations include internal rotation of the femurs and external rotation of the tibias, and the hips may be adducted in the coronal plane. The typical equino-valgus foot deviation seen in spastic diplegia includes hind-foot valgus, breaching of the mid-foot, abduction of the forefoot and consequent hallux valgus (6,14).

Possible causes for the typical gait deviations can be primary, secondary or tertiary. Primary causes pertain to CNS pathology. Secondary causes are due to progressive musculo-skeletal pathology, including muscle shortening, bony torsion, joint instability and degenerative arthritis. Tertiary coping responses can be either compensatory (helpful) or pathological (detrimental) (6). For example, excessive ankle plantar-flexion in mid-stance may be due to a primary cause such as ankle plantar-flexor spasticity or a secondary cause such as myostatic ankle plantar-flexor contracture. Additionally, a tertiary response may be adopted to cope with excessive plantar-flexion such as knee hyper-extension in mid-stance (excessive plantar-flexion/knee extension couple), which can be pathological, or posterior trunk tilt in mid-stance, which can be compensatory.

Clinical management requires the identification of movement abnormalities and their causes. Once this has been performed, the appropriate management options can be considered. Primary abnormalities are likely to respond to spasticity management whether systemic (intrathecal or oral anti-spasmodic drugs and selective dorsal rhizotomy) or focal (Botulinum Toxin A). Secondary abnormalities will require orthopedic intervention (bony or soft-tissue surgery or both). No direct attempt should be made

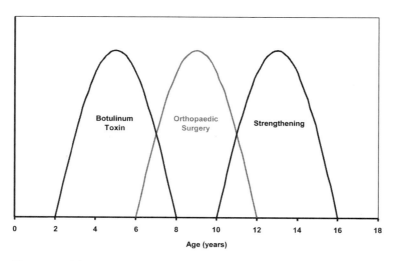

Figure 1 Three phases of management of children with impaired locomotor function as a result of CP.

to "correct" tertiary abnormalities as they resolve when the primary and secondary issues are overcome (Fig. 1).

Because the relative balance of primary and secondary abnormalities is a consequence of development, the management of children with CP is related to age. In the early years, the primary abnormalities and the primary goal is spasticity management, most commonly now with Botulinum Toxin. The increasing severity of musculoskeletal abnormalities then often demands orthopedic intervention, which is best reserved until the skeleton is reasonably mature. Modern surgical techniques now allow for definitive surgery in mid-childhood leading to optimal function in late childhood. Many children, however, will find increasing difficulties in locomotor function accompanying rapid growth in early adolescence. There is thus a third phase during which management must focus on maintaining adequate muscle strength and general fitness.

Three-dimensional gait analysis (3-DGA) is only of limited use in the first phase of management, because the tools for spasticity management are fairly blunt and there is little need for detailed assessment and because children are generally too young to comply with the demands of the assessment itself. It is in the second, orthopedic, phase of management that a detailed assessment of locomotor impairment is necessary and gait analysis is most frequently used. Weakness, in the third phase of management, is assumed to be a generalized problem with management not requiring the specificity gait analysis can offer.

There is now a fairly widespread consensus on the procedures for gait analysis for children with CP. Almost all major centers conduct a thorough clinical examination and collect three-dimensional kinematic and kinetic data (17–20). Surface electromyography (EMG) is only slightly less common and fine-wire EMG may be required for some of the deeper or smaller muscles of the leg. Although collecting data reliably is a considerable skill, the biggest challenge in gait analysis is the interpretation of the data. Expertise in surgical and physiotherapy management of children with CP, gait analysis data collection techniques, and musculoskeletal biomechanics is required. Because it is rare to find an individual possessing all of these skills, interpretation of gait analysis data is generally a team activity. There are two stages to the analysis—identification of abnormalities and attribution of causes. Depending on the composition of the interpretation team, clinical decision-making can be considered either as a third component of the analysis or as separate to the process. Equal in importance to the role of gait analysis in biomechanical analysis and surgical decision-making is its role in clinical audit of surgery. The term "clinical audit" refers to retrospective but systematic analysis of the outcomes of routine clinical services.

Many of the improvements in surgery for children with CP over the last two decades have arisen as a direct result of the increased understanding of these conditions and the effects of orthopedic intervention that gait analysis has enabled. There are some who would argue that with the increased understanding of locomotor pathology in CP, gait analysis of individual children may eventually be no longer required. In fact, recently, there has been some quite severe criticism of the role of gait analysis in children with CP. This has focused on two issues. Noonan et al. (21) and Gorton et al. (22,23) have shown that gait analysis data varies considerably from one laboratory to another. Assuring the quality of data is undoubtedly the biggest challenge facing gait analysis for children with CP, but it is illogical to conclude that collecting no data would be preferable. Noonan et al. (21) and Skaggs et al. (24) have also shown variability to exist in surgical decision-making, based on gait analysis data. In both of these studies there was no consideration as to whether decision-making was more or less consistent in the absence of gait analysis data. The appropriate conclusion is probably that more intensive study of locomotor impairment and orthopedic intervention using objective techniques is required and not less.

II. CLASSIFICATIONS OF GAIT PATTERNS USING GAIT ANALYSIS IN CP

3-DGA promotes understanding of the variable range of gait deviations seen in children with CP and highlights the heterogeneity of gait even within well-defined populations such as spastic hemiplegia or diplegia. The expertise required in the interpretation of 3-DGA data and the difficulties with summarizing the variable range of possible gait deviations in children with

CP have lead to attempts to develop classification systems. Previous classifications of gait in CP using 3-DGA have either been based on a quantitative approach (9,25–27), a qualitative approach (16,28) or combined quantitative data with qualitative pattern recognition (7,10,11,15). Other classifications of gait in CP have been based on observational-rating scales (29–34). A major limitation of classifications based on pure quantitative approach is their limited acceptance and utilization in both clinical and research communities.

The Winters and Gage (1987) classification of spastic hemiplegic gait is one of the most widely used classifications of CP gait using 3-DGA (11). This classification, which is based on sagittal plane kinematics, combines the use of qualitative and quantitative data to construct four groups of gait deviations with a graduated distal to proximal involvement. Thus, Grade I indicates that the only gait anomaly is a foot drop during swing, whereas a Grade IV indicates involvement of the hip, knee, and ankle in swing and stance phases. Accordingly, it helps to simplify a wide variety of gait deviations into four manageable categories and assists with communication of gait dysfunction amongst clinicians with and without direct access to 3-DGA. In addition, the classification has been used to assist with intervention planning and a management algorithm for focal spasticity and contractures requiring orthopedic surgery in children with spastic hemiplegia (10,35).

Although this practical and rather simple classification has been widely utilized by clinicians and researchers, there are some limitations to consider. Like other gait classifications in CP, the Winters and Gage classification applies only to deviations in the sagittal plane. Although such deviations are usually most relevant to the management of spasticity and contracture (35), deviations in the transverse plane resulting from pelvic rotation or bony torsion, or in the coronal plane secondary to limb length discrepancy and/or hip subluxation, are not only common but also important in clinical decision-making and intervention planning (3,12,35). In addition to this issue of content validity, the classification was constructed on a sample of convenience. The possible shortcoming of this approach is a skewed representation towards the more extreme gait deviations and an underestimation of milder dysfunction.

Although the Winters and Gage classification patterns are assumed to be easily recognizable by any clinician (7,9), inter-rater agreement of the classification has never been formally tested. Additionally, the ability to use the classification patterns to visually rate gait deviations, without reference to the kinematic information, would be extremely useful to the majority of clinicians without ready access to complex 3-DGA systems. This criterion-related validity is yet to be explored within this existing classification of hemiplegic gait.

A more recent classification of gait patterns in children with spastic diplegia, by Rodda et al. (15) at the Hugh Williamson Gait Laboratory in Australia, combined the use of qualitative pattern recognition and quantitative kinematic data. This large cross-sectional study devised a five-group classification of gait patterns with a focus on clinical applicability and practical clinical management, in particular to clinicians without access to gait laboratories. Thus, one of the clear distinctions it makes is between patients in "true equinus," where the heel does not make contact with the ground because the ankle is plantarflexed in mid-stance, and "apparent equinus," where the ankle is actually in dorsiflexion, but the heel still does not make contact with the ground because of the position of the hip and knee. Although also limited to the sagittal plane, it was the first CP gait classification to include repeatability studies as part of the tool development. Like the Winters and Gage (1987) classification, a management algorithm has also been devised for children with diplegia using this classification (10,15).

The other main rating scales for CP, based on OGA, are the Physician Rating Scale (PRS) (32,33), the modified PRS (30), and the Observational Gait Scale (OGS) (29). These can be seen as different stages in the development of the same scale and are based on assigning a score to various elements of the gait pattern and taking the total as indicative of the quality of walking. Thus, for example, in the OGS, initial contact with the toe scores 0, with the forefoot 1, with a flat foot 2, and with the heel 3. The original PRS appeared to lack sensitivity and reliability in detecting changes to gait following treatment (30), and the modified PRS only found satisfactory agreement and discrimination in two of the four sections of the scale. The OGS was developed to improve the sensitivity of the PRS and this was found to have acceptable inter-rater (wk 0.43–0.86) and intra-rater reliability (wk 0.53–0.91), and criterion validity was demonstrated by comparison with 3-DGA (34). Recently, a new Functional Mobility Scale (36) was devised to describe functional mobility in children with CP over three distinct distances. This scale has been shown to have high test–retest and inter-rater reliability (ICC: 0.94–0.95, 95% CI: 0.88–0.99) and construct, content, and concurrent validity was demonstrated (36).

One of the main challenges in the development of a classification tool of gait in CP lies in the balance between qualitative and quantitative data that can reliably distinguish gait patterns into identifiable groups. Obtaining a classification that is useful to clinicians with and without direct access to 3-DGA and gaining wide acceptance of the classification present as further challenges. A classification possessing the foregoing qualities, which is successfully able to incorporate gait deviations in all three planes of motion, would be invaluable to clinicians and researchers alike.

III.   GAIT ANALYSIS IN PD AND HD

Basal ganglia diseases such as PD and HD inevitably result in gait disorders (see Chapters 14 and 15 for further details), with a large proportion of patients also experiencing postural instability and an increased rate of falls (37). Locomotor disturbance is a key feature of PD and is one of the major determinants of activity limitation in people with this disabling neurological condition (37–39). The aim of clinical gait analysis in PD is to determine whether the patient has hypokinesia, ignition disturbance, freezing, or dyskinesia, as well as to ascertain the relative contribution of these movement disorders to gait disability at different phases of the anti-parkin-sonian medication cycle. The severity of gait disorders in PD also varies according to disease duration, the environmental context in which walking occurs, the type of locomotor task being performed, the presence of external cues, and the extent to which the person uses attentional strategies to bypass the defective basal ganglia in order to regulate the walking pattern.

Gait hypokinesia is by far the most common gait deviation in PD. A small number of 3-DGA studies have documented typical deviations in the kinetics and kinematics of gait (See Ref. 40 for a summary, and Refs. 41 and 42). These have shown a deficit in "push-off" power generation by the triceps surae at late stance phase, which in turn reduces step length. In addition, hip flexor "pull-off" power is increased (41), presumably as a compensatory mechanism to help lift the leg into swing phase and to ensure adequate hip flexion during swing in order to minimize the risk of tripping on surface objects. Although anti-parkinsonian medication appears to increase the size of the agonist muscle burst at push-off, it does not always normalize power generation (41). Therefore, rehabilitation strategies are recommended as an adjunct to medication in order to increase stride length (36). Strategies can include such things as the use of white cardboard "cues" on the floor to help focus the person's attention on generating long steps (44), teaching the person to think about walking with long steps in order to walk faster (44) and breaking long or complex locomotor sequences down into component parts, such as the initiation of walking, acceleration phase, steady-state walking, turning, and veering (37). Avoiding simultaneous task performance whenever possible is another strategy used to optimize walking performance (37).

Because 3-DGA requires the resources of a fully equipped gait laboratory, together with the need for patients to perform in a highly "artificial" environment, there have been relatively few reports of gait kinetics and kinematics in PD. One of the problems with laboratory studies of this type is that patients often concentrate on their movement patterns more than usual, thereby bypassing the defective basal ganglia control centers and utilizing the frontal cortical regions of the brain to control movement. It is well established that people with PD can perform movements at near normal speed and amplitude when they use the frontal cortices in this way (45). Clinically, it can also be observed that gait disorders in people with PD are accentuated in complex natural environments such as the home setting, work-places, busy shopping centers, and train stations, where there is a frequent need to turn, avoid obstacles, and divert attention to cognitive tasks such as reading signs or answering a mobile cell phone. Therefore, it is recommended that, where possible, clinical gait analysis takes place in "real" world settings while patients perform functional activities of daily living.

The majority of investigations on hypokinesia have reported the manner in which PD affects the spatial (distance) and temporal (timing) parameters of the footstep pattern (38,39,46–51). These have shown the key clinical features of hypokinesia to be reduced step length, reduced ground clearance, and reduced speed (37,38). In addition, the amplitude of arm swing is less than usual and the person typically walks with diminished trunk rotation. These gait deviations appear to result from neurotransmitter imbalances in the output projections from the internal globus pallidus (Gpi) in the basal ganglia to the pedunculopontine nucleus and other brainstem nuclei sub-serving stepping responses and extensor tone. In addition, the basal ganglia projections from the Gpi to the supplementary motor area and premotor cortex are disrupted, which impair motor planning (52) and the regulation of movement amplitude.

It is relatively easy to measure the spatial and temporal parameters of gait in the clinical setting using a 10-m walkway and stopwatch. While the person walks the length of the walkway at preferred, fast, or slow speeds, the clinician times the walk and counts the number of footsteps. The mean cadence (stepping rate) is the number of steps per minute and the mean step length (m) is calculated by dividing the length of the walkway in metres (10) by the number of steps. A computerized version of this method is available in the Clinical Stride Analyser (CSA) (B & L Engineering, Santa Fe, California, U.S.A.) (53). The retest reliability of the CSA for measuring gait speed and stride length in PD is good, with one study showing it to range from ICC = 0.84–0.88 when patients were tested from 1 day to the next at the same locus of the PD medication cycle (53). Urquhart et al. (54) also showed good retest reliability when patients with PD were repeat tested with a 1-week interval. However, performance varies markedly from peak dose in the PD medication cycle to when the person is "off" (usually in the 30-min period prior to the next dose), and repeat measures across these intervals are not reliable (53,54). The CSA does not enable the clinician to measure stride width or step-to-step changes in the footstep pattern. In situations where a need exists to account for sources of step-to-step variability and map gait changes in performance over time, instrumented walkways such as the GAITRite® can be used to measure variability in all footstep parameters for each step in the series. This includes the measurement of stride width, which Gabell and Nayak (55) argue provides an indicator of balance impairment, on the basis of the assumption that people widen their base of support when unsteady in order to gain stability. In the absence of instrumented walkways, clinicians have used inkpad and moleskins attached to patients heels to record the width and size of steps in a walking sequence (56). This is, however, a cumbersome and time-consuming method of charting changes in performance over time and not practical in most clinical settings.

Ignition disturbance, whereby the person experiences difficulty initiating the first steps in the locomotor sequence, is common in people with PD akinesia. The term "akinesia" refers to an absence of movement. Ignition disturbance is context specific, which means that it is exacerbated in environments where there are multiple competing stimuli, such as busy corridors, narrow passages, or cluttered bedrooms (57). Ignition disturbance is also accentuated when the person has to perform more than one motor or cognitive task at a time (57). People with akinesia can also experience freezing part-way through a locomotor sequence, particularly when the sequence requires the person to turn, negotiate an obstacle, or negotiate doorways and other changes in sensory context. Only one 3-DGA study has reported the biomechanics of akinesia in PD (58). Burleigh-Jacobs et al. (58) showed a disorder of weight transference in order to unload one leg, enabling it to step forward. This was overcome when the patients were provided with auditory cues to trigger the action. Patients report anecdotally that "blocking" of this type can also be temporarily overcome by using tricks such as stepping over a matchbox, an upturned walking stick or their partner's leg, thinking about stepping over a log or listening to a musical beat and trying to step in time to it. Further research is needed to explore the mechanisms by which these strategies enable the person to ignite the walking sequence, as well as to explore how other task and environmental constraints affect ignition disturbance and freezing in people with PD. In the meantime, clinical gait assessment should incorporate a range of environmental settings (e.g., walking in open areas, narrow corridors, through doorways), speeds (preferred, fast, and slow), and tasks (e.g., stand and walk, walk and turn, walk from floorboards to carpet, walk from wide to narrow pathways) and monitor how akinesia is presented according to each constraint.

Dyskinesia during gait occurs in a small proportion of people with PD, after many years on anti-parkinsonian medication. It appears to be particularly common in younger adults with early-onset PD. No research data has yet been reported on the kinetics, kinematics, or spatio-temporal parameters of gait in dyskinesia. OGA is therefore the major method used to evaluate therapy outcomes, even though its reliability and validity are yet to be established for this particular movement disorder. Because dyskinesia can involve the head, trunk, and limbs and varies in amplitude and frequency over time, it is important for clinicians to observe total-body performance on a range of locomotor tasks at frequent intervals in a given time period. The dyskinesia sub-section of the United Parkinson's Disease Rating Scale (59) is a common measurement tool used to quantify the severity and location of this movement disorder.

IV. HUNTINGTON'S DISEASE

Less common than PD yet just as disabling, HD is a basal ganglia disorder that leads to progressive impairments of gait (60–64) and postural stability (65,66). The purpose of clinical gait analysis in HD is to determine the extent to which co-existing voluntary and involuntary movement disorders contribute to the locomotor disorder.

Chorea is the most overt involuntary movement disorder in HD and may cause excessive movements of the head and trunk, upper and lower limbs during the performance of functional tasks such as walking, moving from sitting to standing, and rolling over in bed. The presence of chorea also results in frequent changes in hip, knee, and ankle joint velocities during gait (67). Nevertheless, Koller and Trimble (61) found that reduction of chorea does not necessarily lead to improvements in walking speed, stride length, or footstep cadence. Dystonia is also common in HD. It may cause excessive plantar-flexion and inversion during the stance phase of gait, as well as excessive trunk flexion (63). In addition, knee flexion is often increased during the stance phase of gait, which may be due to dystonia of the hamstring muscles or, more commonly, chorea.

Voluntary movement disorders affecting gait in people with HD include hypokinesia, akinesia, and postural instability. Increased variability of movement is also characteristic of this progressive basal ganglia disease. Recent research by Churchyard et al. (60) has shown that people with HD have reduced walking speed due to shortened stride length and reduced footstep cadence. Gait cycle duration is extended; yet single limb and double limb support times are within normal limits (60). Visual observation reveals that many people with HD also walk with increased step width (61,68,69).

Increased variability in walking speed, cadence, and stride length occurs in the majority of people as the disease progresses (60,61). Because an increase in variability is a marker of disease severity, it needs to be carefully monitored over time. The exact factors contributing to increased variability are not well understood, although within-group variability may reflect the severity of striatal and palladial dysfunction (43). Previous observational gait analysis studies of people with HD have shown that variability of walking speed and stride length increase not only over extended periods such as months and years, but also within a single walking trial (61). Within trial variability of temporal footstep variables has been shown to be 2 to 3 times greater in people with HD than for comparison subjects (43). This suggests that over time, people with HD become progressively more impaired in their ability to regulate footstep timing. The clinical significance of increased variability within footstep patterns of people with HD has not yet been established. However, there is some evidence that excessive footstep variability may be related to an increased risk of falls in the elderly (43,55). The ability to change the relationships between spatial and temporal footstep variables from one step to the next and from one stride to the next on command is retained in people with HD, even though the basic parameters remain abnormal.

As well as pinpointing the sources of variability in locomotor performance, clinical gait analysis in people with HD should be directed towards the identification of factors that reduce safety, independence, or walking speed. This can include identifying the extent to which reduced cadence and step length contribute to reduced gait speed; establishing the relationship between chorea, postural instability, and movement variability; and examining the ways in which the secondary effects of dystonia may cause muscle shortening. The extent to which these factors increase the risk of falls is another key consideration during OGA.

V. GAIT ANALYSIS IN STROKE

Clinical gait analysis is an integral component of stroke rehabilitation, with assessment and analysis of gait dysfunction providing direction to treatment planning and evaluation of gait-training outcomes. Gait deviations occur in around 70% of people following stroke, with up to 86% of patients admitted for rehabilitation unable to ambulate independently (71,72). Recovery of gait following stroke is a primary goal for patients and their rehabilitation teams (73,74). Around 50–80% of survivors achieve independent gait (75,76). As physiotherapists in rehabilitation settings spend around half the available therapy time treating gait disorders, the practice of clinical gait analysis warrants close attention (77).

Gait deviations in stroke vary according to the site, size, and type of lesion and also vary according to the length of time following the event (71). Biomechanical impairments that affect gait immediately following stroke include an inability to generate muscle contractions, as well as inappropriately timed or graded muscle contractions. In the initial weeks following the event, spasticity and alterations to the mechanical properties of muscles may also contribute to gait deviations (78). Muscle weakness, soft tissue contracture, and loss of cardiovascular fitness become apparent, particularly when the ability to walk is not regained quickly (79). Depending on the site of the brain lesion, additional factors such as sensory impairment, cognitive dysfunction, perceptual disorders, and behavioral deficits can adversely affect a person's capacity to ambulate quickly, easily, safely, and with a normal gait pattern.

The abnormal walking patterns resulting from stroke have been described and reviewed in detail (78,80,81). After stroke, people commonly walk very slowly, with a shorter step and stride length and an increased double support phase. They are able to walk faster on demand but are limited to speeds lower than unimpaired adults (82). Timing and step asymmetry are usually present, with the lower limbs exhibiting altered gait phase durations and uneven step sizes. Swing phase of the affected limb is prolonged, with the unaffected limb spending proportionately longer in stance phase (83).

Although the term "hemiparetic" gait pattern is often used in clinical practice, it is recognized that heterogenous and variable pattern of gait disturbances result from stroke (81). Several authors have described common kinematic disorders in stroke, which may be identified by visual analysis of gait (84,85). Studies of joint angular excursion have shown both specific deviations and reduced joint motion in general. Specific sagittal plane kinematic deviations vary but commonly include reduced knee motion in swing and early stance, reduced ankle dorsiflexion in swing and at initial contact, and reduced hip extension in late stance (83, 86–89, 94). Common coronal plane abnormalities of hip hiking and circumduction have also been defined (90). EMG recordings in a number of studies have also shown abnormal muscle activation and control, with variable patterns of reduced activation, excessive and prolonged activation, and co-activation reported (89,91). Joint moment and ground reaction force curves during gait after stroke differ in magnitude from those of unimpaired subjects (83,88,92,94) Power profiles are generally diminished in size, relative to unimpaired subjects, with the degree of amplitude reduction broadly correlated with walking speed (83).

Although stroke causes a primarily unilateral motor impairment, there is increased awareness of the bilateral nature of the gait deviations. Reduced joint amplitude and altered kinetics are evident in the non-affected limb (83),(93), across a range of gait speeds. Biomechanical evaluation of the unaffected limb in stiff-legged gait after stroke has suggested that clinicians must consider the possibility that compensations in the sound limb may have adverse consequences (94). Recent studies also highlight the functional difficulties that people after stroke have with more complex gait tasks such as obstacle crossing (95) or walking while talking (96) or performing cognitive tasks.

Clinical gait analysis after stroke has an important role in assessment of gait ability and planning and in evaluation of gait-training programs. Although many physiotherapy approaches to gait training after stroke have been proposed (79,97,98), all are reliant upon accurate and reliable assessment and analysis of the individual's gait dysfunction. After stroke, different levels of gait analysis are described, varying in complexity and instrumentation required. In clinical settings, the most common form of assessment is OGA, where gait is observed for the presence of specific gait deviations. It can be considered as a diagnostic tool, aiding identification of areas needing intervention (99,100). Despite the widespread use of OGA, there is little consensus about what gait components should be observed and only limited evidence supporting the reliability and validity of this assessment tool (101,102). The few existing studies of the measurement properties of OGA in stroke populations are of limited quality, with no decisive evidence available to support the use of OGA as it routinely occurs in clinical practice (100,103–107).

Gait analysis after stroke also commonly includes simple spatio-temporal measures and functional assessment tools in conjunction with OGA. Gait speed, in particular, has been found to be an important outcome measure as it is being sensitive to change during rehabilitation, correlating with lower limb strength and function, and being related to discharge destination (108,109). Specific scales and ambulation profiles are also available to measure gait outcomes after stroke in terms of independence, functional ability, activity, and participation. Common examples of these include the Motor Assessment Scale (110), the modified Hoffer Functional Ambulation Scale (111) and the Modified Emory Functional Ambulation Profile (112). Recognition of activity limitations after stroke has further prompted clinicians to more carefully and systematically analyze gait ability in wider community contexts and with altering task conditions. These include a challenging terrain such as uneven surfaces or surfaces in motion (e.g., escalators, buses) and tasks such as negotiating obstacles, walking while carrying or talking, or walking through crowds (113).

Recent reports also describe the use of more sophisticated laboratory-based measures such as 3-DGA to evaluate gait dysfunction after stroke. The major role of this technology in gait after stroke has been as a research tool to either describe the biomechanical changes or evaluate efficacy of interventions. Insights gained from biomechanical analysis have clearly identified a need for clinicians to consider the underlying forces (kinetics) that cause the observable kinematic gait pattern. For example, identification of abnormalities in power generation after stroke has challenged therapists to consider training of specific muscle groups such as the ankle plantar-flexors (83). Similarly, the increased knowledge of the complex biomechanics underlying spastic paretic stiff-legged gait provides assistance to clinicians seeking to analyze an individual's gait dysfunction (91,93,94). Three-dimensional motion analysis has also provided evidence about therapy efficacy, including specific therapy programs (114), ankle–foot orthoses (115), and medical interventions such as intrathecal baclofen (116). As 3-DGA is expensive, time consuming, and difficult to access, it is unlikely that this form of measurement will become routine for evaluation of gait disorders post-stroke. However, experts in rehabilitation now suggest that 3-DGA analysis may be useful to assist clinical decision-making for selected patients after stroke (83,117,118).

There are several typical gait disorders that frequently occur following stroke. Three common deviations are knee hyper-extension, abnormal patterns of lateral pelvic displacement (LPD), and reduced push-off power of the triceps surae at late-stance phase. For example, knee hyper-extension occurs in more than 40% of ambulant stroke patients and results in a cosmetically unacceptable limp, damage to the anterior cruciate ligament and posterior capsule of the knee joint and, eventually, pain and disability. Morris et al. (70) showed that knee hyper-extension values ranged from 5° to 20° in acute-rehabilitation phase patients and noted that it can range up to 40° in chronic stroke patients. Although therapy based on a motor relearning approach and the use of electrogoniometric biofeedback reduced the amplitude of knee hyper-extension in most patients, ongoing disability was noted in some. Because knee hyper-extension is essentially a sagittal-plane amplitude regulation disorder, it can easily be observed in the clinical setting using simple visual analysis procedures. The clinician views the person from the side while they perform several gait trials at different speeds, with and without orthoses, and the maximum and typical hyper-extension values at heel strike, mid-stance, and terminal stance are documented.

In the early rehabilitation phase, some stroke patients also exhibit increased amplitude of LPD, such as patients who walk with a wide base of support that requires the pelvis to laterally displace further in order to balance over the weight-bearing foot. A recent study of 15 people (mean age: 77.2 years; SD: 8.1) assessed soon after their stroke (mean time since stroke: 28.3; SD: 15.4 days) confirmed that the amplitude of LPD was significantly larger than demonstrated by unimpaired matched controls (120). Other patients demonstrate decreased amplitude of LPD, as occurs in people who over-constrain pelvic motion due to a fear of falling. A separate study of 20 chronic stroke patients (mean: 61 years; SD: 6.5 years; stroke duration median before testing: 10 months) showed that abnormal patterns of LPD could persist long after the stroke (121). Compared with controls, stroke patients had large amplitudes of LPD and reduced displacement of the pelvis toward the paretic side (i.e., more asymmetry) (121). These gait deviations have the potential to increase energy expenditure and the risk of falls and can result in a walking pattern that some people find cosmetically unacceptable.

Another common gait deviation after stroke is reduced ankle power generation of the triceps surae at push-off. Ankle power generation in late stance provides the single largest burst of power generation in the gait cycle of unimpaired adults and has been found to be reduced in gait dysfunction after stroke (83). The magnitude of ankle power generated by individuals after stroke is also highly correlated with gait speed, an established outcome measure of gait performance for this population (109). Impaired push-off is associated with reduced peak knee flexion during swing phase, which is assumed to be related to increased risk of tripping and reduced gait efficiency (94). Push-off has also been identified by physiotherapists as one of the most relevant components of gait analysis (119). As ready access to 3-DGA is impractical or unavailable in rehabilitation, clinicians currently rely upon observation to infer forces associated with push-off. Encouraging recent evidence suggests that therapists can be both reliable and accurate when observing push-off in gait after stroke (107). Eighteen rehabilitation physiotherapists observed videotaped gait performances from 11 subjects after stroke. A high correlation ($r = 0.84$) was obtained between the observations and a concurrent criterion measure of ankle power generation. As yet, the ability of therapists to accurately infer kinetic variables from gait observations, as they routinely occur in clinical settings, is unknown.

VI. SUMMARY AND CONCLUSIONS

Gait deviations are common in people with neurological conditions such as CP, PD, HD, and stroke. OGA is routinely used to assess the severity of neurological deficits in people with these conditions, as well as to monitor the outcomes of therapeutic interventions. To a lesser extent, 3-DGA is used to determine the underlying biomechanical factors that contribute to the abnormal movement pattern. Because gait deviations show wide variation according to the type of neurological condition, disease duration, the effects of medication, and constraints afforded by the environment, task, and therapy, clinical gait analysis needs to take these factors into account during the clinical decision-making process.

ACKNOWLEDGMENTS

The authors of this chapter are members of the National Health and Medical Research Council of Australia, CCRE in Clinical Gait analysis and Gait Rehabiltation. They acknowledge the support of the CCRE in preparing this work.

REFERENCES

1. Toro B, Nester C, Farren P. A review of observational gait assessment in clinical practice. Physiother Theory Practice 2003; 19:137–149.
2. Stanley F, Blair E, Alberman E. Cerebral palsies: epidemiology and causal pathways. Clin Developmental Med. Vol. 151. London: MacKeith Press, 2000: 14–39.
3. Gage JR. Gait Analysis in Cerebral Palsy. London: MacKeith, 1991.
4. Graham HK, Selber P. Musculoskeletal aspects of cerebral palsy. J Bone Joint Surg 2003; 85(Series B):157–166.

5. Scutton D. Physical assessment and aims of treatment. In: Neville B, Goodman R, eds. Congenital Hemiplegia. Clinics in Developmental Medicine. Vol. 15. London: MacKeith Press, 2000:65–80.

6. Bache CE, Selber P, Graham HK. The management of spastic diplegia. Curr Orthop 2003; 17:88–104.

7. Hullin MG, Robb JE, Loudon IR. Gait patterns in children with hemiplegic spastic cerebral palsy. J Pediatr Orthop Part B 1996; 5:247–251.

8. Knutsson E, Richards C. Different types of disturbed motor control in gait of hemiparetic patients. Brain 1979; 102:405–430.

9. O'Byrne JM, Jenkinson A, O'Brien TM. Quantitative analysis and classification of gait patterns in cerebral palsy using a three-dimensional motion analyzer. J Child Neurol 1998; 13:101–108.

10. Rodda J, Graham HK. Classification of gait patterns in spastic hemiplegia and spastic diplegia: a basis for a management algorithm. Eur J Neurol 2001; 8: 98–108.

11. Winters T, Gage J, Hicks R. Gait patterns in spastic hemiplegia in children and adults. J Bone Joint Surg Am 1987; 69A:437–441.

12. Ounpuu S, Deluca P, Davis RB. Gait analysis. In: Neville B, Goodman R, eds. Congenital Hemiplegia. Clinics in Developmental Medicine. Vol. 150. London: MacKeith Press, 2000:81–97.

13. Novacheck TF. Management options for gait abnormalities. In: Neville B, Goodman R, eds. Congenital Hemiplegia. Clinics in Developmental Medicine. Vol. 150. London: MacKeith Press, 2000:98–112.

14. Bennet GC, Rang M, Jones D. Varus and valgus deformities of the foot in cerebral palsy. Develop Med Child Neurol 1982; 24:499–503.

15. Rodda JM, Carson L, Graham HK, Galea MP, Wolfe R. Sagittal gait patterns in spastic diplegia. J Bone Joint Surg Br 2004; 86B:251–258.

16. Sutherland DH, Davids JR. Common gait abnormalities of the knee in cerebral palsy. Clin Orthop Relat Res 1993; March 288:139–147.

17. Davis R, Ounpuu S, Tyburski D, Gage J. A gait analysis data collection and reduction technique. Hum Mov Sci 1991; 10:575–587.

18. Kadaba M, Ramakrishnan H, Wootten M. Measurement of lower extremity kinematics during level walking. J Orthop Res 1990; 8:383–391.

19. Kadaba M, Ramakrishnan H, Wootten M, Gainey J, Gorton G, Cochran G. Repeatability of kinematic, kinetic, and electromyographic data in normal adult gait. J Orthop Res 1989; 7:849–860.

20. Ounpuu S, Gage J, Davis R. Three-dimensional lower extremity joint kinetics in normal pediatric gait. J Pediatr Orthop 1991; 11:341–349.

21. Noonan K, Halliday S, Browne R, O'Brien S, Kayes KJF. Inter-observer variability of gait analysis in patients with cerebral palsy. J Pediatr Orthop 2003; 23:279–287.

22. Gorton G, Hebert D, Goode B. Assessment of the kinematic variability between 12 Shriners motion analysis laboratories. Gait Posture 2001; 13:247.

23. Gorton G, Hebert D, Goode B. Assessment of kinematic variability between 12 Shriners motion analysis laboratories part 2: short term follow up. Gait Posture 2002; 6(suppl 1):S65–S66.

24. Skaggs DL, Rethlefsen S, Kay RM, Dennis S, Reynolds RA, Tolo VT. Variability in gait analysis interpretation. J Pediatr Orthop 2000; 20: 759–764.

25. Kadaba MP, Ramakrishnan HK, Jacobs D, Wootten ME, Chambers C, Scarborough C, Goode B. Quantitative gait analysis pattern recognition in spastic diplegia. In: Proceedings of the 6th Annual East Coast Clinical Gait Analysis Conference. East Lansing, MI: Michigan State University, 1990:9–12.

26. O'Malley MJ, Abel MF, Damiano DL, Vaughan CL. Fuzzy clustering of children with cerebral palsy based on temporal-distance gait parameters. IEEE Trans Rehabil Eng 1997; 5:300–309.

27. Wong MA, Simon S, Olshen RA. Statistical analysis of gait patterns of persons with cerebral palsy. Stat Med 1983; 2:345–354.

28. Rang M, Silver R, De La Garza J. Cerebral palsy. In: Lovell WW, Winter RB, eds. Pediatric Orthopaedics. 2d ed. Philadelphia: JB Lippincott Company, 1986:345–396.

29. Boyd RN, Graham HK. Objective measurement of clinical findings in the use of Botulinum toxin A for the management of children with cerebral palsy. Eur J Neurol 1999; 6:S23–S35.

30. Corry IS, Cosgrove AP, Duffy CM, McNeill S, Taylor TC, Graham HK. Botulinum toxin A compared with stretching casts in the treatment of spastic equinus: a randomised prospective trial. J Pediatr Orthop 1998; 18:304–311.

31. de Bruin H, Russell DJ, Latter JE, Sadler JT. Angle–angle diagrams in monitoring and quantification of gait patterns for children with cerebral palsy. Am J Phys Med 1982; 61:176–192.

32. Koman LA, Mooney JF III, Smith BP, Goodman A, Mulvaney T. Management of spasticity in cerebral palsy with botulinum-A toxin: report of a preliminary, randomized, double-blind trial. J Pediatr Orthop 1994; 14:299–303.

33. Koman LA, Mooney JF III, Smith BP, Walker F, Leon JM. Botulinum toxin type A neuromuscular blockade in the treatment of lower extremity spasticity in cerebral palsy: a randomized, double-blind, placebo-controlled trial. BOTOX Study Group. J Pediatr Orthop 2000; 20:108–115.

34. Mackey AH, Lobb GL, Walt SE, Stott NS. Reliability and validity of the observational gait scale in children with spastic diplegia. Develop Med Child Neurol 2003; 45:4–11.

35. Preiss RA, Condie DN, Rowley DI, Graham HK. The effects of Botulinum toxin (BTX-A) on spasticity of the lower limb and on gait in cerebral palsy. J Bone Joint Surg Br 2003; 85B:943–948.

36. Pirpiris M, Rodda J, Nattrass GR, Graham HK. The functional mobility scale. J Pediatr Orthop. 2004; Sept.–Oct.; 24(5):514–520.

37. Morris ME. Movement disorders in people with Parkinson's disease: a model for physical therapy. Phys Ther 2000; 80:578–597.

38. Morris ME, Iansek R, Matyas TA, Summers JJ. The pathogenesis of gait hypokinesia in Parkinson's disease. Brain 1994; 117:1169–1181.

39. Morris ME, Iansek R, Matyas T, Summers J. Abnormalities in the stride length–cadence relation in parkinsonian gait. Mov Disord 1998; 13(1): 61–69.

40. Morris ME, Huxham F, McGinley J, Dodd K, Iansek R. The biomechanics and motor control of gait in Parkinson's disease. Clin Biomechan 2001; 16:459–470.
41. Lewis GN, Byblow WD, Walt SE. Stride length regulation in Parkinson's disease: the use of extrinsic, visual cues. Brain 2000; 123(Pt 10):2077–2090.
42. Morris ME, McGinley J, Huxham F, Collier J, Iansek R. Constraints on the kinetic, kinematic and spatiotemporal parameters of gait in Parkinson's disease. J Hum Mov Sci 1999; 18:461–483.
43. Hausdorff JM, Cudkowicz ME, Firtion R, Wei JY, Goldberger AL. Gait variability and basal ganglia disorders: stride-to-stride variations of gait cycle timing in Parkinson's disease and Huntington's disease. Mov Disord 1998; 13(3):428–437.
44. Morris ME, Iansek R, Matyas TA, Summers JJ. Stride length regulation in Parkinson's disease. Normalization strategies and underlying mechanisms. Brain 1996; 119(Pt 2):551–568.
45. Cunnington R, Iansek R, Bradshaw JL. Movement-related potentials in Parkinson's disease: external cues and attentional strategies. Mov Disord 1999; 14(1):63–68.
46. Stolze H, Kuhtz-Buschbeck JP, Drucke H, Johnk K, Illert M, Deuschl G. Comparative analysis of the gait disorder of normal pressure hydrocephalus and Parkinson's disease. J Neurol Neurosurg Psychiatry 2001; 70(3):289–297.
47. O'Sullivan JD, Said CM, DillonLC, Hoffman M, Hughes AJ. Gait analysis in patients with Parkinson's disease and motor fluctuations: influence of levodopa and comparison with other measures of motor function. Mov Disord 1998; 13(6):900–906.
48. Murray MP, Sepic SB, Gardner GM, Downs WJ. Walking patterns of men with parkinsonism. Am J Phys Med 1978; 57(6):278–294.
49. Ebersbach GM, Heijmenberg H, et al. Interference of rhythmic constraint on gait in healthy subjects and patients with early Parkinson's disease: evidence for impaired locomotor pattern generation in early Parkinson's disease. Mov Disord 1999; 14(4):619–625.
50. Blin O, Ferrandez AM, Serratrice G. Quantitative analysis of gait in Parkinson patients: increased variability of stride length. J Neurol Sci 1990; 98(1): 91–97.
51. Pedersen SW, Eriksson T, Oberg B. Effects of withdrawal of antiparkinson medication on gait and clinical score in the Parkinson patient. Acta Neurol Scand 1991; 84(1):7–13.
52. Marsden CD. Slowness of movement in Parkinson's disease. Mov Disord 1989; 4(suppl 1):S26–S37.
53. Morris ME, Matyas TA, Summers JJ, Iansek R. Temporal stability of gait in Parkinson's disease. Phys Ther 1996; 76:763–777.
54. Urquhart DM, Morris ME, Iansek R. Gait consistency over a 7-day interval in people with Parkinson's disease. Arch Phys Med Rehabil 1999; 80: 696–701.
55. Gabell A, Nayak US. The effect of age on variability in gait. J Gerontol 1984; 39:662–666.

56. Cerny K. A clinical method of quantitative gait analysis. Phys Ther 1983; 63:1125–1126.
57. Giladi N, Kao R, Fahn S. Freezing phenomenon in patients with parkinsonian syndromes. Mov Disord 1997; 12:302–305.
58. Burleigh-Jacobs A, Horak FB, et al. Step initiation in Parkinson's disease: influence of levodopa and external sensory triggers. Mov Disord 1997; 12(2):206–215.
59. Fahn S, Elton RL. Unified Parkinson's disease rating scale. In: Fahn S, ed. Recent Developments in Parkinson's Disease. New York: MacMillan, 1987:153–163.
60. Churchyard A, Morris M, et al. Gait dysfunction in Huntington's disease: In: Ruzicka E, Hallett M, Jankovic J, eds. Parkinsonism and a Disorder of Timing. Adv Neurol Philadelphia: Lippincott Williams & Wilkins, 2001.
61. Koller WC, Trimble J. The gait abnormality of Huntington's disease. Neurology 1985; 35:1450–1454.
62. Hausdorff JM, Edelberg HK, et al. Increased gait unsteadiness in community-dwelling elderly fallers. Arch Phys Med Rehabil 1997; 78:278–283.
63. Louis ED, Lee P, et al. Dystonia in Huntington's disease: prevalence and clinical characteristics. Mov Disord 1999; 14(1):95–101.
64. Thaut MH, Miltner R, et al. Velocity modulation and rhythmic synchronization of gait in Huntington's disease. Mov Disord 1999; 14(5):808–819.
65. Tian J, Herdman SJ, et al. Postural stability in patients with Huntington's disease. Neurology 1992; 42:1232–1238.
66. Tian J, Herdman SJ, et al. Postural control in Huntington's disease (HD). Acta Otolaryngol Suppl 1991; 481:333–336.
67. Reynolds NC, Myklebust JB, et al. Analysis of gait abnormalities in Huntington's disease. Arch Phys Med Rehabil 1999; 80(1):59–65.
68. Folstein S. Huntington's Disease. A Disorder of Families. Baltimore: The John Hopkins University Press, 1989.
69. Maki BE. Gait changes in older adults: predictors of falls or indicators of fear? J Am Geriatr Soc 1997; 45:313–320.
70. Morris ME, Matyas TA, Bach TA, Goldie PA. Electrogoniometric feedback: its effect on knee hyperextension in stroke. Arch Phys Med Rehabil 1992; 73:1147–1154.
71. Jorgensen HS, Nakayama H, Raashou HO, Olsen TS. Recovery of walking function in stroke patients: the Cohenhagen stroke study. Arch Phys Med Rehabil 1995; 76:27–32.
72. Wade DT, Wood VA, Heller A, Maggs J, Langton Hewer R. Walking after stroke. Measurement and recovery over the first 3 months. Scand J Rehabil Med 1987; 19:25–30.
73. Mulder T, Pauwels F, Nienhuis B. Motor recovery following stroke: towards a disability-orientated assessment of motor dysfunction. In: Harrison M, ed. Physiotherapy in Stroke Management. Edinburgh, UK: Churchill-Livingstone Inc, 1995:275–282.
74. Bohannon R, Andrews A, Smith M. Rehabilitation goals of patients with hemiplegia. Int J Rehabil Res 1988; 11:181–183.

75. Greveson GC, Gray CS, French JM, James OFW. Longterm outcome for patients and carers following hospital admission for stroke. Age Ageing 1991; 20:337–344.
76. Chin P, Rosie A, Irving M, Smith R. Studies in hemiplegic gait. In: Rose F, ed. Advances in stroke therapy. New York: Raven Press, 1982.
77. Goldie PA, Matyas TA, Evans OM. Deficit and change in gait velocity during rehabilitation after stroke. Arch Phys Med Rehabil 1996; 10:1074–1082.
78. Olney SJ, Richards C. Hemiparetic gait following stroke. Part 1: characteristics. Gait Posture. 1996; 4:136–148.
79. Carr J, Shepherd R. Stroke Rehabilitation. Guidelines for Exercise and Training to Optimise Motor Skill. Butterworth-Heinemann, 2003.
80. Bohannon R. Gait after stroke. Orthop Phys Ther Clin North America 2001; 10:151–171.
81. Woolley SM. Characteristics of gait in hemiplegia. Topics Stroke Rehabil 2001; 7:1–18.
82. Bohannon R. Walking after stroke: comfortable vs. maximum safe speed. Int J Rehabil Res 1992; 15:246–248.
83. Olney SJ, Griffin MP, Monga TN, McBride ID. Work and power in stroke gait. Arch Phys Med Rehabil 1991; 72:309–314.
84. Moseley A, Wales A, Herbert R, Schurr K, Moore S. Observation and analysis of hemiplegic gait: Stance phase. Austr J Physiother 1993; 39:259–267.
85. Moore S, Schurr K, Wales A, Moseley A, Herbert R. Observation and analysis of hemiplegic gait: swing phase. Austr J Physiother 1993; 39:271–278.
86. Kuan T, Tsou J, Su F. Hemiplegic gait of stroke patients: the effect of using a cane. Arch Phys Med Rehabil 1999; 80:777–784.
87. Kramers-de Quervain IA, Simon SR, Leurgans S, Pease WS, McAllister D. Gait recovery in the early recovery period after stroke. J Bone Joint Surg 1996; 78A:1506–1514.
88. Lehman JF, Condon SM, Price R, deLateur BJ. Gait abnormalities in hemiplegia: their correction by ankle–foot orthoses. Arch Phys Med Rehabil 1987; 68:763–771.
89. Knuttson E. Gait control in hemiparesis. Scand J Rehabil Med 1981; 13:101–108.
90. Kerrigan D, Frates E, Rogan S, Riley P. Hip hiking and circumduction: quantitative definitions. Am J Phys Med Rehab 2000; 79:247–252.
91. Kerrigan D, Gronley J, Perry J. Stiff-legged gait in spastic paresis. A study of quadriceps and hamstring muscle activity. Am J Phys Med Rehabil 1991; 70:294–300.
92. Carlsoo S, Dahllof A, Holm J. Kinetic analysis of the gait in patients with hemiparesis and in patients with intermittent claudication. Scand J Rehabil Med 1974; 6:166–179.
93. Kerrigan D, Frates EP, Rogan S, Riley PO. Spastic paretic stiff-legged gait: biomechanics of the unaffected limb. Am J Phys Med Rehabil 1999; 78:354–360.
94. Kerrigan D, Karvosky M, Riley P. Spastic paretic stiff-legged gait joint kinetics. Am J Phys Med Rehabil 2001; 80:244–249.

95. Said C, Goldie P, Patla A, Sparrow W. Effect of stroke on step characteristics of obstacle crossing. Arch Phys Med Rehabil 2001; 82:1712–1719.
96. Bowen A, Wenman R, Mickelborough J, Foster J, Hill E, Tallis R. Dual-task effects on talking while walking on velocity and balance following a stroke. Age Ageing 2001; 30:319–323.
97. Bobath B. Adult hemiplegia: Evaluation and Treatment. 3rd ed. Oxford: Butterworth-Heinemann, 1990.
98. Davies P. Steps to Follow. A Guide to the Treatment of Adult Hemiplegia. Berlin: Springer-Verlag, 1985.
99. Pathokinesiology Service and Physical Therapy Department (Rachos Los Amigos). Ranchos Los Amigos Medical Centre, Observational Gait Analysis Handbook, Downey, CA. 1989.
100. Lord S, Halligan P, Wade D. Visual gait analysis: the development of a clinical assessment and scale. Clin Rehabil 1998; 12:107–119.
101. Malouin F. Observational gait analysis. In: Craik R, Oatis C, eds. Gait Analysis: Theory and Applications. St Louis: Mosby, 1995:112–124.
102. Toro B, Nestor CJ, Farren PC. The status of gait assessment among physiotherapists in the United Kingdom. Arch Phys Med Rehabil 2003; 84: 1878–1884.
103. Miyazaki S, Kubota T. Quantification of gait abnormalities on the basis of a continuous foot-force measurement: correlation between quantitative indices and visual rating. Med Biol Eng Comput 1984; 22:70–76.
104. Hughes K, Bell F. Visual assessment of hemiplegic gait following stroke: a pilot study. Arch Phys Med Rehabil 1994; 75:1100–1107.
105. Goodkin R, Diller L. Reliability among physical therapists in diagnosis and treatment of gait deviations in hemiplegics. Percept Mot Skills 1973; 37: 727–734.
106. Riley M, Goodman M, Fritz V. A comparison between observational analysis and temporal distance measurements. S Afr J Physiother 1996; 52:27–30.
107. McGinley JL, Goldie PA, Greenwood KM, Olney SJ. Accuracy and reliability of observational gait analysis data: judgments of push-off in gait following stroke. Phys Ther 2003; 83:146–160.
108. Friedman P. Gait recovery after hemiplegic stroke. Int Disabil Stud 1990; 12:119–122.
109. Richards CL, Malouin F, Dumas F, Tardif D. Gait velocity as an outcome measure of locomotor recovery after stroke. In: Craik R, Oatis C, eds. Gait Analysis: Theory and Application. Mosby: St Louis, 1995:355–364.
110. Carr J, Shepherd R, Nordholm L, Lynne D. Investigation of a new motor assessment scale for stroke patients. Phys Ther 1985; 65:175–180.
111. Perry J, Garrett M, Gronley J, Mulroy S. Classification of walking handicap in the stroke population. Stroke 1995; 26:982–989.
112. Baer H, Wolf S. Modified emory functional ambulation profile. An outcome measure for the rehabilitation of post-stroke gait dysfunction.. Stroke 2001; 32:973–979.
113. Gentile AM. Skill acquisition; action, movement and neuromotor processes. In: Carr J, ed. Movement Science: Foundations for Physical Therapy in Rehabilitation. London: Heinemann Physiotherapy, 1987.

114. Teixeira-Salmela LF, Nadeau S, McBride I, Olney S. Effects of muscle strengthening and physical conditioning training on temporal, kinematic and kinetic variables during gait in chronic stroke survivors. J Rehabil Med 2001; 33:53–60.
115. Gok H, Kucukdeveci A, Altinkaynak H, Yavuzer G, Ergin S. Effects of ankle–foot orthoses on hemiparetic gait. Clin Rehabil 2003; 17:137–139.
116. Remy-Neris O, Tiffreau V, Bouilland S, Bussel B. Intrathecal Baclofen in subjects with spastic hemiplegia: assessment of the antispastic effect during gait. Arch Phys Med Rehabil 2003; 84:643–650.
117. Carr J, Shepherd R. Neurological Rehabilitation: Optimising Motor Performance. Oxford: Butterworth Heinemann, 1998.
118. Olney S, Colborne G. Assessment and treatment of gait dysfunction in the geriatric stroke patient. Topics Geriatr Rehabil 1991; 7:70–78.
119. Patla A, Proctor J, Morson B. Observation of aspects of visual gait assessment: a questionnaire study. Physiother Can 1987; 39(5):311–316.
120. Dodd KJ, Morris ME. Lateral pelvic displacement during gait: abnormalities after stroke and changes during the first month of rehabilitation. Arch Phys Med Rehabil 2003; 84:1200–1205.
121. Tyson SF. Trunk kinematics in hemiplegic gait and the effect of walking aids. Clin Rehabil 1999; 13:295–300.
122. Bohannon R. Gait after stroke. Orthop Phys Ther Clin North America 2001; 10:151–171.
123. Woolley SM. Characteristics of gait in hemiplegia. Topics Stroke Rehabil 2001; 7:1–18.
124. Bohannon R. Walking after stroke: comfortable vs. maximum safe speed. Int J Rehabil Res 1992; 15:246–248.
125. Olney SJ, Griffin MP, Monga TN, McBride ID. Work and power in stroke gait. Arch Phys Med Rehabil 1991; 72:309–314.
126. Moseley A, Wales A, Herbert R, Schurr K, Moore S. Observation and analysis of hemiplegic gait: Stance phase. Austr J Physiother 1993; 39:259–267.
127. Moore S, Schurr K, Wales A, Moseley A, Herbert R. Observation and analysis of hemiplegic gait: swing phase. Austr J Physiother 1993; 39:271–278.
128. Kuan T, Tsou J, Su F. Hemiplegic gait of stroke patients: the effect of using a cane. Arch Phys Med Rehabil 1999; 80:777–784.
129. Kramers-de Quervain IA, Simon SR, Leurgans S, Pease WS, McAllister D. Gait recovery in the early recovery period after stroke. J Bone Joint Surg 1996; 78A:1506–1514.
130. Lehman JF, Condon SM, Price R, deLateur BJ. Gait abnormalities in hemiplegia: their correction by ankle–foot orthoses. Arch Phys Med Rehabil 1987; 68:763–771.
131. Knuttson E. Gait control in hemiparesis. Scand J Rehabil Med 1981; 13:101–108.
132. Kerrigan D, Frates E, Rogan S, Riley P. Hip hiking and circumduction: quantitative definitions. Am J Phys Med Rehab 2000; 79:247–252.
133. Kerrigan D, Gronley J, Perry J. Stiff-legged gait in spastic paresis. A study of quadriceps and hamstring muscle activity. Am J Phys Med Rehabil 1991; 70:294–300.

134. Carlsoo S, Dahllof A, Holm J. Kinetic analysis of the gait in patients with hemiparesis and in patients with intermittent claudication. Scand J Rehabil Med 1974; 6:166–179.
135. Kerrigan D, Frates EP, Rogan S, Riley PO. Spastic paretic stiff-legged gait: biomechanics of the unaffected limb. Am J Phys Med Rehabil 1999; 78: 354–360.
136. Kerrigan D, Karvosky M, Riley P. Spastic paretic stiff-legged gait joint kinetics. Am J Phys Med Rehabil 2001; 80:244–249.
137. Said C, Goldie P, Patla A, Sparrow W. Effect of stroke on step characteristics of obstacle crossing. Arch Phys Med Rehabil 2001; 82:1712–1719.
138. Bowen A, Wenman R, Mickelborough J, Foster J, Hill E, Tallis R. Dual-task effects on talking while walking on velocity and balance following a stroke. Age Ageing 2001; 30:319–323.
139. Bobath B. Adult hemiplegia: Evaluation and Treatment. 3rd ed. Oxford: Butterworth-Heinemann, 1990.
140. Davies P. Steps to Follow. A Guide to the Treatment of Adult Hemiplegia. Berlin: Springer-Verlag, 1985.
141. Pathokinesiology Service and Physical Therapy Department, Observational Gait Analysis Handbook, Downey, CA:Rachos Los amigos Medical Centre. 1989.
142. Lord S, Halligan P, Wade D. Visual gait analysis: the development of a clinical assessment and scale. Clin Rehabil 1998; 12:107–119.
143. Malouin F. Observational gait analysis. In: Craik R, Oatis C, eds. Gait Analysis: Theory and Applications. St Louis: Mosby, 1995:112–124.
144. Toro B, Nestor CJ, Farren PC. The status of gait assessment among physiotherapists in the United Kingdom. Arch Phys Med Rehabil 2003; 84: 1878–1884.
145. Miyazaki S, Kubota T. Quantification of gait abnormalities on the basis of a continuous foot-force measurement: correlation between quantitative indices and visual rating. Med Biol Eng Comput 1984; 22:70–76.
146. Hughes K, Bell F. Visual assessment of hemiplegic gait following stroke: a pilot study. Arch Phys Med Rehabil 1994; 75:1100–1107.
147. Goodkin R, Diller L. Reliability among physical therapists in diagnosis and treatment of gait deviations in hemiplegics. Percept Mot Skills 1973; 37: 727–734.
148. Riley M, Goodman M, Fritz V. A comparison between observational analysis and temporal distance measurements. S Afr J Physiother 1996; 52: 27–30.
149. McGinley JL, Goldie PA, Greenwood KM, Olney SJ. Accuracy and reliability of observational gait analysis data: judgments of push-off in gait following stroke. Phys Ther 2003; 83:146–160.
150. Friedman P. Gait recovery after hemiplegic stroke. Int Disabil Stud 1990; 12:119–122.
151. Richards CL, Malouin F, Dumas F, Tardif D. Gait velocity as an outcome measure of locomotor recovery after stroke. In: Craik R, Oatis C, eds. Gait Analysis: Theory and Application. Mosby: St Louis, 1995:355–364.

152. Carr J, Shepherd R, Nordholm L, Lynne D. Investigation of a new motor assessment scale for stroke patients. Phys Ther 1985; 65:175–180.
153. Perry J, Garrett M, Gronley J, Mulroy S. Classification of walking handicap in the stroke population. Stroke 1995; 26:982–989.
154. Baer H, Wolf S. Modified emory functional ambulation profile. An outcome measure for the rehabilitation of post-stroke gait dysfunction.. Stroke 2001; 32:973–979.
155. Gentile AM. Skill acquisition; action, movement and neuromotor processes. In: Carr J, ed. Movement Science: Foundations for Physical Therapy in Rehabilitation. London: Heinemann Physiotherapy, 1987.
156. Teixeira-Salmela LF, Nadeau S, McBride I, Olney S. Effects of muscle strengthening and physical conditioning training on temporal, kinematic and kinetic variables during gait in chronic stroke survivors. J Rehabil Med 2001; 33:53–60.
157. Gok H, Kucukdeveci A, Altinkaynak H, Yavuzer G, Ergin S. Effects of ankle–foot orthoses on hemiparetic gait. Clin Rehabil 2003; 17:137–139.
158. Remy-Neris O, Tiffreau V, Bouilland S, Bussel B. Intrathecal Baclofen in subjects with spastic hemiplegia: assessment of the antispastic effect during gait. Arch Phys Med Rehabil 2003; 84:643–650.
159. Carr J, Shepherd R. Neurological Rehabilitation: Optimising Motor Performance. Oxford: Butterworth Heinemann, 1998.
160. Olney S, Colborne G. Assessment and treatment of gait dysfunction in the geriatric stroke patient. Topics Geriatr Rehabil 1991; 7:70–78.
161. Patla A, Proctor J, Morson B. Observation of aspects of visual gait assessment: a questionnaire study. Physiother Can 1987; 39(5):311–316.
162. Dodd KJ, Morris ME. Lateral pelvic displacement during gait: abnormalities after stroke and changes during the first month of rehabilitation. Arch Phys Med Rehabil 2003; 84:1200–1205.
163. Tyson SF. Trunk kinematics in hemiplegic gait and the effect of walking aids. Clin Rehabil 1999; 13:295–300.

14

Treatment of Parkinsonian Gait Disturbances

Nir Giladi and Yacov Balash

Movement Disorders Unit, Department of Neurology, Tel Aviv Sourasky Medical Center and Sackler School of Medicine, Tel Aviv University, Tel Aviv, Israel

I. INTRODUCTION

Gait disturbances are among the most important motor problems associated with Parkinson's disease (PD). They are the presenting symptom in 12–18% of the cases and will affect all patients as the disease progress (1,2). Gait disturbances can lead to falls, insecurity, fear, and loss of mobilization and independence, and institutionalization (3). The possibility of losing the ability to walk and the need for a wheelchair is one of the compelling concerns and fears of patients when they are first informed that they have PD. "When will I need a wheelchair?" is one of the most common questions asked by a recently diagnosed PD patient.

The treatment of parkinsonian-gait disturbances should start straightaway at the time of diagnosis and continue throughout the course of the disease. The therapeutic strategy should be based on the concept that walking safely and effectively requires the patient to have a regular exercise program directed to support effective postural responses and avoid falls, to preserve locomotion ability at a reasonable speed, and to have general confidence in the ability to maintain balance as well as relatively preserved mental function. Insecurity combined with fear of falling can lead to loss of independent walking unrelated to the patient's physiological status. Cognitive decline can cause misjudgment of real obstacles in the environment as well as diminish the patient's actual abilities to maintain an effective walking pattern. Assessing and treating affective and cognitive states can play a vital role in the fight to keep patients walking independently and effectively.

The therapeutic strategies in parkinsonian-gait disturbances should take into consideration the stage of the disease and the degree of disability. As such, this chapter will first deal with the clinical approach to the parkinsonian patient at the early stages of the disease when there are objective gait disturbances but their impact on daily function is still between minor and moderate. All patients at these stages are fully independent but are understandably worried about the future. The second part of this chapter will discuss the therapeutic approach for an advanced PD patient when all effort is focused on the need to prevent falls and maintain independence. The under-cited therapeutic studies strategies were rated according to evidence-based criteria proposed by the American Academy of Neurology (4). For orientation in the current levels of evidence, class I provides the strongest evidence.

II. TREATMENT OF GAIT DISTURBANCES IN THE EARLY STAGES OF PARKINSONISM

A. Gait Disturbances Typical to the Early Stages of the Disease

At the time of diagnosis of PD, the most common presentations are complaints of slowness of locomotion, shuffling gait (also noting the sounds of shoes or slippers being dragged on the floor), and decreased arm swing, mainly on the more affected side of the body. These symptoms develop slowly and, as a result, most patients are not aware of the growing problem. It is frequently the spouse who first notices such changes and organizes the first appointment with the doctor. The fact that there is no significant disability and that the patient can adjust his/her daily activities according to his/her altered walking speed (such as leaving the house several minutes earlier in order not to be late for a meeting) is an important element in the mapping out of current patient management.

Other more significant gait disturbances which can be experienced during the early stages of PD but are less frequently seen include: freezing of gait (FOG) in up to 7.1% of the patients prior to initiation of any treatment (5), postural instability and falls [seen in 1.3% of 800 patients (5) and more commonly among older patients (14)], and leg dystonia with pain [observed in 0.4% of the same 800 patients (5)].

General fatigue reported by [50%] of 66 patients (6), low-back pain due to rigidity of lumbar muscles [42.9% of 14,530 patients (7)], and orthostatic hypotension (14%) of 51 patients with de novo PD (8), can also contribute to walking difficulties.

Based on our own clinical experience, we propose to subdivide progressive gait deterioration in the following stages with respective approach to the treatment (Table 1). (Compare with Tables 1–3 in Chapter 1.)

B. Long-term Prevention Approach

Based on the general knowledge that as PD progresses gait and balance problems will inevitably develop, a "delaying" approach should be taken from the time of diagnosis. The therapeutic plan should be geared to deal with the patient's general physical condition, general affective and cognitive aspects, strategies for the prevention of falls and associated injuries, as well as adopting a positive attitude of being active and taking responsibility in the fight for independence and mobility.

Many nonneurological problems can affect mobility and balance among these adult patients. They should be urged to aggressively treat any existing hyperlipidemia, diabetes, cardiac problems, and hypertension (10). They should be encouraged from the very early stages of the disease to keep their body weight down to BMI = 25 or less, considering the deleterious contribution of overweight to instability and immobilization (11) as well as to brain dysfunction and the development of dementia (12). Special attention should be given to the condition of the feet, joints, and spinal column because of the affect of orthopedic problems upon general mobility (13). In general, patients in the early stages of the disease do not realize the extent to which their general health status will impact their future mobility, and it is the responsibility of the neurologist to make the patient aware of these dynamics. This approach should be maintained throughout the course of the disease, and every visit should start with a discussion on the assessment and control of nonneurological issues.

Gait disturbances and falls are closely related to the individual's affective state and cognition (10,15–18). Depressed people fall and break bones as a result of their falls more frequently than nondepressed people (16–18). Aggressive treatment of depression can have a significant impact on the willingness of the PD patient to exercise and take steps to enhance his/her physical fitness. It is vitally important to treat depression either medically or by psychosocial support or both. Among its many benefits, physical activity can also improve mood with its recognized positive consequences. Dementia is a widespread complication of advanced PD and a significant contributing factor to the occurrence of falls (19,21). Dementia is the end result of many solely progressive pathological processes, such as atherosclerosis, hyperhomocysteinemia, obesity, depression, lack of cognitive stimulation, or head trauma (16,22,24–27), in addition to primary neurodegeneration. Treating all secondary risk factors can delay or slow down the rate of cognitive decline, with significant impact on the mental

Table 1 Stages of Gait Deterioration in PD Progression (9)

Stage	Degree of disability	Clinical features	Treatment
I	Negligible functional significance	Decreased arm(s) swing; decreased gait speed, short steps; increased stride-to stride variability	No need for drug treatment. Daily walking for 30–45 min
II	Mild-moderate functional disturbance	Slow and shuffling gait, flexed posture, short stride; short-lasting turning and starting hesitations. Festinations	Selegiline, rasagiline, amantadine, L-dopa, dopamine agonists, physiotherapy, daily walking for 30–45 min
III	Severe functional disturbance	Unable to walk during "OFF" state Dyskinetic gait during "ON" state Insecure gait Ataxic gait Long-lasting freezing episodes Recurrent falls Significant fear of falling Orthostatic hypotension	Fine adjustment of medications Treatment of orthostatic hypotension Teaching of cueing Intensive physiotherapy Improvement of alertness and mentation Treatment of depression and anxiety Deep brain stimulation
IV	No independent walking	Severe postural instability Frequent falls Severe fear of falling—phobia Cognitive decline or dementia Severe flexed posture, unable to straighten knees, feet contractions Severe orthostatic hypotension	Walker with constant support Physiotherapy Training for improvement of alertness and cognition Treatment of orthostatic hypotension Wheelchair Better adjustment of medications

and gait performance of PD patients in the more advanced stages of the disease (20).

Another aspect of delaying potential consequences of PD is the early detection and aggressive treatment of osteoporosis. Osteoporotic bone is significantly more vulnerable to injury, and even minor trauma can sometimes cause fractures that require surgery and lead to loss of mobility. All PD patients should be educated to assess their bone density continuously throughout the course of the disease and follow professional advice to attempt to ward it off or treat it.

Following a disciplined regimen of daily exercise has many positive outcomes, several of which were mentioned above. It is common belief that exercise during the early stages of PD will delay or slow down physical deterioration and loss of mobility. The few studies that have evaluated this have shown that the condition of patients with PD who suffer from FOG could be improved by balance training and high-intensity resistance training as well as increase the perceived functional independence and quality of life in individuals with PD (23), class III study (24–26).

C. Symptomatic Medical Treatment

Symptomatic medical treatment aimed specifically for gait disturbances in the early stages of PD should be given only if it causes significant disability. The main concern for considering the initiation of anti-parkinsonian treatment is the risk of falls. Another common cause to weigh drug initiation is painful rigidity of one leg as well as dystonic posturing while walking. A mildly to moderately slow gait or a decreased arm swing do not justify the use of drugs, unlike a history of frequent falls or shuffling gait with low ground clearance for which drugs should be given. The 4 major groups of medications are: amantadine, MAO-B inhibitors, dopamine agonists, and levodopa. The first 2 have mild to modest symptomatic effect and are given mainly for patients with FOG or other episodic gait disturbances (e.g., festination). Selegiline has been shown to be possibly effective for the treatment of FOG in the DATATOP study [5, 27] class I studies). Similarly, rasagiline (a second generation MAO-B inhibitor) was shown to be of significant benefit over placebo for the treatment of FOG in PD [28] class I study). Amantadine has also been reported in open studies to be of some benefit for the treatment of FOG as well as for general parkinsonian gait (29–31).

Both dopamine agonists and levodopa were effective for the treatment of gait by improving gait stride and speed as well as gait rhythmicity [32,33] class II study). Some prospective studies been suggested, however, that dopamine agonists might increase FOG ([34–36] class I studies).

D. Symptomatic Nonmedical Treatment

The role of physiotherapy in the early stages of PD is questionable. A daily walk for 30–45 min is probably the best recommendation one can give to a recently diagnosed parkinsonian patient. Special attention should be given to posture. Some patients develop a stooping posture at very early stages and their camptocormia (bent spine) is almost predictable. Those patients should receive specific instructions and physical treatment from the early stages of the disease and pay strict attention to his/her posture. It is our experience that hydrotherapy has a specific beneficial effect on posture, and patients who tend to bend forward or to one side (Pisa syndrome) should be recommended to try it. Patients with early postural instability as a major symptom can benefit from physical exercise by improving postural control and reflexes as well as by learning and practicing strategies for avoiding falls and identifying and responding appropriately to situations that pose some risk to them.

One common gait-related question concerns the need to intentionally swing the nonswinging arm while walking. No quantitative study has looked into that question, but one of the undesirable outcomes of walking while intentionally swinging one or two arms is the development of unnatural nonautomatic locomotion. We instruct our patients to walk as naturally as possible and practice an automatic mode, paying no attention to arm swing.

III. TREATMENT OF GAIT DISTURBANCES IN THE ADVANCED STAGES OF PARKINSONISM

A. Gait Disturbances Characteristic to the Advanced Stages of the Disease

Disturbed gait and postural control represent major and very disabling aspects of advanced parkinsonism affecting all patients (37). Walking becomes difficult and patients tend to fall and so they either actually suffer fractures or develop a fear of falling and avoidance strategies with loss of mobility and independence. Gait disturbances initially appear at the "Off" state, when dopaminergic treatment is less effective. As the disease progresses, even the "On" state is associated with gait disturbances and postural instability which manifest as a very short stride while drugging the feet on the ground, a conspicuously stooped posture and a frequent feeling that the feet become glued to the ground (FOG) or a tendency for propulsion and festinations. In addition, significant gait dysrhythmicity with increased stride-to-stride variations can develop and this itself becomes a significant risk factor for falls (38). These symptoms can initially be improved up to the level of a normal gait during the "On" state when medications are effective. Other common problems of advanced parkinsonian stages are involuntary leg movements in the form of "Off" dystonia and "On" dyskinesia. Those involuntary movements are the result of disease progression or long-term dopaminergic treatment. At the advanced stages of parkinsonism, cognitive disturbances play a major role in the fight for mobility and independence without falls. Dementia and psychosis can significantly influence the therapeutic options with regard to both drugs and nonmedical interventions. Other nonmotor symptoms that can significantly affect gait are orthostatic hypotension, leg weakness, general fatigue, and leg or low back pain (see Table 1).

At the advanced stages, treatment is aimed at maintaining mobilization and avoiding falls. When instability becomes a major risk for falls, walking aids can decrease the risk and preserve mobility. Use of a wheelchair is a practical and effective option when all others fail: it affords the patient much safer and easier mobilization.

B. Medical Treatment of Gait Disturbances

Gait disturbances are much more significant during the "Off" state. Fine-tuning of the medical regimen by decreasing the total daily "Off" time and decreasing the severity of "On" dyskinesia can significantly improve mobility and general stability. A combination of 4 to 8 daily dosages of levodopa treatment in combination with dopamine agonist and amantadine can frequently achieve this goal. Subcutaneous injections of apomorphine (another dopamine agonist which acts within 2–3 min) can alleviate "Off" periods and maintain mobility even when "Offs" are unpredictable. Controlled release and long-acting drugs can contribute significantly to the goal of as many "Ons" as possible throughout the day.

Aside from optimal control and fine-tuning of "Off" and "On" periods, specific treatments can improve local problems and nonmotor disturbances. Leg dystonia (painful or nonpainful) can be treated with local injections of botulinum toxin, which has been reported to be of significant clinical benefit (39–41).

General fatigue, weakness, and apathy have been treated with methylphenidate with some benefit (42–44). Ritalin has also been reported to improve gait speed when added to levodopa (43).

Orthostatic hypotension is a common cause of disability, which can present as leg weakness, freezing episodes or light-headedness and instability. The alpha agonist midodrine and the mineralo-corticoid fludrocortisone are very effective in the treatment of orthostatic hypotension in addition to nonmedical treatments such as high elastic socks and high fluid intake.

Medical treatment of depression and dementia can have a significant symptomatic effect on confidence during mobility. It is our common clinical experience that treatment of depressed PD patients who frequently experience FOG with antidepression drugs from the serotonin reuptake inhibitors

(SSRIs group) can dramatically alleviate FOG, however, this has never been assessed systematically. Dementia in PD has improved in response to acetylcholine esterase inhibitors (AChE-I) (45–47). The main improvement with AChE-I concerns cognitive features associated with attention (46,48). Considering the importance of attention to the avoidance of falls (49), it stands to reason that gait and posture can benefit from improved cognition and attention.

Low back pain or referred radicular pain to one or both legs can frequently lead to loss of mobilization and severe stress. Uncontrolled pain can cause considerable stress and worsening of parkinsonian symptoms, including those involving gait and locomotion. Any pain should be treated aggressively by medications or (preferably) locally. Pain can be caused centrally by parkinsonism (50–52). Better adjustment of medications and higher dosages of dopaminergic treatment can lead to significant amelioration of pain even if degenerative changes have been demonstrated on imaging studies of the spine or joints (53).

C. Surgical Treatment of Gait Disturbances in Parkinsonism

At the most advanced stages of PD when drugs are no longer effective and side effects such as dyskinesias are causing major disability, functional neurosurgery at the level of the basal ganglia in the brain has been used successfully over the past 15 years (54). Pallidotomy was the first procedure to be carried out, and deep brain stimulation of the subthalamic nucleus (STN) and the internal globus pallidum (GPi) have been very effective in avoiding motor response fluctuations with the elimination of "Off" periods for the past 10 years. In addition, the ability to decrease medications in patients who have bilateral STN stimulation could stop dyskinesias dramatically. Similarly, bilateral GPi stimulation could also stop dyskinesias but it did so with no decrease of dopaminergic drugs.

Both STN and GPi stimulations have been shown to improve spatio-temporal gait parameters in patients with advanced disease at the "Off" medication state to a level of almost normal walking (55,56).

Other surgical interventions that should be considered on a case-to-case basis are laminectomy in patients with lumbar spinal stenosis or disc hernia, hip or knee replacement in severe degenerative joint disease, and revascularization of the legs in cases of severe peripheral vascular disease.

If a PD patient cannot walk and complains of pain, a differential diagnosis needs to be undertaken, taking into account that other nonparkinsonian causes may be responsible for the disability.

D. Nonmedical Treatment of Parkinsonian Gait Disturbances

Posture, balance, gait, and transfers could be targeted by physiotherapists (57,58). Physical therapy may induce small but significant improvements in gait speed and stride length (57). A sensory, cue-enhanced physical therapy program showed improvements lasting up to 3 months after the therapy had ended (57,59). Examples of possibly useful interventions also include teaching of alternative motor strategies in order to make safer transfers (60), gait training with external weight support (61) and the use of exercises to improve stability, spinal flexibility, and general fitness (62). Patients with FOG should be taught not to try and overcome their motor block during walking, as this may increase the risk of a fall. Physical therapy is best delivered in the domestic situation, as the effects of home treatment exceeded those of hospital-based interventions (63). However, recent meta-analyses concluded that there is little evidence to support or refute the use of physical therapy, because of methodological flaws in published studies (26,57,64). While there is much potential, further study is needed.

Other nonmedical treatments should be focused on preservation of general physical fitness for maintaining good stride and walking speed and educating the patient how to overcome specific difficulties, such as walking in a crowd or avoiding or overcoming a freezing or festinating episode. Specific attention should be given to posture and postural reflexes in order to avoid falls and the development of a fear of falling.

General fitness can be maintained by daily exercise which should be recommended to every patient but even more persuasively to those at the more advanced stages of PD. A daily walk for 30 to 45 minutes during the "On" period is highly recommended for general health as well as for specific physical and mental needs. Patients should be encouraged to walk at their own most comfortable pace, although it is better to avoid frequent stops as much as possible in order to practice the automatic mode. Falling is the most serious complication of a daily walk. Patients should be instructed to walk with comfortable and closed shoes, in daylight, in an open space and avoid obstacles. Walking outdoors has the advantage of practicing locomotion and entails cognitive aspects, such as strategic planning, avoiding obstacles, and interacting with the environment. On the other hand, walking on a treadmill can be safer and has the advantage of introducing external rhythm (sensory cue), although balance is not practiced if the patient holds the bars and the upper body does not move. Still, walking either outdoors or on a treadmill is better than not walking at all. Daily exercise is of great importance to preserve the range of motion of joints, muscle strength, and an upright posture. A decreased range of ankles, knees or hips motion as well as a stooped posture with flexed shoulders can significantly impede the ability to walk. Muscle strength, especially of the legs, plays a major role in maintaining stride length, walking speed, balance, and confidence. As a result, daily exercises should include both stretching as well as strengthening programs. Daily walking has been shown to improve stride length and walking speed with a carryover effect of several months, even when the exercise was stopped (65–67).

Much of the parkinsonian gait can be dramatically improved by focused attention of the patient to the upright posture, stride length and locomotion rhythm (68). Similarly, motor or sensory cues have been shown to be highly effective for the treatment of the parkinsonian gait (57). Stripes on the floor, marching and following external commands or the presence of an external rhythm is commonly used cues (tricks) to maintain mobility in difficult "Off" periods (69). This improvement is maintained, however, only as long as attention is focused upon the act of walking and shortly thereafter (carryover effect), but not for a longer period of time (59). As a result, cues are used to overcome difficult periods but are less effective for normal daily functioning. Since not all patients are aware of the dramatic and clinically significant effect of cueing on parkinsonian-gait disturbances, it is very important to teach them this skill and how to use cues in difficult situations. Having such an easy-to-use and always available solution on hand can improve the PD patient's confidence and, as a result, his/her mobility and independence.

Dysrhythmic locomotion with increased stride-to-stride variation in time is a primary disturbance of parkinsonian gait (70,71) and is associated with increased falls in patients with PD (38). Walking on a treadmill with a fixed speed can improve stride-to-stride variation with a short-term [15 min] carryover effect (72). Similarly, rhythmic auditory stimulation (RAS) has been shown to improve gait rhythmicity as another effective and easy-to-use mode of intervention (73–75). The long-term effect of RAS or treadmill exercise on locomotion has never been studied objectively, but there is good reason to speculate that it should have a positive effect.

Special attention should be given to the episodic gait disturbances of start hesitation and freezing in narrow places and in stressful situations as well as while reaching the destination (76). These episodes can be the result of hypo-dopaminergic treatment but also of a hyper-dopaminergic state. Most FOG episodes are caused by a hypo-dopaminergic state, and enhanced treatment of "Off" periods will decrease their severity (38). When a patient can walk slowly but with no freezing before he/she takes the first morning dose of dopaminergic drugs, and FOG develops shortly after the first morning dose of medications has time to take effect, the patient is experiencing the relatively rare "On" freezing phenomenon and the levodopa dose—especially dopamine agonists—should be tapered down.

FOG can be avoided behaviorally or overcome by cues (57,77). Teaching the patient about FOG and its consequences is the first step to avoid it. Patients should be taught and practice to use the cues at the right time and, more importantly, to deliberately relax during the freezing episode. Only by relaxing can the patient use cues effectively. RAS has been demonstrated to be effective in decreasing FOG frequency (59,60). Similarly, increased visual flow was shown to improve gait velocity and prevent or overcome FOG episodes (78).

Mobilization should be maintained for as long as possible but not at the price of exposing the individual to dangerous falls. Walking aids should be considered if drugs and behavioral treatment cannot maintain safe walking. Only rarely will the patient be the first to suggest the use of walking aids, so the obligation of raising this issue falls upon the doctor or the physical therapist. It is a process that has to be introduced tactfully and requires support and encouragement: this is what all patients fear and dread from the moment they learn that they are affected by PD and represents a turning point in the individual's process of coping with the development of the disease.

A rollator (walker with 3 or 4 wheels) can improve security and balance while maintaining locomotion. Ambulation with a walker has recently been shown to improve internal rhythmicity of gait (72). A classical walker is the next step in order to maintain short distance mobilization, mainly at home. When walking becomes extremely difficult and dangerous and demands much effort and energy but does not substantially improve the patient's quality of life, it is time to switch the patient's mindset to start looking on walking as an exercise without any mobilization goal. This is the time to introduce the use of a wheelchair for actual mobilization and represents the end of the fight for ambulatory independence.

IV. CONCLUSIONS

Walking is a very important motor function for an individual's independence. It is affected by parkinsonism throughout the course of the disease. Gait disturbances are common, easily measured, and observable during the early stages of the disease, but they have minor to moderate functional significance. Treatment is usually not directed towards improvement of locomotion at Hoehn and Yahr (37) stages 1 and 2. The early stages of the disease should be used for the adaptation of a healthy lifestyle, and for aggressively treating all risk factors for atherosclerosis, dementia, and deterioration of physical fitness. Daily exercise can be adopted at this stage to prepare for the future when physical deterioration is inevitable. At the more advanced stages of the disease, walking independently and effectively becomes the main target as a sign of functioning. Medical, surgical, mental, and physical interventions are now focused towards the preservation of independent mobilization. It is a long-term task, which needs a multidisciplinary team of neurologists, internists, ophthalmologists, physical therapists, and many others.

REFERENCES

1. Martin WE, Loewenson RB, Resch JA, Baker AB. Parkinson's disease. Clinical analysis of 100 patients. Neurology 1973; 23:783–790.
2. Pahwa R, Koller W. Gait disorders in parkinsonism and other movement disorders. In: Masdeu JC, Sudarsky L, Wolfson L, eds. Gait Disorders

of Aging. Falls and Therapeutic Strategies. Philadelphia: Lipincott-Raven Publishers, 1997:209–220.

3. Martignoni E, Godi L, Citterio A, Zangaglia R, Riboldazzi G, Calandrella D, Pacchetti C, Nappi G. Comorbid disorders and hospitalisation in Parkinson's disease: a prospective study. Neurol Sci 2004; 25:66–71.

4. Miyasaki JM, Martin W, Suchowersky O, Weiner WJ, Lang AE. Practice parameter: initiation of treatment for Parkinson's disease: an evidence-based review: report of the Quality Standards Subcommittee of the American Academy of Neurology. Neurology 2002; 58:11–17.

5. Giladi N, McDermott MP, Fahn S, Przedborski S, Jankovic J, Stern M, Tanner C, Parkinson Study Group. Freezing of gait in PD: prospective assessment in the DATATOP cohort. Neurology 2001; 56:1712–1721.

6. Herlofson K, Larsen JP. The influence of fatigue on health-related quality of life in patients with Parkinson's disease. Acta Neurol Scand 2003; 107:1–6.

7. Gage H, Hendricks A, Zhang S, Kazis L. The relative health related quality of life of veterans with Parkinson's disease. J Neurol Neurosurg Psychiatry 2003; 74:163–169.

8. Bonuccelli U, Lucetti C, Del Dotto P, Ceravolo R, Gambaccini G, Bernardini S, Rossi G, Piaggesi A. Orthostatic hypotension in de novo Parkinson disease. Arch Neurol 2003; 60:1400–1404.

9. Balash Y, Hausdorff JM, Giladi N. Clinical evaluation and treatment of gait disorders in Parkinson's disease. In: Ebadi M, Pfeiffer R, eds. "Parkinson's disease." In press.

10. Skoog I, Gustafson D. Hypertension, hypertension-clustering factors and Alzheimer's disease. Neurol Res 2003; 25:675–680.

11. McGraw B, McClenaghan BA, Williams HG, Dickerson J, Ward DS. Gait and postural stability in obese and nonobese prepubertal boys. Arch Phys Med Rehabil 2000; 81:484–489.

12. Gustafson D, Rothenberg E, Blennow K, Steen B, Skoog I. An 18-year follow-up of overweight and risk of Alzheimer disease. Arch Intern Med 2003; 163:1524–1528.

13. Bloem BR. Postural instability in Parkinson's disease. Clin Neurol Neurosurg 1992; 94(suppl):S41–S45.

14. Bloem BR, Grimbergen YA, Cramer M, Willemsen M, Zwinderman AH. Prospective assessment of falls in Parkinson's disease. J Neurol 2001; 248:950–958.

15. Adkin AL, Frank JS, Jog MS. Fear of falling and postural control in Parkinson's disease. Mov Disord 2003; 18:496–502.

16. Jantti PO, Pyykko I, Laippala P. Prognosis of falls among elderly nursing home residents. Aging 1995; 7:23–27.

17. Whooley MA, Kip KE, Cauley JA, Ensrud KE, Nevitt MC, Browner WS. Depression, falls, and risk of fracture in older women. Study of Osteoporotic Fractures Research Group. Arch Intern Med1999; 159:484–490.

18. Lenze EJ, Munin MC, Dew MA, Rogers JC, Seligman K, Mulsant BH, Reynolds CF III. Adverse effects of depression and cognitive impairment on rehabilitation participation and recovery from hip fracture. Int J Geriatr Psychiatry 2004; 19:472–478.

19. Anderson KE. Dementia in Parkinson's disease. Curr Treat Options Neurol 2004; 6:201–207.

20. Haan MN, Wallace R. Can dementia be prevented? Brain aging in a population-based context. Annu Rev Public Health 2004; 25:1–24.
21. Camicioli R, Fisher N. Progress in clinical neurosciences: Parkinson's disease with dementia and dementia with Lewy bodies. Can J Neurol Sci 2004; 31:7–21.
22. Sachdev P. Homocysteine and neuropsychiatric disorders. Rev Bras Psiquiatr 2004; 26:50–56.
23. Hirsch MA, Toole T, Maitland CG, Rider RA. The effects of balance training and high-intensity resistance training on persons with idiopathic Parkinson's disease. Arch Phys Med Rehabil 2003; 84:1109–1117.
24. Van Vaerenbergh J, Vranken R, Baro F. The influence of rotational exercises on freezing in Parkinson's disease. Funct Neurol 2003; 18:11–16.
25. Baatile J, Langbein WE, Weaver F, Maloney C, Jost MB. Effect of exercise on perceived quality of life of individuals with Parkinson's disease. Rehabil Res Dev 2000; 37:529–534.
26. De Goede CJ, Keus SH, Kwakkel G, Wagenaar RC. The effects of physical therapy in Parkinson's disease: a research synthesis. Arch Phys Med Rehabil 2001; 82:509–515.
27. Shoulson I, Oakes D, Fahn S, Lang A, Langston JW, LeWitt P, Olanow CW, Penney JB, Tanner C, Kieburtz K, Rudolph A, Parkinson Study Group. Impact of sustained deprenyl (selegiline) in levodopa-treated Parkinson's disease: a randomized placebo-controlled extension of the deprenyl and tocopherol antioxidative therapy of parkinsonism trial. Ann Neurol 2002; 51:604–612.
28. Giladi N, Rascol O, Brooks DJ, Melamed E, Oertel WH, Poewe W, Stocchi F, Tolosa E, LARGO Study Group. Rasagiline treatment can improve freezing of gait in advanced Parkinson's disease: a prospective, randomized, double blind, placebo- and entacapone-controlled study. Neurology 2004; 62(suppl 5):A329–A330.
29. Yoritaka A, Hattori T, Hattori Y, Mori H, Matsuoka S, Shirai T, Kondo T, Mizuno Y. A 85-year-old woman with the onset of progressive gait disturbance at 80 years of the age. No To Shinkei. 1997 ;49:379–389.
30. Ahlskog JE. Medical treatment of later-stage motor problems of Parkinson disease. Mayo Clin Proc 1999; 74:1239–1254.
31. Manek S, Lew MF. Gait and balance dysfunction in adults. Curr Treat Options Neurol 2003; 5:177–185.
32. Kemoun G, Defebvre L. Gait disorders in Parkinson disease. Gait freezing and falls: therapeutic management. Presse Med 2001; 30:460–468.
33. Shan DE, Lee SJ, Chao LY, Yeh SI. Gait analysis in advanced Parkinson's disease—effect of levodopa and tolcapone. Can J Neurol Sci 2001; 28:70–75.
34. Ahlskog JE, Muenter MD, Bailey PA, Stevens PM. Dopamine agonist treatment of fluctuating parkinsonism. D-2 (controlled-release MK-458) vs combined D-1 and D-2 (pergolide). Arch Neurol 1992; 49:560–568.
35. Rascol O, Brooks DJ, Korczyn AD, De Deyn PP, Clarke CE, Lang AE. A five-year study of the incidence of dyskinesia in patients with early Parkinson's disease who were treated with ropinirole or levodopa. 056 Study Group. N Engl J Med 2000; 342:1484–1491.
36. Holloway R, Shoulson I, Kieburtz K, Parkinson Study Group. Pramipexole vs. levodopa as initial treatment for Parkinson disease: a randomized controlled trial. Parkinson Study Group. JAMA 2000; 284:1931–1938.

37. Hoehn MM, Yahr MD. Parkinsonism: onset, progression and mortality. Neurology 1967; 17:427–442.
38. Schaafsma JD, Giladi N, Balash Y, Bartels AL, Gurevich T, Hausdorff JM. Gait dynamics in Parkinson's disease: relationship to Parkinsonian features, falls and response to levodopa. J Neurol Sci 2003; 212:47–53.
39. Giladi N, Meer J, Kidan C, Greenberg E, Gross B, Honigman S. Interventional neurology: botulinum toxin as a potent symptomatic treatment in neurology. Isr J Med Sci 1994; 30:816–819.
40. Dowsey-Limousin P. Parkinsonian dystonia. Rev Neurol 2003; 159:928–931.
41. Tsui JK. Treatment of dystonia in Parkinson's disease. Adv Neurol 2003; 91:361–364.
42. Nutt JG, Carter JH, Sexton GJ. The dopamine transporter: importance in Parkinson's disease. Ann Neurol 2004; 55:766–773.
43. Camicioli R, Lea E, Nutt JG, Sexton G, Oken BS. Methylphenidate increases the motor effects of L-Dopa in Parkinson's disease: a pilot study. Clin Neuropharmacol 2001; 24:208–213.
44. Chatterjee A, Fahn S. Methylphenidate treats apathy in Parkinson's disease. J Neuropsychiatry Clin Neurosci 2002; 14:461–462.
45. Bullock R, Cameron A. Rivastigmine for the treatment of dementia and visual hallucinations associated with Parkinson's disease: a case series. Curr Med Res Opin 2002; 18:258–264.
46. Giladi N, Shabtai H, Gurevich T, Benbunan B, Anca M, Korczyn AD. Rivastigmine (Exelon) for dementia in patients with Parkinson's disease. Acta Neurol Scand 2003; 108:368–373.
47. Fogelson N, Kogan E, Korczyn AD, Giladi N, Shabtai H, Neufeld MY. Effects of rivastigmine on the quantitative EEG in demented Parkinsonian patients. Acta Neurol Scand 2003; 107:252–255.
48. Leitner Y, Barak R, Giladi N, Gruendlinger L, Hausdorff JM. Attention: regulation of stride-to-stride variability of gait may require attention. Mov Disord 2004; 19:S414.
49. Hausdorff JM, Balash J, Giladi N. Effects of cognitive challenge on gait variability in patients with Parkinson's disease. J Geriatr Psychiatry Neurol 2003; 16:53–58.
50. Ford B. Pain in Parkinson's disease. Clin Neurosci 1998; 5:63–72.
51. Waseem S, Gwinn-Hardy K. Pain in Parkinson's disease. Common yet seldom-recognized symptom is treatable. Postgrad Med 2001; 110:33–46.
52. Sage JI. Pain in Parkinson's disease. Curr Treat Options Neurol 2004; 6: 191–200.
53. Waters CH. Treatment of advanced stage patients with Parkinson's disease. Parkinsonism Relat Disord 2002; 9:15–21.
54. Giladi N, Melamed E. The role of functional neurosurgery in Parkinson's disease. Isr Med Assoc J 2000; 2:455–461.
55. Allert N, Volkmann J, Dotse S, Hefter H, Sturm V, Freund HJ. Effects of bilateral pallidal or subthalamic stimulation on gait in advanced Parkinson's disease. Mov Disord 2001; 16:1076–1085.
56. Ferrarin M, Rizzone M, Lopiano L, Recalcati M, Pedotti A. Effects of subthalamic nucleus stimulation and L-dopa in trunk kinematics of patients with Parkinson's disease. Gait Posture 2004; 19:164–171.

57. Rubinstein TC, Giladi N, Hausdorff JM. The power of cueing to circumvent dopamine deficits: a review of physical therapy treatment of gait disturbances in Parkinson's disease. Mov Disord 2002; 17:1148–1160.
58. Plant RD, Jones D, Ashburn A, et al. Physiotherapy for people with Parkinson's disease: UK Best Practice. Short Report. Newcastle upon Tyne: Institute of Rehabilitation, 2001.
59. Nieuwboer A, Feys P, de Weerdt W, Dom R. Is using a cue the clue to the treatment of freezing in Parkinson's disease? Physiother Res Int 1997; 2:125–132.
60. Kamsma YP, Brouwer WH, Lakke JP. Training of compensation strategies for impaired gross motor skills in Parkinson's disease. Physiother Theory Pract 1995; 11:209–229.
61. Schenkman M, Cutson TM, Kuchibhatla M, et al. Exercise to improve spinal flexibility and function for people with Parkinson's disease: a randomised, controlled trial. J Am Geriatr Soc 1998;46:1207–1216.
62. Morris ME. Movement disorders in people with Parkinson disease: a model for physical therapy. Phys Ther 2000; 80:578–597.
63. Nieuwboer A, de Weerdt W, Dom R, et al. The effect of a home physiotherapy program for persons with Parkinson's disease. J Rehabil Med 2001; 33: 266–272.
64. Deane KH, Ellis-Hill C, Jones D, et al. Systematic review of paramedical therapies for Parkinson's disease. Mov Disord 2002;17:984–991.
65. Sunvisson H, Lokk J, Ericson K, Winblad B, Ekman SL. Changes in motor performance in persons with Parkinson's disease after exercise in a mountain area. J Neurosci Nurs 1997; 29:255–260.
66. Lokk J. The effects of mountain exercise in Parkinsonian persons—a preliminary study. Arch Gerontol Geriatr 2000; 31:19–25.
67. Scandalis TA, Bosak A, Berliner JC, Helman LL, Wells MR. Resistance training and gait function in patients with Parkinson's disease. Am J Phys Med Rehabil 2001; 80:38–43.
68. Morris ME, Huxham F, McGinley J, Dodd K, Iansek R. The biomechanics and motor control of gait in Parkinson disease. Clin Biomech 2001; 16:459–470.
69. Burleigh-Jacobs A, Horak FB, Nutt JG, Obeso JA. Step initiation in Parkinson's disease: influence of levodopa and external sensory triggers. Mov Disord 1997; 12:206–215.
70. Baltadjieva R, Giladi N, Balash Y, Herman T, Hausdorff JM. Gait changes in de novo Parkinson's disease patients: A force/rhythm dichotomy. Mov Disord 2004; 19:S138.
71. Hausdorff JM, Cudkowicz ME, Firtion R, Wei JY, Goldberger AL. Gait variability and basal ganglia disorders: stride-to-stride variations of gait cycle timing in Parkinson's disease and Huntington's disease. Mov Disord 1998; 13:428–437.
72. Toledo-Frankel S, Giladi N, Gruendlinger L, Baltadjieva R, Herman T, Hausdorff JM. Treadmill walking as an external pacemaker to improve gait rhythm and stability in Parkinson's disease. Mov Disord 2005; in press.
73. McIntosh GC, Brown SH, Rice RR, Thaut MH. Rhythmic auditory-motor facilitation of gait patterns in patients with Parkinson's disease. J Neurol Neurosurg Psychiatry 1997; 62:22–26.
74. Freedland RL, Festa C, Sealy M, McBean A, Elghazaly P, Capan A, Brozycki L, Nelson AJ, Rothman J. The effects of pulsed auditory stimulation on various

gait measurements in persons with Parkinson's disease. NeuroRehabilitation 2002; 17:81–87.
75. Lowenthal J, Gruedlinger L, Baltadjieva R, Herman T, Hausdorff JM, Giladi N. Effects of rhythmic auditory stimulation on gait dynamics in Parkinson's disease. Mov Disord 2004; 19:S139.
76. Giladi N, Kao R, Fahn S. Freezing phenomenon in patients with parkinsonian syndromes. Mov Disord 1997; 12:302–305.
77. Stern GM, Lander CM, Lees AJ. Akinetic freezing and trick movements in Parkinson's disease. J Neural Transm Suppl 1980; 16:137–141.
78. Ferrarin M, Brambilla M, Garavello L, Di Candia A, Pedotti A, Rabuffetti M. Microprocessor-controlled optical stimulating device to improve the gait of patients with Parkinson's disease. Med Biol Eng Comput 2004; 42:328–332.

15

Treatment of Axial Mobility Deficits in Movement Disorders

Bastiaan R. Bloem and Frank-Erik De Leeuw

Department of Neurology, Radboud University Nijmegen Medical Center, Nijmegen, The Netherlands

Elif K. Orhan

Department of Neurology, Medical School, University of Istanbul, Istanbul, Turkey

I. INTRODUCTION

Axial mobility deficits include difficulties with balance, gait, posture, and transfers. Such mobility deficits are common features of many different basal ganglia disorders (1). Furthermore, axial mobility deficits may occur in patients with cortical lesions, in particular when these involve the frontal lobes or their connecting tracts in subcortical areas. For both groups of patients, these axial mobility deficits can be the sole or predominant sign, but may also coincide with "appendicular" signs (in the hands). For most patients, axial mobility deficits are difficult to treat using standard medical management, including pharmacotherapy and stereotactic neurosurgery. Alternative treatment strategies are now beginning to emerge, including physiotherapy, occupational therapy, and cognitive rehabilitation to reduce fear of falling. Here, we will provide a structured review of the possible treatments for mobility deficits in several common basal ganglia disorders (Table 1), excluding idiopathic Parkinson's disease, which is discussed in Chapter 14.

Table 1 Classification of the Mobility Disorders Discussed in this Chapter

---

Extrapyramidal syndromes
Progressive supranuclear palsy
Multiple system atrophy (MSA-P and MSA-C phenotype)[a]
Huntington's disease
Primary orthostatic tremor
Cerebrovascular disorders
Senile gait disorder
Primary progressive freezing gait
Vascular "lower-body half" parkinsonism
Normal pressure hydrocephalus[b]

---

[a]MSA-P when parkinsonian features predominate (previously also termed striatonigral degeneration), and MSA-C when cerebellar features predominate (previously also termed olivo-ponto-cerebellar atrophy).
[b]Classified separately because the underlying pathophysiology is imprecisely understood.

II. EXTRAPYRAMIDAL SYNDROMES

A. Progressive Supranuclear Palsy (PSP)

1. Mobility Deficits

Postural instability and recurrent falls are important features of PSP that occur early in the course of the disease, often within the first year of onset of first symptoms or even as the initial symptom (2,3). In a recent questionnaire survey (4), we showed that at least one prior fall had occurred since disease onset in no less than 97% of PSP patients (all members of the PSP Association in the UK), as opposed to "only" 65% of patients with idiopathic Parkinson's disease (significant difference at $p < 0.001$). Daily falls were present in some 23% of PSP patients who were still mobile, compared to only 6% of Parkinson patients. Injuries had occurred in 90% of PSP, and this often included fractures (mainly of the arms and hips) and head injuries. PSP patients typically report seemingly "spontaneous" or unprovoked falls, and they usually fall backwards (4,5). Contributing factors include the severity of the balance deficit, freezing of gait, blepharospasm (leading to temporary visual impairment, thereby hampering route finding and scanning of the environment), as well as the retrocollis and vertical gaze palsy which may both lead to falls while climbing or descending stairs (4,6). These physical problems are compounded by "motor recklessness," characterized by an inability to properly judge the risk of e.g., sudden turning movements or transfers.

2. Pharmacotherapy

Treatment options for falls in PSP are summarized in Table 2 and Fig. 1. In the aforementioned questionnaire survey, patients themselves considered

Table 2 Specific Causes and Circumstances of Falls in PSP, as well as Possible Treatment Strategies (Modified from Ref. 1.)

Cause	Treatment
Severe postural instability	Levodopa; amitriptyline; walking aids; physiotherapy
Blepharospasm	Botulinum toxin; prostheses (crutches) mounted on glasses
Vertical gaze palsy	Spectacles fitted with prism glasses
Diplopia	Eye patch
Retrocollis	Botulinum toxin
Motor recklessness	Restriction of activities
Backward falls	Shoes with heightened heels
Indoor falls	Structuring the house; remove domestic hazards
Injurious falls	Hip/wrist protectors; safety helmets; shock absorbing floors

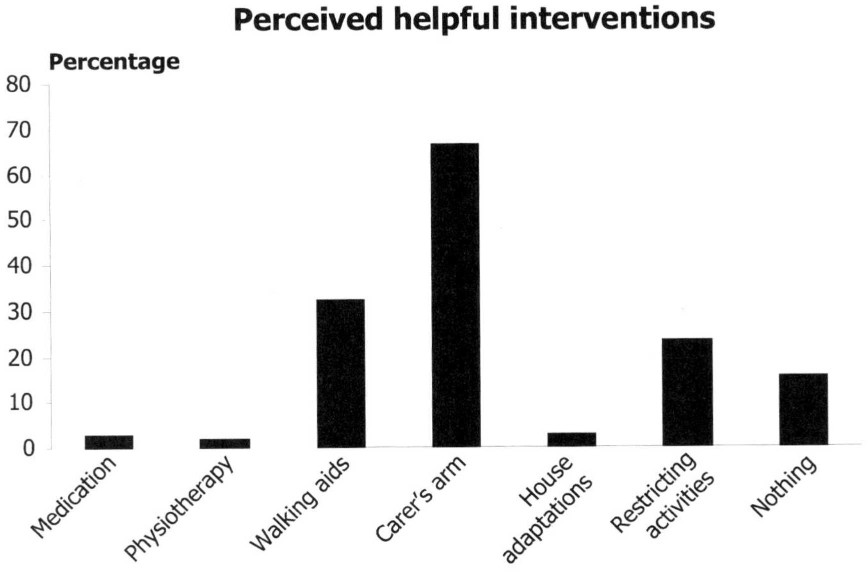

Figure 1 Interventions that patients with PSP perceived to be helpful in reducing their number of falls (From Ref. 4.). Note the high proportion of patients for which only the carer's support, or restriction of activities, or even nothing at all seemed beneficial.

traditional antiparkinson drugs to be rarely helpful (4). Adequate doses of levodopa (up to 1 g/day, if needed) are occasionally effective for a brief period, but most patients have dopa-resistant balance problems. Such patients sometimes benefit from a dopamine receptor agonist (7,8), but some reports failed to observe a response to dopamine agonists in PSP (9,10). Retrospective studies suggest that combinations of different drugs may be more effective than monotherapy (11).

Theoretically, drugs aimed at restoring nondopaminergic deficits might alleviate some balance deficits in PSP patients. Postural control can improve quite dramatically in some patients taking tricyclic antidepressants such as amitriptyline or desipramine (12–14), perhaps by correcting the cholinergic deficit caused by cell loss in the PPN or basal nucleus of Meynert. However, these observations must be corroborated by controlled studies involving large numbers of patients. Involvement of the locus coeruleus may explain the observed therapeutic effects of idazoxan, a selective alpha-2 adrenoreceptor inhibitor that restores the central norepinephrine deficit. Treatment with idazoxan during four weeks in a double-blind crossover study of nine patients with PSP improved clinical ratings of gait and postural instability (15). This drug has been withdrawn because of toxicity.

Several other drugs have been tried, but failed to improve axial motor symptoms in PSP or showed at best brief and inconsistent effects. This included cholinergic agents such as physostigmine or donezepil (16–18) and the serotonin antagonist methysergide (prescribed to correct an assumed overcompensation in the serotonergic system) (19,20). Patients with PSP are overly sensitive to anticholinergics, so their use should be avoided (18).

3. Physiotherapy and Occupational Therapy

Various case reports have suggested that patients with PSP might benefit from active rehabilitation strategies (21–24). Examples of delivered interventions include gait training on a treadmill under conditions of weight support (to reduce "loading" of the legs), exercises to improve strength and coordination, or balance training. Although promising, these findings require confirmation from controlled studies. Pending further studies, we believe a trial of physiotherapy is justified for individual patients with PSP, aiming to maintain independence for as long as possible in mobile patients, and to avoid the secondary consequences of immobilization in severely affected patients.

Occupational therapy has not been studied formally in patients with PSP. Expectations should not be too high because many patients are cognitively impaired, and this may interfere with active participation in the therapeutic process (the same concern also applies to many aspects of physiotherapy). Also, additional disabilities are likely to emerge before new skills have been properly trained because of the usually rapid disease progression. For this reason, occupational therapy might cause frustration for some patients and their carers.

4. Other Measures

One uncontrolled study showed that nine sessions of electroconvulsive therapy [aimed to increase central neurotransmitter sensitivity] improved balance and gait in two out of five patients, but this came at the expense of treatment-related complications such as confusion or leg dystonia (25). The side-effects and intensive treatment regime prohibit more widespread use of electroconvulsive therapy in routine management of PSP. Blepharospasm and neck dystonia (retrocollis) may be alleviated by botulinum toxin injections (23,26). Prostheses (crutches) attached to spectacles can also reduce blepharospasm. Some patients benefit from the use of spectacles fitted with prism glasses, which may help to prevent falls related to vertical gaze palsy. Walking aids can be helpful in the early stages of the disease, but cognitively impaired patients are often unable to use them properly. According to many patients, the supporting arm of the partner or other carer is the only helpful measure to reduce falls (4). If nothing really helps, the focus should shift to injury prevention and activities without strict supervision must be avoided.

B. Multiple System Atrophy (MSA)

1. Mobility Deficits

MSA is characterized clinically by a variable combination of autonomic failure, parkinsonism, cerebellar ataxia and pyramidal signs. The cerebellar features may predominate in some patients (MSA-C phenotype), whereas in others the parkinsonian features predominate (MSA-P phenotype). For both phenotypes, gait and balance disorders are important features, even early in the course of the disease (27,28). Cerebellar ataxia seems to play an important role in causing balance and gait problems (29), leading to a staggering but not necessarily wide-based gait. Patients with the MSA-P phenotype have a shuffling gait with festination and a reduced arm swing, and eventually a mixed pattern of hypokinetic-rigid and cerebellar features can be observed in most patients. Freezing of gait is not uncommon in MSA-P patients (30,31). About 15% of patients suffer syncopal falls due to symptomatic orthostatic hypotension (29).

2. Pharmacotherapy

Antiparkinson medication is generally ineffective and not tolerated well. Particularly patients with post-synaptic striatal lesions or cerebellar pathology respond poorly to dopaminergic treatment (27,32,33). However, some patients can respond favorably for several years (34,35). High dosages of levodopa are usually required, if needed up to 1 g/day. Oftentimes patients deny having improved with levodopa, but report worsening of their symptoms following subsequent withdrawal of levodopa, suggesting mild dopa-responsiveness. A dopamine receptor agonist can be tried next, and some patients respond transiently. Patients should be monitored for aggravation of postural hypotension when dopaminergic therapy is started. If present, orthostatic hypotension can be treated using fludrocortisone (combined with an adequate salt intake) or sympathicomimetics such as midrodine (36). This may cause supine hypertension, but this is generally acceptable in light of the reduced survival. The compound (D) L-threo-dihydroxyphenylserine (DOPS), a synthetic precursor of norepinephrine, may reduce orthostatic hypotension by restoring plasma norepinephrine levels. In one small study of four patients with MSA, DOPS increased the upright blood pressure (37). Finally, one study reported beneficial effects of octreotide on orthostatic hypotension in MSA (38).

The cerebellar components of balance and gait impairment are very difficult to treat. In a randomized double-blind study of seven MSA patients, ondansetron (a serotonergic antagonist) failed to reduce gait and balance ataxia (39).

3.   Stereotactic Neurosurgery

Most patients with MSA are deemed unsuitable candidates for neurosurgery because of the rapid progression, limited survival, and widespread pathology in this disease. However, one uncontrolled study recently examined the effects of bilateral high-frequency stimulation of the subthalamic nucleus in four MSA-P patients who were unresponsive to levodopa (40). The gait item of the UPDRS improved by one point (on a score of 0–4) in three patients one month after surgery, but this was maintained in only one patient at longer follow-up. The improvement was due to reduction of extrapyramidal gait features (such as slowness and reduced stride length), whereas gait ataxia was unaffected. These pilot observations require confirmation in larger and controlled series.

4.   Physiotherapy and Occupational Therapy

These interventions have not been studied formally in patients with MSA.

5.   Other Measures

Falls due to symptomatic orthostatic hypotension can be reduced using various nonpharmacological interventions (41). This includes avoiding undesirable behavior such as rapid changes in posture or prolonged episodes of quiet stance. Adequate intake of salt and fluids should be encouraged. Raising the cranial end of the bed leads to a smaller drop in blood pressure when standing up in the morning, and helps to reduce nocturia, thereby restricting volume depletion. Specific antiorthostatic manoeuvres, such as standing with crossed legs or squatting (42,43), are effective but can be too demanding for patients with severe balance impairment. Elastic compression stockings are variably effective and treatment compliance is suboptimal because of discomfort. Finally, electroconvulsive therapy has been tried in an open-label fashion for a few MSA patients. Although concurrent depression may get better, gait and balance impairment remained unchanged or showed at best a transient mild improvement (44).

C. Huntington's Disease

1. Mobility Deficits

Huntington's disease is an autosomal dominant disorder characterized by chorea, behavioral changes, and frontostriatal cognitive impairment, culminating in dementia. Recent studies underscore the important contribution of bradykinesia to the movement abnormalities in this disorder (45). Gait has a rather unique presentation, with a mixture of chorea, "ataxia" (broad based; swaying) and parkinsonism (shuffling; reduced arm movements; propulsion; festination) (46). The disease is invariably progressive and eventually leads to loss of independence, often necessitating nursing home admission. The prevalence of gait impairment and falls has not been studied formally, but clinical experience suggests these are not rare in Huntington's disease. Their importance is underscored by the fact that gait impairment and poor tandem walking are leading markers of nursing home admission (47). At least four different factors might contribute to falls in this disorder. First, falls may be related to severe choreatic movements of the limbs or trunk, leading to precipitous excursions of the center of gravity beyond the patient's limits of stability. Indeed, postural sway (recorded during stance on a stable or tilting support surface) is increased in Huntington's disease (48,49). The unpredictable and jerky choreatic movements could also explain why gait variability is increased in Huntington patients (50), and this is associated with falls in this disorder. Second, the concurrent bradykinesia may be involved, as this leads to slowness of corrective stepping responses or stumbling over small obstacles. Indeed, careful gait analysis reveals bradykinetic features in most patients, including a reduced gait velocity and a shortened stride length (51). Third, automatic postural responses in leg muscles are delayed in onset and abnormally sized in Huntington's disease (48). Finally, in some patients, the frontostriatal cognitive impairment can lead to reckless behavior and thereby contribute to falls.

2. Pharmacotherapy

The effects of drug therapy on gait and balance have not been studied specifically. Chorea can be reduced by "abusing" the extrapyramidal side-effects of classic neuroleptics or other antidopaminergic agents. However, this often leads to worsening of voluntary motor performance by aggravating the pre-existent bradykinesia. In one study (46), neuroleptics decreased chorea but failed to improve gait in patients with Huntington's disease.

Patients with prominent bradykinesia—as might occur in juvenile or late onset Huntington's disease—may benefit from levodopa or dopamine receptor agonists. Even postural instability can improve in such patients, and levodopa does not necessarily aggravate the chorea (52–54).

Riluzole might afford symptomatic relief in Huntington's disease by decreasing glutamatergic neurotransmission or by improving mitochondrial energy metabolism. Two small open label studies suggested that riluzole may reduce chorea and improve psychomotor speed and behavior, but the effects on balance and gait were not specifically reported (55,56).

3. Neurosurgery

Fetal striatal transplantation has been proposed for use in Huntington's disease. Immature fetal striatal tissue can survive and differentiate into mature striatal tissue following transplantation into the striatum of patients with Huntington's disease, as demonstrated in a post-mortem report of a single case who died 18 months after surgery (57). In a pilot clinical trial, this was clinically associated with motor, cognitive, and functional improvement in three out of five grafted patients (58). However, the effects on balance or gait were not examined specifically, and these results require confirmation in larger groups who are followed over several years after grafting. Many technical issues remain to be resolved before this experimental procedure can be used in routine clinical practice.

4. Physiotherapy and Occupational Therapy

Physiotherapy—including gait rehabilitation, exercise training, falls prevention strategies, and relaxation therapy—is expected to be helpful (51), but the available scientific evidence is too weak to make strong recommendations (59). The same applies to occupational therapy (provision of walking aids; wheelchair education).

D. Primary Orthostatic Tremor

1. Mobility Deficits

Patients with primary orthostatic tremor complain of a subjective feeling of *increasing* instability that develops seconds after assuming quiet stance. For this reason, patients can only stand upright for brief periods of time, and subjects are forced to sit down or walk away to relieve this subjective instability. Actual falls are rare, but the condition can be very disabling for patients (60). Clinical inspection typically reveals few discernable abnormalities. Upon prolonged standing, a low-frequency tremor of the legs or trunk can develop. An unequivocal diagnosis can be established using surface EMG, which can detect the pathognomonic 16 Hz (range: 12–18 Hz) tremor with alternating bursts in antagonistic leg muscles, even during walking (61). This same tremor can be identified using auscultation over the muscles of the thigh and calf, which can disclose a characteristic thumping sound.

2. Pharmacotherapy

Benzodiazepines—in particular clonazepam—are most effective in reducing orthostatic tremor, but tolerance can be problematic and an initially good response may taper off over time (61). Other drugs such as primidone, phenobarbitone, and sodium valproate are occasionally effective (62). More recent studies suggest that gabapentin may be a useful treatment for orthostatic tremor (63,64). Some patients respond partially to levodopa or a dopamine receptor agonist such as pramipexole, but a clinically relevant response seems rare (65–67). Unlike essential tremor, propanolol and alcohol are rarely helpful.

3. Other Measures

Patients should plan to avoid prolonged quiet stance, for example by placing chairs in the kitchen or by taking along shooting sticks with rubber ends when they need to stand in line for long periods of time (62).

III. CEREBROVASCULAR DISORDERS

- "Senile" or "cautious" gait disorder.
- Primary progressive freezing gait.
- Vascular "lower-body half" parkinsonism.

A. Mobility Deficits

Gait and balance disorders that are related to cerebrovascular disease may present in several different forms. The first and mildest type is that of an isolated and slowly progressive mixture of extrapyramidal features (small and slow steps, en bloc turns) and ataxic features (staggering with a wide base) in otherwise physically intact elderly persons (68,69). Start hesitation, shuffling, or overt freezing are rare, but balance reactions can be mildly impaired. A fear of falls is common. Signs of pyramidal tract lesions—including the presence of pathological reflexes (glabella, snout, or palmo-mental reflex) or a Babinski's sign—are frequently observed in these patients. No apparent vestibular or orthopaedic cause can be found upon clinical examination. However, neuroimaging studies may reveal diffuse white matter vascular lesions (70–72). This syndrome is commonly referred to as the "senile gait disorder." This terminology continues to be popular, partly for "historical" reasons and partly also for lack of a better term, but may cause confusion as it suggests that gait disorders are an inevitable result of aging in the absence of disease, which is not proven and in fact unlikely. While using the term senile gait disorder, one must realize that the underlying cerebrovascular lesions are a disease associated with aging and not an inevitable progression of aging. In other words, the nonspecific extrapyramidal and ataxic gait associated with cerebrovascular disease is just that, nonspecific gait findings associated with cerebrovascular disease, and not a true senile gait disorder. Others use the term "cautious gait disorder" because the walking pattern somewhat resembles the way that even healthy people move while walking on e.g., a slippery surface such as an icy floor (73). Indeed, some "active" or self-chosen adaptation in gait due to real or imagined threats may play a role in some subjects, but for most individuals the cerebrovascular gait disorder that we now allude to is—at least in part—simply a defective gait because the underlying neural machinery is damaged.

The second type also presents with an isolated and gradually progressive gait disorder, but now freezing of gait dominates the picture ("primary progressive freezing gait" or "gait ignition failure"). The severity of freezing ranges from occasional motor blocks to being wheelchair-bound (74). Start hesitation varies from a slightly delayed initiation to a completely frozen state. Gait is slow and shuffling, but becomes more normal after patients have taken a few steps ("slipped clutch phenomenon"). Patients compensate by using visual cues or by concentrating on walking, so any distraction (e.g., dual tasking) reinstates the underlying gait difficulties. Significantly, the neurological examination is otherwise normal, and patients can imitate normal walking movements as long as they are seated or recumbent. Climbing stairs also causes less problems than simple walking on a flat surface. Most patients have vascular lesions in the basal ganglia (including lacunar infarcts or dilated Virchow–Robin spaces), although others may have cortical atrophy or periventricular white matter lesions (74). Occasionally idiopathic Parkinson's disease presents with isolated gait freezing that responds well to levodopa (75).

The third presentation is usually referred to as "lower body" parkinsonism because the symptoms and signs predominate in the legs. However, others use the terms "arteriosclerotic" or vascular parkinsonism. A gait disorder is again the dominant feature, but (unlike the second presentation type) additional hypokinetic-rigid features can be observed while subjects are seated. Lower body parkinsonism typically presents as a frontal gait disorder (shuffling with short steps), frequent falls, mild extrapyramidal involvement of the upper limbs—including a relatively preserved arm swing during walking—and absent resting tremor. Infarcts in the putamen, globus pallidus, or thalamus are usually responsible when this syndrome develops acutely; more diffuse white matter changes (leukoaraiosis) are more closely associated with an insidious onset (see Fig. 2) (76,77). A stepwise progression is a strong diagnostic hint, but is present in only a proportion of patients.

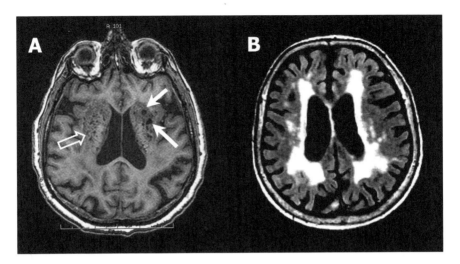

Figure 2 (A) T1-weighted MR image showing multiple dilatations of perivascular spaces (open arrow) and a few lacunar infarcts in the left basal ganglia (closed arrows). (B) Fluid attenuated inversion recovery T2-weighted image showing extensive periventricular white matter lesions in a nondemented elderly patient with lower body parkinsonism.

The fourth and most severe presentation consists of a progressive and incapacitating gait impairment that coincides with dementia, spasticity, and urinary incontinence (78–80). This presentation is related to extensive white matter lesions for which the radiological diagnosis of Binswanger's disease once became fashionable. However, nowadays this dementia syndrome is considered a vascular dementia according to the NINCDS–AIREN criteria (81).

B. Pharmacotherapy

The senile gait disorder is often regarded as an unavoidable (and untreatable!) feature of the "normal" aging process. Consequently, no attempts have been made to treat this gait disorder symptomatically. Levodopa has been tried in patients with primary progressive freezing gait, usually without success (74,82). However, a trial of levodopa should always be given to patients with lower body parkinsonism, as some 25–40% of patients may improve (77,83). Note that levodopa needs to given in adequate doses (if needed, up to 1 g daily for at least one month).

All patients with cerebrovascular gait disorders are at risk of developing other cardiovascular morbidity and mortality, including myocardial infarction or overt strokes. For example, persons with senile gait disorders have an increased risk of cardiovascular mortality compared with age-matched persons who could still walk normally (80). Therefore, a search for potentially treatable cardiac, cerebrovascular, or other vascular diseases seems warranted, and strategies of secondary prevention should be considered (Fig. 3). This includes management of cardiovascular risk factors (for example, hypertension and cholesterol) and prophylactic treatment with antiplatelet agents (84,85). However, the efficacy and cost-efficiency of these interventions remains to be demonstrated in large controlled studies, particularly for the subgroup of very old subjects (in which cardiovascular risk factors may no longer be a threat) and for patients with leukoaraiosis.

C. Physiotherapy

This has not been studied specifically for this group of gait and balance disorders. However, stimulating everyday mobility and use of exercise training

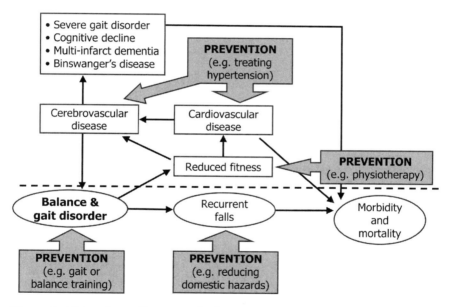

Figure 3 This scheme illustrates the importance of recognizing the presence of underlying cerebrovascular diseases in patients with gait or balance impairment. Physicians who merely pay attention to the easy-to-spot sequelae [*below* the dotted line (circles)] would focus their preventive strategies at symptomatic gait or balance training, or aim at secondary fall prevention. However, recognition of the complex pathophysiology of senile gait disorders (illustrated *above* the dotted line in square boxes) opens additional avenues for the prevention of falls by tackling the underlying disease process and its sequelae (such as reduced fitness). This also helps to reduce the associated morbidity and mortality. (From Ref. 84.)

is felt to be important in arresting further progression of the underlying cerebrovascular (and other cardiovascular) pathology (84).

IV. NORMAL PRESSURE HYDROCEPHALUS

1. Mobility Deficits

It remains unknown whether normal pressure hydrocephalus (NPH) truly exists as a separate entity with its own unique pathophysiology. Classically, the disorder is said to present with a recognizable triad of gait impairment, urinary incontinence, and (frontal) dementia. The gait disorder has a frontal character with marked slowing and small shuffling steps, regular freezing, and an increased stance width, but usually with largely preserved arm movements (6,86). Based on clinical and even neuroradiological grounds, it is often difficult to separate NPH from vascular lower body parkinsonism. The pathophysiology has not been clarified, but may relate to an excessive volume of intraventricular cerebrospinal fluid which is not explained by cerebral atrophy. The classical radiological appearance includes widened lateral ventricles (in particular involving the anterior horns), but this is often accompanied by periventricular white matter lesions. An important question (with direct implications for therapy) is whether these periventricular white matter lesions are the cause or consequence of ventricular widening. Adherents of the latter theory believe that the excessive volume of cerebrospinal fluid is pressed into the periventricular white matter, causing radiological lucencies (87). Why there should be an excessive volume of cerebrospinal fluid is unknown. However, others feel that the periventricular white matter lesions are primarily cerebrovascular in nature, leading to subcortical atrophy and secondary ventricular widening.

2. Pharmacotherapy

Basal ganglia dysfunction may contribute to the pathophysiology of NPH (88), and this could explain the occasional responsiveness to treatment with levodopa.

3. Neurosurgery

Various studies have shown that selected patients with a typical clinical and neuroradiological appearance can benefit from shunting of cerebrospinal fluid, but properly designed randomized controlled studies are still missing (89). The best available evidence to date suggest that single lumbar taps of large cerebrospinal fluid (CSF) volumes can be effective in some patients, but others require prolonged drainage via an external lumbar drain or a permanent ventriculo–peritoneal or ventriculo–atrial shunt. Still others do not respond at all to CSF drainage. In responders, tapping of CSF helps to improve the gait velocity, but step width remains broad (86). The cognitive problems are usually refractory to treatment. It is difficult to predict who will respond best to CSF drainage. Single lumbar punctures are often used for this purpose (90), but these are hampered by high false-positive rates (nonresponders to lumbar puncture may yet improve with an external lumbar drain or permanent internal shunting). Similar problems arise when external lumbar drainage is used to identify responders to shunting (91). The lumbar infusion technique (which documents the pressure response to steady-state infusion of an isotonic saline solution) has been advocated to predict who might respond to therapy (92). Although the positive and negative predictive rate is acceptable, this technique has not been implemented widely because it is cumbersome to use in inexperienced hands. Patients with severe cognitive problems or marked concurrent cerebrovascular disease are no good candidates for CSF drainage (93), suggesting that, at least in this specific subpopulation, ventricular widening is secondary to the periventricular white matter lesions and, as such, is not related to an excess intraventricular CSF.

A recent study showed that patients with vascular parkinsonism may also respond to a lumbar puncture (94). This result once again underscores the overlap between NPH and vascular parkinsonism. Further prospective studies or randomized clinicals trial are needed to determine what patients with vascular parkinsonism might become candidates for shunting.

4. Physiotherapy and Occupational Therapy

External visual or auditory cues are usually not very effective in patients with NPH (86).

V. CONCLUSIONS

Many mobility disorders that were covered in this chapter are generally regarded as difficult to treat. This relates in particular to the balance and gait difficulties that are common in these disorders. However, this chapter illustrates the broad spectrum of possible therapeutic interventions that may become available to alleviate gait and balance problems in affected patients. Therapeutic options range from purely symptomatic to prophylactic strategies, aimed to maintain current functioning and prevent further damage in the future. Unfortunately, the level of supporting scientific evidence was usually insufficient to make very strong recommendations. Therefore, well-designed and adequately powered studies are needed in the next few years to further improve and expand the therapeutic arsenal, focusing in particular on development of simple and easy-to-use screening tools that can help identify those patients that are most likely to benefit from a particular intervention.

ACKNOWLEDGMENTS

Dr. B.R. Bloem was supported by a research grant of the Prinses Beatrix Fonds.

REFERENCES

1. Bloem BR, Bhatia KP. Basal ganglia disorders. In: Bronstein AM, Brandt T, Nutt JG, Woollacott MH, eds. Clinical Disorders of Balance, Posture and Gait. London: Arnold, 2004:173–206.
2. Litvan I, Agid Y, Calne D, et al. Clinical research criteria for the diagnosis of progressive supranuclear palsy (Steele–Richardson–Olszewski syndrome): report of the NINDS-SPSP international workshop. Neurology 1999; 47:1–9.
3. Daniel SE, de Bruin VMS, Lees AJ. The clinical and pathological spectrum of Steele–Richardson–Olszewski syndrome (progressive supranuclear palsy): a reappraisal. Brain 1995; 118:759–770.
4. Bloem BR, Munneke M, Mazibrada G, et al. The nature of falling in progressive supranuclear palsy. Mov Disord 2004; 19:359–360.
5. Maher ER, Lees AJ. The clinical features and natural history of the Steele–Richardson–Olszewski syndrome (progressive supranuclear palsy). Neurology 1986; 36:1005–1008.
6. Giladi N. Freezing of gait. Clinical overview. Adv Neurol 2001; 87:191–197.
7. Jankovic J. Controlled trial of pergolide mesylate in Parkinson's disease and progressive supranuclear palsy. Neurology 1983; 33:505–507.
8. Jackson A, Crossman AR. Nucleus tegmenti pedunculopontinus: efferent connections with special reference to the basal ganglia, studied in the rat by anterograde transport of horseradish peroxidase. Neuroscience 1983; 10:725–765.
9. Neophytides A, Lieberman AN, Goldstein M, et al. The use of lisuride, a potent dopamine and serotonin agonist, in the treatment of progressive supranuclear palsy. J Neurol Neurosurg Psychiatry 1982; 45:261–263.
10. Kappos L, Moeri D, Radue EW, et al. Predictive value of gadolinium-enhanced magnetic resonance imaging for relapse rate and changes in disability or impairment in multiple sclerosis: a meta-analysis. Lancet 1999; 353:964–969.
11. Nieforth KA, Golbe LI. Retrospective study of drug response in 87 patients with progressive supranuclear palsy. Clin Neuropharmacol 1993; 16:338–346.
12. Newman GC. Treatment of progressive supranuclear palsy with tricyclic antidepressants. Neurology 1985; 35:1189–1193.
13. Kvale JN. Amitriptyline in the management of progressive supranuclear palsy. Arch Neurol 1982; 39:387–388.
14. Engel PA. Treatment of progressive supranuclear palsy with amitriptyline: therapeutic and toxic effects. J Am Geriatr Soc 1996; 44:1072–1074.
15. Ghika J, Tennis M, Hoffman E, Schoenfeld D, Growdon J. Idazoxan treatment in progressive supranuclear palsy. Neurology 1991; 41:986–991.
16. Fabbrini G, Barbanti P, Bonifati V, et al. Donepezil in the treatment of progressive supranuclear palsy. Acta Neurol Scand 2001; 103:123–125.
17. Litvan I, Phipps M, Pharr VL, Hallett M, Grafman J, Salazar A. Randomized placebo-controlled trial of donepezil in patients with progressive supranuclear palsy. Neurology 2001; 57:467–473.

18. Litvan I, Blesa R, Clark K, et al. Pharmacological evaluation of the cholinergic system in progressive supranuclear palsy. Ann Neurol 1994; 36:55–61.
19. Rafal RD, Grimm RJ. Progressive supranuclear palsy: functional analysis of the response to methysergide and antiparkinsonian agents. Neurology 1981; 31:1507–1518.
20. Paulson GW, Lowery HW, Taylor GC. Progressive supranuclear palsy: pneumoencephalography, electronystagmography and treatment with methysergide. Eur Neurol 1981; 20:13–16.
21. Izzo KL, DiLorenzo P, Roth A. Rehabilitation in progressive supranuclear palsy: case report. Arch Phys Med Rehabil 1986; 67:473–476.
22. Sosner J, Wall GC, Sznajder J. Progressive supranuclear palsy: clinical presentation and rehabilitation of two patients. Arch Phys Med Rehabil 1993; 74:537–539.
23. Piccione F, Mancini E, Tonin P, Bizzarini M. Botulinum toxin treatment of apraxia of eyelid opening in progressive supranuclear palsy: report of two cases. Arch Phys Med Rehabil 1997; 78:525–529.
24. Suteerawattananon M, MacNeill B, Protas EJ. Supported treadmill training for gait and balance in a patient with progressive supranuclear palsy. Phys Ther 2002; 82:485–495.
25. Barclay CL, Duff J, Sandor P, Lang AE. Limited usefulness of electroconvulsive therapy in progressive supranuclear palsy. Neurology 1996; 46:1284–1286.
26. Polo KB, Jabbari B. Botulinum toxin-A improves the rigidity of progressive supranuclear palsy. Ann Neurol 1994; 35:237–239.
27. Fearnley JM, Lees AJ. Striatonigral degeneration. A clinicopathological study. Brain 1990; 113:1823–1842.
28. Litvan I, Goetz CG, Jankovic J, et al. What is the accuracy of the clinical diagnosis of multiple system atrophy? A clinicopathologic study. Arch Neurol 1997; 54:937–944.
29. Wenning GK, Ben-Shlomo Y, Magalhaes M, Daniel SE, Quinn NP. Clinical features and natural history of multiple system atrophy. An analysis of 100 cases. Brain 1994; 117:835–845.
30. Gurevich T, Giladi N. Freezing of gait in multiple system atrophy (MSA). Parkinsonism Relat Disord 2003; 9:169–174.
31. Muller J, Seppi K, Stefanova N, Poewe W, Litvan I, Wenning GK. Freezing of gait in postmortem-confirmed atypical parkinsonism. Mov Disord 2002; 17:1041–1045.
32. Perani D, Bressi S, Testa D, et al. Clinical/metabolic correlations in multiple system atrophy. A fludeoxyglucose F 18 positron emission tomographic study. Arch Neurol 1995; 52:179–185.
33. Ito H, Kusaka H, Matsumoto S, Imai T. Striatal efferent involvement and its correlation to levodopa efficacy in patients with multiple system atrophy. Neurology 1996; 47:1291–1299.
34. Hughes AJ, Colosimo C, Kleedorfer B, Daniel SE, Lees AJ. The dopaminergic response in multiple system atrophy. J Neurol Neurosurg Psychiatry 1992; 55:1009–1013.
35. Colosimo C, Pezzella FR. The symptomatic treatment of multiple system atrophy. Eur J Neurol 2002; 9:195–199.

36. Mathias CJ, Kimber JR. Treatment of postural hypotension. J Neurol Neurosurg Psychiatry 1998; 65:285–289.

37. Kaufmann H, Oribe E, Yahr MD. Differential effect of L-threo-3,4-dihydroxyphenylserine in pure autonomic failure and multiple system atrophy with autonomic failure. J Neural Transm Park Dis Dement Sect 1991; 3:143–148.

38. Bordet R, Benhadjali J, Libersa C, Destee A. Octreotide in the management of orthostatic hypotension in multiple system atrophy: pilot trial of chronic administration. Clin Neuropharmacol 1994; 17:380–383.

39. Bier JC, Dethy S, Hildebrand J, et al. Effects of the oral form of ondansetron on cerebellar dysfunction. A multi-center double-blind study. J Neurol 2003; 250:693–697.

40. Visser-Vandewalle V, Temel Y, Colle H, van der LC. Bilateral high-frequency stimulation of the subthalamic nucleus in patients with multiple system atrophy—parkinsonism. Report of four cases. J Neurosurg 2003; 98:882–887.

41. Bloem BR, Overeem S, van Dijk JG. Syncopal falls and their mimics. In: Bronstein AM, Brandt T, Nutt J G, Woollacott MH, eds. Clinical Disorders of Balance, Posture and Gait. London: Arnold, 2004:286–316.

42. van Lieshout JJ, ten Harkel AD, Wieling W. Physical manoeuvres for combating orthostatic dizziness in autonomic failure. Lancet 1992; 339:897–898.

43. Krediet CTP, van Dijk N, Linzer M, van Lieshout JJ, Wieling W. Management of vasovagal syncope: controlling or aborting faints by leg crossing and muscle tensing. Circulation 2002; 106:1684–1689.

44. Roane DM, Rogers JD, Helew L, Zarate J. Electroconvulsive therapy for elderly patients with multiple system atrophy: a case series. Am J Geriatr Psychiatry 2000; 8:171–174.

45. van Vugt JP, Roos RA. Huntington's disease—options for controlling symptoms. CNS Drugs 1999; 11:105–123.

46. Koller WC, Trimble J. The gait abnormality of Huntington's disease. Neurology 1985; 35:1450–1454.

47. Wheelock VL, Tempkin T, Marder K, et al. Predictors of nursing home placement in Huntington disease. Neurology 2003; 60:998–1001.

48. Huttunen J, Hömberg V. EMG responses in leg muscles to postural perturbations in Huntington's disease. J Neurol Neurosurg Psychiatry 1990; 53:55–62.

49. Tian J-R, Herdman SJ, Zee DS, Folstein SE. Postural stability in patients with Huntington's disease. Neurology 1992; 42:1232–1238.

50. Hausdorff JM, Cudkowicz ME, Firtion R, Wei JY, Goldberger AL. Gait variability and basal ganglia disorders: stride-to-stride variations of gait cycle timing in Parkinson's disease and Huntington's disease. Mov Disord 1998; 13:428–437.

51. Churchyard AJ, Morris ME, Georgiou N, Chiu E, Cooper R, Iansek R. Gait dysfunction in Huntington's disease: parkinsonism and a disorder of timing. Implications for movement rehabilitation. Adv Neurol 2001; 87:375–385.

52. Racette BA, Perlmutter JS. Levodopa responsive parkinsonism in an adult with Huntington's disease. J Neurol Neurosurg Psychiatry 1998; 65:577–579.

53. Reuter I, Hu MT, Andrews TC, Brooks DJ, Clough C, Chaudhuri KR. Late onset levodopa responsive Huntington's disease with minimal chorea masquerading as Parkinson plus syndrome. J Neurol Neurosurg Psychiatry 2000; 68:238–241.

54. Bonelli RM, Niederwieser G, Diez J, Gruber A, Koltringer P. Pramipexole ameliorates neurologic and psychiatric symptoms in a Westphal variant of Huntington's disease. Clin Neuropharmacol 2002; 25:58–60.
55. Rosas HD, Koroshetz WJ, Jenkins BG, et al. Riluzole therapy in Huntington's disease (HD). Mov Disord 1999; 14:326–330.
56. Seppi K, Mueller J, Bodner T, et al. Riluzole in Huntington's disease (HD): an open label study with one year follow up. J Neurol 2001; 248:866–869.
57. Freeman TB, Cicchetti F, Hauser RA, et al. Transplanted fetal striatum in Huntington's disease: phenotypic development and lack of pathology. Proc Nat Acad Sci USA 2000; 97:13877–13882.
58. Bachoud-Levi AC, Remy P, Nguyen JP, et al. Motor and cognitive improvements in patients with Huntington's disease after neural transplantation. Lancet 2000; 356:1975–1979.
59. Bilney B, Morris ME, Perry A. Effectiveness of physiotherapy, occupational therapy, and speech pathology for people with Huntington's disease: a systematic review. Neurorehabil Neural Repair 2003; 17:12–24.
60. Gerschlager W, Katzenschlager R, Schrag A, et al. Quality of life in patients with orthostatic tremor. J Neurol 2003; 250:212–215.
61. Britton TC, Thompson PD, van der Kamp W, et al. Primary orthostatic tremor: further observations in six cases. J Neurol 1992; 239:209–217.
62. Britton TC, Thompson PD. Primary orthostatic tremor. BMJ 1995; 310:143–144.
63. Evidente VG, Adler CH, Caviness JN, Gwinn KA. Effective treatment of orthostatic tremor with gabapentin. Mov Disord 1998; 13:829–831.
64. Onofrj M, Thomas A, Paci C, D'Andreamatteo G. Gabapentin in orthostatic tremor: results of a double-blind crossover with placebo in four patients. Neurology 1998; 51:880–882.
65. Wills AJ, Brusa L, Wang HC, Brown P, Marsden CD. Levodopa may improve orthostatic tremor: case report and trial of treatment. J Neurol Neurosurg Psychiatry 1999; 66:681–684.
66. Finkel MF. Pramipexole is a possible effective treatment for primary orthostatic tremor (shaky leg syndrome). Arch Neurol 2000; 57:1519–1520.
67. Katzenschlager R, Costa D, Gerschlager W, et al. [123I]-FP-CIT-SPECT demonstrates dopaminergic deficit in orthostatic tremor. Ann Neurol 2003; 53:489–496.
68. Elble RJ, Hughes L, Higgins C. The syndrome of senile gait. J Neurol 1992; 239:71–75.
69. Bloem BR, Haan J, Lagaay AM, van Beek W, Wintzen AR, Roos RA. Investigation of gait in elderly subjects over 88 years of age. J Geriatr Psychiatry Neurol 1992; 5:78–84.
70. Kerber KA, Enrietto JA, Jacobson KM, Baloh RW. Disequilibrium in older people: a prospective study. Neurology 1998; 51:574–580.
71. Tell GS, Lefkowitz DS, Diehr P, Elster AD. Relationship between balance and abnormalities in cerebral magnetic resonance imaging in older adults. Arch Neurol 1998; 55:73–79.
72. Baloh RW, Ying SH, Jacobson KM. A longitudinal study of gait and balance dysfunction in normal older people. Arch Neurol 2003; 60:835–839.

73. Nutt JG, Marsden CD, Thompson PD. Human walking and higher-level gait disorders, particularly in the elderly. Neurology 1993; 43:268–279.
74. Achiron A, Ziv I, Goren M, et al. Primary progressive freezing gait. Mov Disord 1993; 8:293–297.
75. Quinn NP, Luthert P, Honavar M, Marsden CD. Pure akinesia due to lewy body Parkinson's disease: a case with pathology. Mov Disord 1989; 4:85–89.
76. Zijlmans JC, Thijssen HO, Vogels OJ, et al. MRI in patients with suspected vascular parkinsonism. Neurology 1995; 45:2183–2188.
77. Winnikates J, Jankovic J. Clinical correlates of vascular parkinsonism. Arch Neurol 1999; 56:98–102.
78. Thompson PD, Marsden CD. Gait disorder of subcortical arteriosclerotic encephalopathy: Binswanger's disease. Mov Disord 1987; 2:1–8.
79. Kotsoris H, Barclay LL, Kheyfets S, Hulyalkar A, Dougherty J. Urinary and gait disturbances as markers for early multi-infarct dementia. Stroke 1987; 18:138–141.
80. Bloem BR, Gussekloo J, Lagaay AM, Remarque EJ, Haan J, Westendorp RGJ. Idiopathic senile gait disorders are signs of subclinical disease. J Am Geriatr Soc 2000; 48:1098–1101.
81. Roman GC, Tatemichi TK, Erkinjuntti T, et al. Vascular dementia: diagnostic criteria for research studies. Report of the NINDS–AIREN International Workshop. Neurology 1993; 43:250–260.
82. Factor SA, Jennings DL, Molho ES, Marek KL. The natural history of the syndrome of primary progressive freezing gait. Arch Neurol 2002; 59:1778–1783.
83. Demirkiran M, Bozdemir H, Sarica Y. Vascular parkinsonism: a distinct, heterogeneous clinical entity. Acta Neurol Scand 2001; 104:63–67.
84. Boers I, Gerschlager W, Stalenhoef PA, Bloem BR. Falls in the elderly. II. Strategies for prevention. Wien Klin Wochenschr 2001; 113:398–407.
85. Roman GC. New insight into Binswanger disease. Arch Neurol 1999; 56:1061–1062.
86. Stolze H, Kuhtz-Buschbeck JP, Drucke H, Johnk K, Illert M, Deuschl G. Comparative analysis of the gait disorder of normal pressure hydrocephalus and Parkinson's disease. J Neurol Neurosurg Psychiatry 2001; 70:289–297.
87. Tullberg M, Hultin L, Ekholm S, Mansson JE, Fredman P, Wikkelso C. White matter changes in normal pressure hydrocephalus and Binswanger disease: specificity, predictive value and correlations to axonal degeneration and demyelination. Acta Neurol Scand 2002; 105:417–426.
88. Curran T, Lang AE. Parkinsonian syndromes associated with hydrocephalus: case reports, a review of the literature, and pathophysiological hypotheses. Mov Disord 1994; 9:508–520.
89. Esmonde T, Cooke S. Shunting for normal pressure hydrocephalus (NPH). Cochrane Database Syst Rev 2002; CD003157.
90. Sand T, Bovim G, Grimse R, Myhr G, Helde G, Cappelen J. Idiopathic normal pressure hydrocephalus: the CSF tap-test may predict the clinical response to shunting. Acta Neurol Scand 1994; 89:311–316.
91. Walchenbach R, Geiger E, Thomeer RT, Vanneste JA. The value of temporary external lumbar CSF drainage in predicting the outcome of shunting on normal pressure hydrocephalus. J Neurol Neurosurg Psychiatry 2002; 72:503–506.

92. Boon AJ, Tans JT, Delwel EJ, et al. Dutch normal-pressure hydrocephalus study: prediction of outcome after shunting by resistance to outflow of cerebrospinal fluid. J Neurosurg 1997; 87:687–693.
93. Boon AJ, Tans JT, Delwel EJ, et al. Dutch Normal-Pressure Hydrocephalus Study: the role of cerebrovascular disease. J Neurosurg 1999; 90:221–226.
94. Ondo WG, Chan LL, Levy JK. Vascular parkinsonism: clinical correlates predicting motor improvement after lumbar puncture. Mov Disord 2002; 17:91–97.

16

Systems Approach to Gait Rehabilitation Following Stroke

Anouk Lamontagne and Joyce Fung

*School of Physical and Occupational Therapy, McGill University, Montreal,
Jewish Rehabilitation Hospital Research Centre, Laval,
Quebec, Canada*

I. INTRODUCTION AND BACKGROUND

A. Multicausal Nature of Mobility Problems

Stroke is one of the most debilitating diseases, causing 9 million survivors a year around the world (1) to live with some degree of disability and handicap. Among stroke survivors, only 50% will manage to walk in the community (2), but two-thirds will do so with limitations. Most of them are not able, for instance, to walk independently in a crowded shopping center (3). According to Hill et al. (4), only 7% of all stroke clients meet the criteria for independent community ambulation when discharged from rehabilitation.

Walking after stroke is characterized by slow gait speed, poor endurance, and changes in the quality and flexibility of the walking pattern. Average gait speeds for stroke patients reported in the literature vary from 0.23 to 0.73 m/sec (5), which represent 19–60% of the gait speed of healthy elderly subjects in their late sixties (6). The energy demand of hemiparetic gait is higher than that of normal walking (7,8). The endurance of the stroke subjects, as measured by the distance covered during the 6-min walk test, is equivalent to 49.8% of that predicted for healthy individuals with similar physical characteristics (9). The movements of their lower body (10) and upper body (11–13) are both disrupted during walking. Their walking pattern also lacks flexibility and cannot be adapted to environmental demands, such as walking on a slippery surface, or to some new or changing task constraints such as in turning the head while walking (13).

Several factors or systems can interact and lead to poor mobility after stroke. Disrupted motor commands, altered sensory information, and poor sensorimotor integration likely generate uncoordinated and maladaptive movements resulting in poor balance and mobility. As a combined result of the neurological insult and disuse, secondary physiological (e.g., changes in muscle fiber types) and biomechanical changes (e.g., muscle–tendon unit shortening) also take place, thus further modifying the constraint of the body. Adaptive behaviors and compensations usually emerge with recovery. Physical deconditioning and presumably premorbid life habits may concomitantly contribute to poor cardiovascular function, while cognitive and motivational factors may come into play and impact on rehabilitation outcomes. Mobility problems thus appear to be multicausal, resulting from the mutual interaction of multiple systems, both lesioned and intact.

B. Contemporary Systems Approach in Rehabilitation

One of the central assumptions of the systems or task-oriented approach is that normal behavior results from the interaction of different systems (14). The abnormal walking pattern of stroke patients, as outlined in the previous section, thus reflects the interaction of the lesioned and intact systems, from which adaptive or maladaptive behaviors can both emerge. Another assumption of the systems approach is that movements are goal-oriented, constrained not only by the individual or the task characteristics, but also by the environment (14). The interaction of the individual with the task and with the environment suggests that behaviors and tasks need to be adapted in a context-dependent fashion, and that problem-solving skills prevail over practice of stereotyped movement strategies. The emphasis should thus be placed on training patients using functional and meaningful tasks, rather than the practice of sequenced and invariant movement patterns. Hence, gait training should be initiated even in nonambulatory patients, providing them with necessary assistance, rather than training segmented lower limb movements while sitting or lying supine.

Figure 1 schematizes the interface that exist between the individual, the task and the environment. From the interaction of these factors, a context-dependent behavior emerges. Manipulating one or more of these factors allow a "motor problem" to be targeted from multiple angles, while allowing the tasks to be made gradually more complex. For instance in gait training, one may decide to intervene at the individual level, using functional electrical stimulation to favor ankle dorsiflexion during the swing phase of

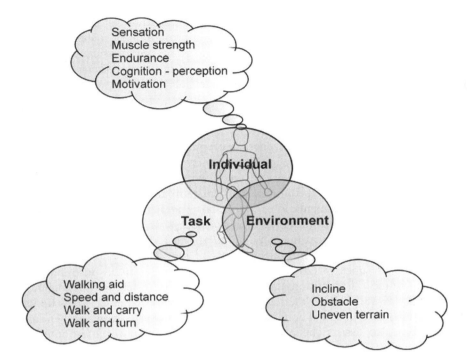

Figure 1 A schematic figure of the interface existing between the individual, the task and the environment, and their influence on the organization of the locomotor behavior. Factors within each of the three components are illustrated in the inserts. From the interaction of these factors, a context-dependent locomotor behavior emerges. In return, manipulating one or more of these factors allow targeting the "problem" from multiple angles, while providing the possibility of grading task complexity. [Adapted from Shumway-Cook and Woollacott (14)]

walking. The task itself can also be modified, such as walking and carrying an object, or turning while walking.

Environmental characteristics such as the incline and texture of the support surface can also be varied. Adjusting gradually the complexity of a task (e.g., walking with and without turning) and the characteristics of environment (e.g., the degree of slope changes) will allow patients to adapt to their individual capability while training their problem-solving skills.

C. Motor Learning in the Framework of the Systems Approach

Motor learning involves processes associated with practice or experience that result in relatively permanent changes (15). In the contexts of gait rehabilitation and systems approach, the processes pertain to the improved capability for producing skilled locomotion through the search for new task solutions that emerge from interactions of the individual with the task and the environment (Fig. 1). Motor learning is promoted by factors such as changing environmental contexts, alterations in the physical demands, problem solving, random presentation of practice tasks, sufficient practice and self-empowerment [see review by Winstein (16)]. The current framework of knowledge in rehabilitation emphasizes the need for intense task-related practice to promote the reacquisition of locomotor skills. As most of the motor recovery of the lower extremity takes place within the first 6 weeks after stroke (17), there is a general acceptance that the training of the locomotor function should be initiated as early as possible (18). The number of repetitions and the specificity of the activities selected for training were found to be critical for promoting cortical reorganization associated with the recovery of movements after a cortical infarct in nonhuman primates [see review by Nudo et al. (19)]. Similar findings were reported in human studies using transcranial magnetic stimulation (TMS), a noninvasive tool to investigate the underlying mechanisms of plasticity associated with the restitution of function (20–23). Results from clinical studies also support the importance of repetition and training specificity in recovery of locomotor skills (17,18,24–26). Practice of different locomotor-related skills under environmentally different conditions not only improves strength and endurance, but also assists the patient in learning to adapt to environmental demands (25,27).

II. TREADMILL TRAINING

A. Rationale

Treadmill training is a task-oriented approach that allows the practice of repetitive and rhythmic stepping. The rationale behind the use of treadmill training is that it would provide repetitive sensory inputs that activate the spinal circuitry involved in the generation of locomotor movements (1). Such premise is based on animal studies, in which spinalized cats were shown to recover the ability to walk on a treadmill with training (28–30). Devoid of supraspinal inputs, the locomotor recovery after a complete spinal cord transection must be mediated through learning or plasticity at the spinal cord level [see review by de Leon et al. (31)].

B. Treadmill vs. Overground Walking

Although treadmill and overground walking are quite similar, they still differ in some of their temporal distance features and movement patterns. For a given gait speed, treadmill walking in healthy subjects has been associated with increased cadence and shorter stride length (32–34), shorter stance duration (33,34), higher heart rate (32), and higher predicted energy cost (35). Subjects demonstrate larger hip flexion at initial contact on the treadmill (32,34). Head movements are modified in the sagittal plane (32), and the spine and pelvis motions in the frontal and transverse planes also differ between the two modes of locomotion (36). Activation of the lower limb muscles (32) and vertical ground reaction forces (32,37) may vary in amplitude between treadmill and overground locomotion, but the electromyographic (EMG) patterns remain identical (38).

Although the treadmill is widely used in gait rehabilitation, little is known about gait adaptation to treadmill walking in stroke subjects. Bayat et al. (39) observed that at similar speeds, stroke subjects displayed shorter stride lengths and higher cadences on the treadmill as compared to overground, as reported for the healthy subjects. Harris-Love et al. (40) also found that the durations of relative stance and single limb support on the paretic side increased during treadmill walking, whereas the reverse occurred in the nonparetic side. This resulted in greater symmetry between the paretic and nonparetic limbs' temporal features. These observations suggest that treadmill training may promote walking with higher cadences and shorter stride lengths, while possibly improving symmetry.

Treadmill also differs from overground walking in terms of sensory information involvement and processing. On the treadmill, the moving surface provides tactile and proprioceptive stimuli that were shown to trigger stepping movements in spinalized animals (28–30). While the limbs are stepping and providing the central nervous system (CNS) with stimuli inherent to locomotor movements, the visual and vestibular systems, on the other hand, are "informing" the CNS that no net forward progression in space occurs. Such conflict in sensory information is apparently well integrated and resolved in healthy subjects, as they can easily walk or run on a treadmill without falling. It may explain, however, why postural sway is momentarily increased after treadmill walking (41) and why an "after-effect" may be perceived after running on a treadmill for several minutes. As stroke subjects present with defective integration of sensory and motor information (42), the conflicting sensory information induced by treadmill walking may impact negatively on their walking balance.

C. Evidence for Efficacy of Treadmill Training

Although treadmill training is commonly used in rehabilitation, the training protocols with respect to belt speed, duration, and frequency of the training sessions vary from study to study. While some training programs are designed to increase walking speed of stroke subjects (43,44), others specially target aerobic capacity and endurance (45,46). Treadmill training is also often used in combination with body weight support (BWS) (44,47–49). Such variability in the training protocols makes it hard to compare the outcomes of the different studies. The next section is dedicated to review studies involving treadmill training with full weight bearing

(FWB) or minimal weight support ($\leq 10\%$), whereas the use of BWS is addressed in a later section in this chapter.

Studies investigating the effect of treadmill training are not so numerous (18,46,50,51), and even fewer incorporated a proper control group receiving conventional overground walking training (17,43,52). In subjects with a recent stroke, Richards et al. (17) and Laufer et al. (52) compared the effects of an early intensive treadmill training regimen to that of conventional therapy including overground walking training. After 3–6 weeks of training, improvements in walking speed were observed (17,52). Laufer et al. (52) also reported improved functional walking ability, as measured by the Functional Ambulation Category (53), improved temporal-distance characteristics and increased activation of the paretic calf muscles.

Richards et al. (17), however, reported only a moderate difference in walking speed increments between the experimental and control groups, yielding a modest effect size of 0.58, which even leveled out during follow-ups at 3 and 6 months' intervals. In Laufer et al. (52), although the improvements in gait speed were greater in the experimental (135%) than in the control (88%) group, post-treatment walking speeds were not significantly different between the two groups. Altogether, the findings from these controlled studies suggest that treadmill training is well tolerated in subjects early after stroke and that it is more effective than conventional gait therapy to improve certain aspects of locomotion. The gains in gait speed provided by treadmill training, however, barely exceed those achieved through conventional training, and they seem not to be retained after a few months. In both studies (17,52), however, subjects were trained at comfortable gait speed. In studies comparing speed-intensive walking to training at slower gait speeds (43,44), it would be later shown that the key for significant improvement and retention of gait speed may lie in the intensity and the belt speed chosen for training (see section IV-C "Intensity: The Key for Improved Speed and Endurance").

D. Weighing Advantages and Limitations of Treadmill Training

As compared to overground walking, treadmill training offers several advantages. It allows subjects to be trained within a confined environment, while facilitating access for manual assistance, or use of external support such as rails or suspended BWS systems. The speed of the treadmill can also be controlled and monitored. It can thus provide subjects with a high-intensity training program designed to increase walking speed (43,44) or a low-intensity aerobic paradigm to improve cardiovascular fitness (45,46). In several studies, however, it can be observed that the gait speed achieved after treadmill training are faster on the treadmill than overground (43,48,52). Table 1 synthesized the gains in speed reported by Visintin et al. (48) for subjects trained on a treadmill with FWB and with partial

Table 1 Overground and Treadmill Speeds Achieved Before and After Training on a Treadmill will Full Weight Bearing (FWB) or Partial Body Weight Support (BWS)

Groups	Training speed on treadmill (m/s)	
	Beginning	End
BWS ($n=43$)	0.23 ± 0.11	0.42 ± 0.22
FWB ($n=36$)	0.19 ± 0.14	0.34 ± 0.19
	Overground walking speed (m/s)	
	Pre-training	Post-training
BWS	0.18 ± 0.17	0.34 ± 0.26
FWB	0.15 ± 0.14	0.25 ± 0.24

Source: Data from Visintin et al. 1998.

weight support. It can be seen that for both groups, the gait speeds achieved at the end of the training were faster on the treadmill than overground, suggesting only a partial carry-over effect. Such an incomplete transfer of the gains in gait speed may be explained by task-specificity or, in other words, by some of the differences inherent to the different tasks of treadmill and overground walking.

III. WEIGHT SUPPORTED LOCOMOTOR TRAINING

A. Rationale

The use of BWS in gait retraining originated from animal studies. Barbeau and Rossignol (28) demonstrated that adult spinalized cats were capable of regaining FWB locomotion through an intensive interactive locomotor training program. The program consisted of appropriately graded weight support that was provided by supporting the cat's tail or hindquarters and allowing the animal to walk on the treadmill with only the amount of weight that it was capable of bearing without an arrest in locomotion. A treadmill apparatus with harness support for evaluation and rehabilitation of gait was thus proposed (28,54) and applied to the neurologic population (47,48,55–61). One major advantage is that gait training can be initiated early in the process of rehabilitation by providing nonambulatory patients as much weight support as needed to compensate for their inability to assume an upright position while stepping forward. The effort required in maintaining upright balance of the trunk can be decreased through the external support provided by BWS. Stroke patients usually have difficulty attending simultaneously to all three essential requirements of locomotion: stepping, weight bearing, and balance (62). With weight bearing and balance being assisted through BWS, patients can focus on stepping movements with or without the assistance from therapists. The posture and limb movements sensed by the patients are specific to the task of locomotion, thus enhancing the proprioception and perception of simulated or real movements without inducing any "learned disuse" of the paretic limb(s) (63,64). Moreover, BWS can minimize the development of compensatory overuse with the nonparetic limb that result in asymmetric gait patterns, as often observed with conventional walking aids.

B. Adaptation to Unloading

1. Treadmill Locomotion

Adaptations to unloading are usually studied by providing different levels of BWS with an overhead suspension system during treadmill walking at constant speed. In healthy subjects, BWS or unloading decreases mechanical work (65,66), energy cost (67–69), activation of antigravity muscles such as ankle extensors (70–72), hip extensors (70), and knee extensors (68), as well as peak ground reaction forces and plantar pressure (70,73). With more substantial levels of unloading, a reorganization of muscle activation also takes place, especially for muscles around the hip joint (70).

Body weight support also modifies the temporal-distance parameters of gait, although different studies have yielded contradictory results in terms of the direction of changes. The most consistent findings include a decrease in stride length (70) and in relative stance time (70,74) and double support time (74) with increasing levels of unloading. Lower limb kinematics are also modified, although the changes are more subtle than for kinetics. For instance, unloading would favor larger amplitude of movement at the ankle (74), but smaller excursions at the hip (72,74). Intersegmental co-ordination of thigh, shank, and foot segments is affected by BWS, and movement variability increases with increasing levels of unloading (70).

Adaptations to BWS in stroke subjects resemble those in the healthy subjects but there were scarcely any in-depth studies. While studies with healthy subjects used a wide range of BWS levels, ranging from 10% to 100%, those with stroke subjects used BWS levels that rarely exceeded 30–40% of body weight (57,59,69,75), exceptionally 60% (76). As compared to walking with full weight, 30–45% of BWS causes stroke subjects to walk with less oxygen consumption and lower heart rate (69), as well as with reduced activation of antigravity muscles such as ankle and knee extensors (76). In contrast to healthy subjects (70), hip extensor (gluteus medius) activation was not found to be significantly reduced in stroke subjects, even at 60% of unloading (76). BWS also reduces relative single support duration and increases double support duration on the paretic side, while having no significant impact on temporal-distance factor symmetry between the lower limbs (76). A more upright posture with BWS is also observed, with increased hip and knee extension in midstance, and less hip and knee flexion in swing (76).

2. Overground Locomotion

In a recent study, we investigated the effect of BWS during overground locomotion in nonchronic stroke subjects (75). In this experiment, subjects ($n = 12$) were walking on a walkway in a body harness suspended overhead from a pressurized constant weight support system. Levels of BWS were set at 30% in all but two subjects for whom 50% of unloading was provided. Levels of BWS were decided based on the ability of the subjects to bear weight on the paretic side during stance, and to advance the same limb during swing. Subjects were assessed either at their comfortable or maximal speeds. Figure 2A illustrates the speed achieved by the stroke subjects while walking with BWS, as a function of their speed during the FWB condition. Based on their initial comfortable walking speed, subjects were stratified as low (< 45 cm/sec) or high functioning (> 45 cm/sec). In the low functioning subjects, walking speed with BWS increased as a function of that adopted when walking with FWB. As compared to walking with FWB, they experienced an overall increase of 21 cm/sec (72%) and 72 cm/sec (263%), respectively, for the comfortable and fast walking speed conditions (Fig. 2B). In the high functioning subjects, walking speed with BWS did not significantly covary with the subjects' speed with FWB, as illustrated by slopes approaching zero (Fig. 2A, right panel). The high functioning subjects also showed no change ($\Delta = -1.0$ cm/sec, -1.69%) in walking speed when asked to walk at their comfortable pace with BWS (Fig. 2B). At fast speed, however, they could benefit from BWS and further increase their speed by 108 cm/sec (95%). These preliminary findings suggest that BWS during overground locomotion can induce changes in walking speed. Low functioning subjects appear to benefit from BWS, whereas higher functioning subjects will benefit from it only when they are required to walk at maximal speed.

Lamontagne and Fung (75) also showed that BWS during overground walking had an effect mainly on proximal lower body kinematics. Both the paretic and nonparetic limbs displayed less circumduction during supported locomotion, with increased hip excursions in the plane of progression due to larger hip extension in late stance and larger hip flexion in swing. Body center of mass (CoM) trajectory is also influenced by BWS. Figure 3 illustrates the CoM trajectory of a stroke subject walking with BWS or FWB, both at comfortable or maximal walking speed. Two main findings emerged, and these were also reflected in the average group data. First, walking faster decreases side-to-side displacements of body CoM of stroke subjects, as reported for healthy subjects (77,78). Second, BWS does not reduce side-to-side displacement of body CoM, but it causes the CoM to cross the body's midline and to move toward the paretic side. This

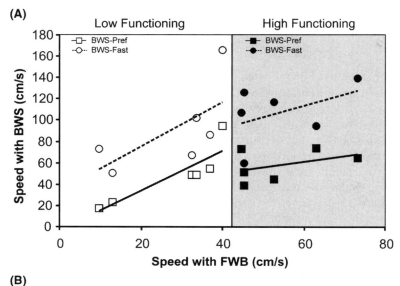

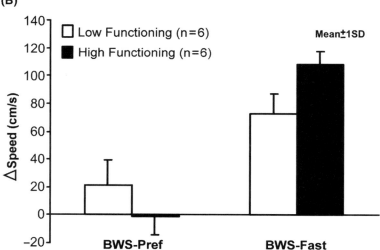

Figure 2 Instantaneous changes in comfortable and fast walking speed of stroke subjects ($n = 12$) in response to unloading through body weight support (BWS) provided during overground locomotion. Based on their initial comfortable walking speed with full weight bearing (FWB), the subjects were stratified as low (< 45 cm/sec) or high functioning (> 45 cm/sec). In (**A**), change in walking speed with BWS as a function of the FWB walking speed is illustrated. In (**B**), absolute and percentage changes in walking speed with BWS as compared to the FWB conditions are shown.

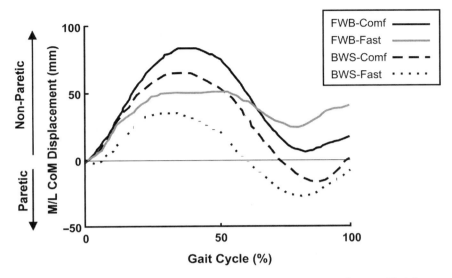

Figure 3 Mediolateral (M/L) trajectory of the body center of mass (CoM) as a function of the gait cycle for one representative stroke subject. The subject was walking either with body weigh support (BWS) or with full weight bearing (FWB), at comfortable or fast speed. A positive lateral displacement of body CoM indicates a displacement toward the nonparetic side.

more centered position of the body CoM is likely due to increased weight bearing of the paretic limb observed during the stance phase of walking with BWS (79).

In contrast to supported treadmill ambulation, overground walking with BWS does not appear to reduce the amplitude of activation of antigravity muscles such as hip extensors or ankle plantarflexors. Instead, bilateral increases in hip flexor activation were observed with overground walking with BWS (75). As BWS during overground locomotion induces changes in walking speed, this increased hip flexor activation may reflect both the larger recruitment of hip flexor muscles with speed (80) and the use of a hip flexor strategy to swing the limb through with BWS. The latter hypothesis would be consistent with the patients' subjective report of less difficulty in moving the paretic limb during swing while walking with BWS.

C. Evidences Supporting the Use of BWS

The combined use of BWS and treadmill ambulation to restore locomotion after stroke has received much attention over the last decade (44,48,56,57) (81–87). In those intervention studies, unloading was usually set at 30–40% of body weight, and progressively adjusted to the patient's walking ability during the course of training (44,47–49,58). As compared to conventional therapy involving no treadmill training, 3 weeks of supported treadmill ambulation training were shown to lead to larger gains in walking ability and gait speed (47), as well as to a tendency for improved walking energy cost (effect size of 0.7) and endurance (effect size of 1.16) (49). Nonambulatory stroke subjects who were plateauing in the improvement of their gait ability were also shown to benefit from 3 weeks of supported treadmill ambulation training, as reflected by significant improvements in their gait speed, temporal-distance factors, and motor function (58). In those studies, however, the effect of BWS could not be separated from that of repetitive treadmill practice, due to either a lack of a control group, or the fact that the control groups were not receiving treadmill training with FWB. In recent trials, Pohl et al. (43) and Sullivan et al. (44) demonstrated impressive increases in walking speed after a supported treadmill ambulation training regime, especially when they were trained at fast walking speeds. As discussed later in this chapter, however, the key element for such improvement could be the walking speed at which these patients were trained, rather than the use of BWS.

Visintin et al. (48) compared 6 weeks of treadmill ambulation training with BWS to treadmill training with full weight in a cohort of a 100 nonchronic (< 6 months) stroke subjects. Post-training (6 weeks) and follow-up (3 months) assessments revealed larger improvements in motor recovery and walking speed in the BWS group, but similar improvements in balance and endurance between the FWB and BWS groups. In Nilsson et al. (83), supported treadmill ambulation training was compared to combined overground gait training and Motor Relearning Programme (MRP) in 73 nonchronic stroke subjects. No post-training differences emerged between the two groups for walking speed, motor control, and balance. It thus seems that BWS combined with treadmill training is preferred over treadmill training alone, yet not superior to overground training. In fact, in the study by Visintin et al. (48), the gain in speeds during treadmill walking was larger than that overground (Table 1), indicating an incomplete carry-over effect to overground locomotion.

In summary, despite the lack of adequate control groups in many BWS studies, it seems that supported treadmill ambulation is preferred over treadmill walking alone to increase walking speed (48), but there is no evidence that it is superior to an intensive overground training. It is also noteworthy to mention that some nonambulatory or very low functioning stroke subject could walk only when provided with BWS (48,58). Moreover, low functioning subjects spontaneously and instantaneously increase their walking speed when walking overground with BWS, which is not the case for high functioning subjects (75). At variance with the conclusions of a recent review on supported treadmill ambulation training (88), these evidences suggest that BWS may be especially useful for low functioning or nonambulatory subjects, providing them with an alternative to practice and develop their walking skills that would otherwise be impossible to achieve.

IV. SPEED-INTENSIVE WALKING

A. Rationale

In sports training paradigms, task-specificity, repetition, and intensity are key elements to skill improvement. Elite athletes not only spend time in general training programs, but also repeatedly practice the specific tasks required for their discipline, such as running or swimming. Their training routine is targeted and graded in such way that it challenges the motor, sensory, and cardiovascular systems to result in task-specific improvements in muscle strength, movement co-ordination, as well as endurance and/or speed of movement execution.

Stroke subjects admitted to rehabilitation spend most of the their time in inactive conditions (89,90). In a recent study, (on average, only 2.8 ± 0.9 and 0.7 ± 0.2 min per session of physical and occupational therapy, respectively, were spent on exercises that increased the heart rate sufficiently to improve cardiovascular function and induce training effect) (91). While recognizing the benefits of current therapies, we may certainly question whether the patients are provided the optimal amount and intensity of training to prevent deconditioning and improve their endurance and walking speed. Based on the principle of task-specificity, should we not train patients at faster speeds of walking if we want them to gain the muscle power, the co-ordination and the postural reactions required in generating and safely maneuvering faster gait speeds? Should we not impose a stress on the muscular and cardiovascular if the goal is to improve endurance? There is no comprehensive information available yet on how a defective "system," such as that affected by a stroke, responds to higher intensity training paradigms. Nonetheless, there are studies showing that muscle strength (25,51), endurance (9,25,46,92), and rapidity of movement execution (25,43,44) can be effectively and safely trained in the stroke population. While the risk of inducing unwanted compensations with high movement speeds or fatigue may also be a concern, we will show results from our recent studies that demonstrate actual improvement of the walking pattern with faster walking speeds.

B. Adaptations to Speed

Adaptations to walking speed are well known in healthy subjects. Higher speeds generally induce increased muscle activation levels (77,93) and larger joint excursions (77,78,94). Speed also impacts on temporal-distance factors such as cadence, stride length, and stance duration (78,94). Optimal head–thorax (95) and thorax–pelvis (96,97) co-ordination profiles are observed at gait speeds within the 1.2 and 1.8 m/sec range. Energy consumption can also be optimized in same bandwidth (65–67).

In a recent study, we investigated the effect of fast overground walking on the walking pattern of hemiparetic subjects early after stroke (75). The objective was twofold: to determine to which extent hemiparetic subjects can increase their walking speed and to identify the changes in muscle activation and joint displacements with speed. Figure 4 illustrates the increase

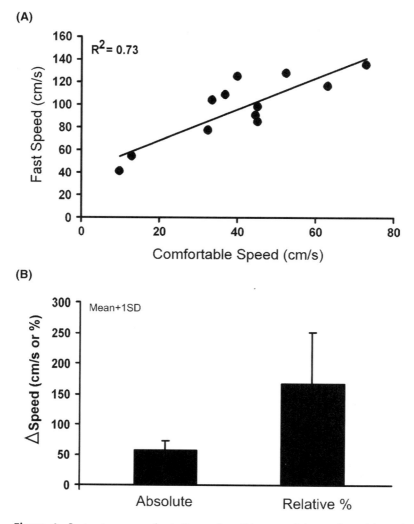

Figure 4 Instantaneous adaptations of walking speed in stroke subjects ($n = 12$) instructed to walk as fast as they could. In (**A**), the relationship between the fast walking speeds and the initial comfortable speeds, as well as the corresponding coefficient of determination (R^2) are represented. In (**B**), the mean absolute and relative (%) changes in walking speed are illustrated.

in speed performed by 12 stroke subjects with initial comfortable walking speeds varying from 9 to 73 cm/sec. Five of those subjects had only started to make steps for less than 1 week. The subjects were walking overground with full weight, secured by a safety harness that was attached to an overhead suspension rail with minimal friction. First, note the dramatic capability of the subjects, even the low functioning ones, to increase their gait speed when instructed to do so in a safe environment. The faster the initial comfortable speed, the faster the fast speed achieved ($R^2 = 0.73$). Surprisingly, the capacity to increase speed in the lower functioning subjects (initial speed < 45 cm/sec) was similar to that of the higher functioning (> 45 cm/sec) ones, with both groups reaching average speed increments of 56 cm/sec. Overall, walking speed was 2–3 times higher than the initial preferred speed. Along with speed changes, symmetry between the paretic and nonparetic sides for double and single limb support phases also improved. As symmetry in variables such as stance and swing durations were reported to remain unchanged with fast treadmill walking (98), it is likely that adaptations to speed differ between overground and treadmill walking.

Figure 5 illustrates the mean changes in muscle activation levels of stroke subjects walking at comfortable and fast speeds. It is evident that faster speed induces larger muscle activation levels, as reported for the healthy subjects (77,93). More specifically, larger muscle activation levels were observed for the ankle plantarflexors at push-off [30–70% of gait cycle] and the hip extensor in early stance [0–30% of gait cycle]. Flexor muscles also followed the same trend, with higher levels of activation on both sides for the ankle dorsiflexors and the hip flexors at toe-off [60–80% of gait cycle]. Similar dependency of lower limb muscle activation was reported in stroke subjects during fast treadmill walking (98). More timely onsets of muscle activation were also observed with fast walking (98), suggesting improvement in the quality of the muscle activation patterns.

Movement patterns of the lower limbs also improve with faster walking speed in hemiparetic subjects (39). Bilateral and symmetrical increases in hip and knee excursions are observed with faster walking speeds (75). Improved thorax–pelvis co-ordination in the horizontal plane emerges when stroke subjects are required to walk at speeds approaching those of healthy subjects (12).

Another important outcome to consider for stroke subjects is their energy expenditure during walking. Interestingly, although stroke subjects display higher heart rates at faster walking speeds, their overall walking energy cost (J m^{-1} kg^{-1}) and heart rate (beats m^{-1}) correlate negatively with speed ($r = -0.51$ to $r = -0.55$), indicating greater efficiency at faster walking speeds (98). Improved co-ordination and facilitation of interjoint and inter-limb energy transfers during fast walking could partly explain this lower energy cost. In summary, fast walking appears to "normalize" temporal-distance factors, increase muscle activation levels and enhance movement

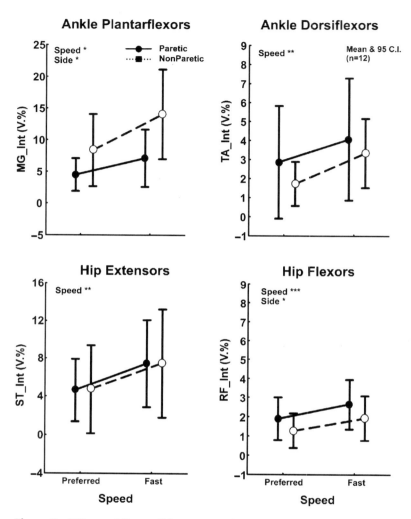

Figure 5 Effects of fast walking on muscle activation of the medial gastrocnemius (MG), tibialis anterior (TA), semitendinosus (ST), and rectus femoris of the paretic and nonparetic limbs of stroke subjects. Amplitudes of muscle activation were measured using integrals (int) over the muscle linear envelopes for functionally relevant time windows of the gait cycle (%): MG activation at push-off [30%:70%], TA activation at toe-off [60%:80%], ST activation in early stance [0%:30%], and RF activation at toe-off [60%:80%]. Main effects resulting from the analyses of variance are indicated, with levels of significance at $*p < 0.05$, $**p < 0.01$, and $***p < 0.001$. There were no significant interaction effects.

co-ordination. This is done at a lower energy expenditure and with no deleterious effects on gait quality.

C. Intensity: The Key for Improved Speed and Endurance

Based on the task-specificity paradigm and on sports physiology principles, new speed-intensive training programs started to emerge and were tested in the stroke subject population. Sullivan et al. (44), in a group of chronic stroke subjects having mild to severe gait disabilities, studied the effect of a 4-week high-speed training program. Subjects were trained on a treadmill at a preset fast speed of 0.89 m/sec. The fast-speed training group was compared to a group trained at slow (0.22 m/sec) and variable (0.22–0.89 m/sec) speeds. The subjects were walking with partial BWS, which was gradually reduced as their walking capacity improved. After 4 weeks, the fast-speed training group showed the largest improvement in overground self-selected walking speed ($\Delta = 0.15$ m/sec), as compared to the slow ($\Delta = 0.06$ m/sec) and the variable ($\Delta = 0.07$ m/sec) training groups. The gains in speed were also retained at 3-months' follow-up. It is worth noting that even severely disabled subjects improved and could handle the fast-training program when provided with the necessary help (BWS and manual assistance). In a cohort of 60 stroke subjects, Pohl et al. (43) compared the effectiveness of a 4-week structured speed-dependent treadmill training to that of limited progressive treadmill training and conventional gait therapy. In the speed-dependent group, subjects were required to walk at maximal speed for preset intervals. Treadmill belt speed was thereafter increased by steps of 10% upon successful completion of each walking trial. The speed-dependent group scored significantly higher than the other two groups in overground walking speed and Functional Ambulation Category scores. In fact, the speed-dependent group increased their overground fast walking speed by 1.0 m/sec (from 0.61 to 1.63 m/sec), as compared to a gain of 0.31 and 0.56 m/sec for the limited progressive and the conventional gait therapy groups, respectively.

A pilot study was carried out by Dean et al. (25) to examine the efficacy of a 4-week task-related circuit-training program in a group of chronic stroke subjects ($n = 12$). The task-circuit consisted of an exercise class with 10 workstations incorporating locomotor-related activities such as side stepping, sit-to-walk, and walking over obstacles, as well as walking races and relays. As compared to the control group, who practiced upper limb tasks, the circuit-training group demonstrated improvements in walking speed, endurance, force production through the affected limb and the ability to balance on the affected limb. The effects were retained at the 2-months' follow-up. Once again, despite the variability of functional abilities among the subjects, they all showed improvements. This pilot study provides evidence for the use of class exercises incorporating task-circuit training to improve locomotor function after stroke. Such a training paradigm based on task-specificity also incorporates the principles of intensity, repetition, graded task complexity, and flexibility. It provides the patient with a motivating environment with meaningful tasks and teamwork with other patients.

Training protocols that specifically target aerobic capacity were also developed and tested in chronic hemiparetic subjects (45,46,92). In contrast to the speed-intensive programs, the aerobic training programs usually involve longer durations of training, such as weekly sessions over 6 months, and require the subjects to walk or exercise within 50–60% of heart rate reserve. Such protocols, although time consuming, yielded very positive results, increasing aerobic capacity, lowering energy cost of walking and increasing workload capacity (45,46,92). Fatigue is reported by 68% of stroke subjects and is perceived as one of the worst of their symptoms that also impacts negatively on functional abilities (99). One may thus suspect that aerobic training most likely enhances functional abilities and quality of life (46), although this has not been formerly studied. How subjects with a recent stroke respond to aerobic training and how such training can be incorporated within rehabilitation programs that are under pressure to be shortened is yet to be determined. A good alternative may be to provide the subjects with outpatient services through the format of class exercises, as in Dean et al. (25).

In summary, gait speed and endurance can improve markedly beyond expectations in stroke subjects, when provided with speed-specific or intensity-specific training. Within the present review, little if no deterioration in walking quality could be observed with fast walking. Due to proper screening of the patients and monitoring of cardiac function during the intensive training protocols (43,44,46,92), no inadvertent cardiopulmonary events were induced, indicating that such training programs can be administered safely. Risks of falls must also be minimized by providing the required assistance and/or supervision throughout the training sessions. Faster walking speed and greater endurance may induce the most important changes in the patient's daily life, allowing the patient, for instance, to cross the street within the required time, or to participate in community activities.

V. SENSORY CUES AND BALANCE ADJUSTMENT DURING LOCOMOTION

A. Balance Control During Locomotion

Functional locomotion involves not only moving from one place to another but also treading on changing and uneven terrains without falling. Thus, appropriate motor strategies must be executed by the CNS, based on the sensory information gathered from the visual, vestibular, and somatosensory systems, to counteract unexpected surface changes during locomotion. Locomotion is often challenged under unpredictable situations in daily activities. The CNS must adapt the locomotor pattern to the environmental changes so that locomotion continues and equilibrium is maintained. Such adaptation requires supraspinal control of goal-directed behavior (100,101). Uneven weight bearing is a common characteristic of stroke patients during standing with more body weight borne on the nonparetic than the paretic limb (102,103). It has been shown that the asymmetrical limb-loading pattern is associated with excessive body sway in the frontal plane and a decrease in lateral stability (103,104), leading to frequent falls towards the affected side (105). Quick and unconscious muscle activations with specific spatio-temporal patterns are prerequisites of the postural responses triggered by an unexpected movement of the support surface. Recent results by Fung et al. (106) demonstrated that the postural responses triggered by surface perturbations in healthy subjects, as measured by the changes in center of pressure, body kinematics, and EMG activation were markedly reduced during walking, as compared to standing. In contrast, stroke patients had difficulty maintaining balance when exposed to perturbations during standing or walking (107).

B. Sensory Cues in the Control of Balance

Motor learning in stroke patients can be compromised by reduced sensory feedback. Various forms of sensory feedback given to hemiplegic patients have successfully improved the performance. For example, the combined use of biofeedback and functional electrical stimulation to tibialis anterior and gastrocnemius muscles improves flexion of the knee and ankle during the swing phase of walking (108). This improvement in gait function is also shown in the increased gait velocity. Sensory feedback has also been used to improve postural control in stroke patients. Hemiplegic patients who are provided with auditory (109) or visual feedback (110) about their relative weight distribution (paretic vs. nonparetic limb) during standing demonstrate a significant improvement in weight symmetry. Karnath et al. (111) have shown that the combination of galvanic stimulation and vibration of neck muscles can improve visual verticality in stroke patients manifesting hemineglect.

Somatosensory information from the fingertip, or haptic cues, is an important source of sensory feedback in the control of balance. Tactile information provided through lightly touching a rigid surface has been shown to decrease postural sway during quiet stance (112,113) and reduce the anticipatory postural adjustments from trunk and leg muscles during a unilateral shoulder flexion task (114). Even passive light touch delivered to the shoulder or leg by an object fixed to the environment can stabilize the body during standing (115). Light touch provided information on the position and velocity of the body in relation to the external objects or surface (116,117).

C. Tactile Sensory Feedback Improves Balance During Walking in Stroke Patients

A recent study was conducted to examine the effects of light touch on postural responses triggered by unexpected surface perturbation in the toes-up direction walking in 11 stroke patients and 8 healthy age-matched subjects. A 5-m wide wood plank was mounted firmly beside the walkway to provide somatosensory information from the environment through the fingertip (on the nonparetic for stroke subjects and on the right side for healthy controls). The top of the rail was adjusted at the level of each individual's hip level. A thin strip of load sensors ($0.15 \, \text{m} \times 2.45 \, \text{m}$ dimension) was secured on the surface of the plank to measure the amount of force exerted by the fingertip. A force that exceeded $4 \, \text{N}$ would trigger a beep and subjects were habituated to walk while sliding the tip of their index finger along the sensor strip without triggering the sound.

Figure 6A compares the instantaneous CoM velocity in the A/P direction during walking between the groups of stroke and healthy subjects. In the absence of tactile cue, the speed of forward progression as measured by the CoM velocity was slightly decreased in the control subjects and markedly reduced in the stroke subjects when walking was perturbed by a sudden toes-up surface tilt. Generally, the stroke subjects demonstrated an average of 60% decrease in the CoM velocity when walking was perturbed in the absence of tactile cue. While tactile cue did not affect the change in the forward progression of the control subjects during perturbed walking, it significantly increased the speed of forward progression in all stroke subjects ($p < 0.005$), even though stroke patients still walked slower than control subjects. In the absence of tactile sensory feedback, the decrease in forward CoM velocity was associated with postural instability induced by perturbations during quiet stance in stroke patients, as shown by the increased RMS of CoM trajectory in the anteroposterior (AP) direction (Fig. 6B). The group of healthy subjects did not exhibit any significant relation of postural sway with decreased CoM velocity during perturbed walking ($R^2 = 0.1$), but when pooled with the group of stroke patients, a strong linear relation emerged (Fig. 6B, solid line, $R^2 = 0.72$). In the presence of tactile cue, this relation became weakened (Fig. 6B, dotted line, $R^2 = 0.4$) with decreased trunk instability in stroke patients. In addition, the deviations of the trunk and pelvis and the excursion of compensatory movements of the free arm in stroke patients during perturbed walking were significantly decreased when tactile cue was provided. The abnormal and asymmetric muscle activations used by stroke subjects in restoring equilibrium also improved significantly with light touch. The effects of light touch were more prominent in stroke

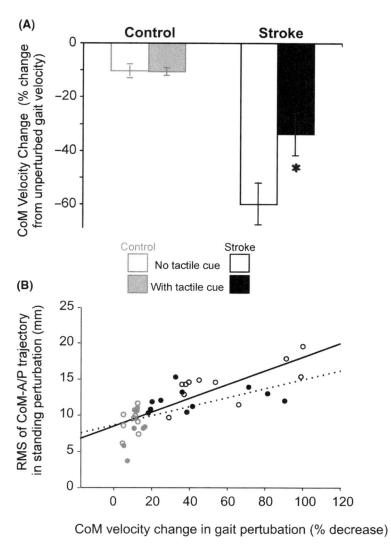

Figure 6 (**A**) Change in instantaneous velocity of the anteroposterior (AP) CoM during toes-up perturbation in walking; and (**B**) correlation of the RMS of CoM-AP trajectory during toes-up perturbations quiet stance with the percentage decrease in instantaneous CoM velocity during perturbed walking; in 11 stroke subjects (black) and 8 age-matched healthy controls (gray), in the presence (filled bars) or absence (open bars) of tactile cue provided through the nonparetic (stroke) or right (healthy) index fingertip. The CoM velocity is expressed as the average change from the instant of toes-up surface perturbation during double limb support to the next initial foot contact in the gait cycle, as a percentage of the baseline CoM velocity averaged over 10 unperturbed gait cycles.

subjects, possibly due to the different degree of sensory information available to the two subject groups. These results suggest that tactile sensory feedback can be used for gait rehabilitation following stroke to improve equilibrium reactions during walking.

VI. CONCLUDING REMARKS

A contemporary approach to gait disorders and rehabilitation is the use of systematic analyses and task-specific locomotor training paradigms. We have presented a comprehensive review of the efficacy of different modes of locomotion (treadmill vs. overground), partial weight support, and speed-intensive training on gait outcomes following stroke. Of particular interest is the potential of speed-intensive training overground with partial weight support that targets low-level functioning stroke patients in the early phase of rehabilitation, as shown by the promising results from our laboratory. We have also investigated the control of balance during locomotion in stroke patients and explored the use of sensory feedback to improve postural adjustment during gait. Recent results have shown that light touch through the nonparetic fingertip can facilitate the recovery of upright balance when gait is perturbed in stroke patients. These new and encouraging findings have advanced our understanding of how motor learning concepts can be extended to gait retraining following stroke.

ACKNOWLEDGMENTS

We acknowledge the skilful assistance of our graduate students, especially Roain Bayat and Rumpa Boonsinsukh, in data collection and analysis. We appreciate the help of Eric Johnstone in designing and fabricating the overground constant weight support system, made possible through the funding of the JRH Foundation and the Canada Foundation for Innovation. We thank the physiotherapists of the JRH neurology program for their help in screening and referring patients for our experiments. A. Lamontagne is a New Investigator supported by the Canadian Institutes of Health Research. J. Fung is a William Dawson Scholar of McGill University and a research scholar of the Fonds de Recherche en Santé du Québec. The JRH Research Center is a site of the Centre de Recherche Interdisciplinaire en Réadaptation of Montreal, Canada.

REFERENCES

1. Wolfe CD, Giroud M, Kolominsky-Rabas P, Dundas R, Lemesle M, Heuschmann P, Rudd A. Variations in stroke incidence and survival in 3 areas of Europe. European Registries of Stroke (EROS) Collaboration. Stroke 2000; 31:2074–2079.

2. Keenan MA, Perry J, Jordan C. Factors affecting balance and ambulation following stroke. Clin Orthop 1984; 182:165–171.
3. Perry J, Garrett M, Gronley JK, Mulroy SJ. Classification of walking handicap in the stroke population. Stroke 1995; 26:982–989.
4. Hill K, Ellis P, Bernhardt J, Maggs P, Hull S. Balance and mobility outcomes for stroke patients: a comprehensive audit. Aust J Physiother 1997; 43:173–180.
5. von Schroeder HP, Coutts RD, Lyden PD, Billings E Jr, Nickel VL. Gait parameters following stroke: a practical assessment. J Rehabil Res Dev 1995; 32:25–31.
6. Murray MP, Kory RC, Clarkson BH. Walking patterns in healthy old men. J Gerontol 1969; 24:169–178.
7. Gersten JW, Orr W. External work of walking in hemiparetic patients. Scand J Rehabil Med 1971; 3:85–88.
8. Corcoran PJ, Jebsen RH, Brengelmann GL, Simons BC. Effects of plastic and metal leg braces on speed and energy cost of hemiparetic ambulation. Arch Phys Med Rehabil 1970; 51:69–77.
9. Dean CM, Richards CL, Malouin F. Walking speed over 10 metres overestimates locomotor capacity after stroke. Clin Rehabil 2001; 15:415–421.
10. Olney SJ, Richards CL. Hemiparetic gait following stroke. Part I: Characteristics. Gait Posture 1996; 4:136–148.
11. Donker SF, Beek PJ, Wagenaar RC, Mulder T. Coordination between arm and leg movements during locomotion. J Mot Behav 2001; 33:86–102.
12. Wagenaar RC, Beek WJ. Hemiplegic gait: a kinematic analysis using walking speed as a basis. J Biomech 1992; 25:1007–1015.
13. Lamontagne A, De Serres S, Fung J, Paquet N. Stroke affects the coordination and stabilization of head, thorax and pelvis during voluntary horizontal head motions performed in walking. Clin Neurophysiol 2005; 116:101–111.
14. Shumway-Cook A, Woollacott M. Motor Control: Theory and Practical Applications. 2nd ed. Maryland: Williams & Wilkins, 2001.
15. Schmidt RA. Motor Control and Learning: A Behavioral Emphasis. 2nd ed. Champaign, IL: Human Kinetics, 1988.
16. Winstein CJ. Knowledge of results and motor learning—implications for physical therapy. Phys Ther 1991; 71:140–149.
17. Richards CL, Malouin F, Wood-Dauphinee S, Williams JI, Bouchard JP, Brunet D. Task-specific physical therapy for optimization of gait recovery in acute stroke patients. Arch Phys Med Rehabil 1993; 74:612–620.
18. Malouin F, Potvin M, Prevost J, Richards CL, Wood-Dauphinee S. Use of an intensive task-oriented gait training program in a series of patients with acute cerebrovascular accidents. Phys Ther 1992; 72:781–789; discussion 789–793.
19. Nudo RJ, Plautz EJ, Frost SB. Role of adaptive plasticity in recovery of function after damage to motor cortex. Muscle Nerve 2001; 24:1000–1019.
20. Traversa R, Cicinelli P, Bassi A, Rossini PM, Bernardi G. Mapping of motor cortical reorganization after stroke. A brain stimulation study with focal magnetic pulses. Stroke 1997; 28:110–117.
21. Liepert J, Bauder H, Wolfgang HR, Miltner WH, Taub E, Weiller C. Treatment-induced cortical reorganization after stroke in humans. Stroke 2000; 31:1210–1216.

22. Liepert J, Miltner WH, Bauder H, Sommer M, Dettmers C, Taub E, Weiller C. Motor cortex plasticity during constraint-induced movement therapy in stroke patients. Neurosci Lett 1998; 250:5–8.
23. Liepert J, Terborg C, Weiller C. Motor plasticity induced by synchronized thumb and foot movements. Exp Brain Res 1999; 125:435–439.
24. Kwakkel G, Wagenaar RC, Twisk JW, Lankhorst GJ, Koetsier JC. Intensity of leg and arm training after primary middle-cerebral-artery stroke: a randomised trial. Lancet 1999; 354:191–196.
25. Dean CM, Richards CL, Malouin F. Task-related circuit training improves performance of locomotor tasks in chronic stroke: a randomized, controlled pilot trial. Arch Phys Med Rehabil 2000; 81:409–417.
26. Dean CM, Shepherd RB. Task-related training improves performance of seated reaching tasks after stroke. A randomized controlled trial. Stroke 1997; 28:722–728.
27. Carr JH, Shepherd RB. A Motor Relearning Programme for Stroke. 2nd ed. Oxford: Butterworth-Heinemann, 1987.
28. Barbeau H, Rossignol S. Recovery of locomotion after chronic spinalization in the adult cat. Brain Res 1987; 412:84–95.
29. Lovely RG, Gregor RJ, Roy RR, Edgerton VR. Weight-bearing hind limb stepping in treadmill-exercised adult spinal cats. Brain Res 1990; 514:206–218.
30. de Leon RD, Hodgson JA, Roy RR, Edgerton VR. Locomotor capacity attributable to step training versus spontaneous recovery after spinalization in adult cats. J Neurophysiol 1998; 79:1329–1340.
31. de Leon RD, Roy RR, Edgerton VR. Is the recovery of stepping following spinal cord injury mediated by modifying existing neural pathways or by generating new pathways? A perspective. Phys Ther 2001; 81:1904–1911.
32. Murray MP, Spurr GB, Sepic SB, Gardner GM, Mollinger LA. Treadmill vs. floor walking: kinematics, electromyogram, and heart rate. J Appl Physiol 1985; 59:87–91.
33. Stolze H, Kuhtz-Buschbeck JP, Mondwurf C, Boczek-Funcke A, Johnk K, Deuschl G, Illert M. Gait analysis during treadmill and overground locomotion in children and adults. Electroencephalogr Clin Neurophysiol 1997; 105:490–497.
34. Alton F, Baldey L, Caplan S, Morrissey MC. A kinematic comparison of overground and treadmill walking. Clin Biomech (Bristol, Avon) 1998; 13:434–440.
35. Pearce ME, Cunningham DA, Donner AP, Rechnitzer PA, Fullerton GM, Howard JH. Energy cost of treadmill and floor walking at self-selected paces. Eur J Appl Physiol Occup Physiol 1983; 52:115–119.
36. Vogt L, Pfeifer K, Banzer W. Comparison of angular lumbar spine and pelvis kinematics during treadmill and overground locomotion. Clin Biomech (Bristol, Avon) 2002; 17:162–165.
37. White SC, Yack HJ, Tucker CA, Lin HY. Comparison of vertical ground reaction forces during overground and treadmill walking. Med Sci Sports Exerc 1998; 30:1537–1542.
38. Arsenault AB, Winter DA, Marteniuk RG. Treadmill versus walkway locomotion in humans: an EMG study. Ergonomics 1986; 29:665–676.

39. Bayat R, Barbeau H, Lamontagne A. Speed and temporal distance adaptations during treadmill and overground walking following stroke. Neurorehabil Neural Repair. In press.
40. Harris-Love ML, Forrester LW, Macko RF, Silver KH, Smith GV. Hemiparetic gait parameters in overground versus treadmill walking. Neurorehabil Neural Repair 2001; 15:105–112.
41. Derave W, Tombeux N, Cottyn J, Pannier JL, De Clercq D. Treadmill exercise negatively affects visual contribution to static postural stability. Int J Sports Med 2002; 23:44–49.
42. Lamontagne A, Paquet N, Fung J. Postural adjustments to voluntary head motions during standing are modified following stroke. Clin Biomech (Bristol, Avon) 2003; 18:832–842.
43. Pohl M, Mehrholz J, Ritschel C, Ruckriem S. Speed-dependent treadmill training in ambulatory hemiparetic stroke patients: a randomized controlled trial. Stroke 2002; 33:553–558.
44. Sullivan KJ, Knowlton BJ, Dobkin BH. Step training with body weight support: effect of treadmill speed and practice paradigms on poststroke locomotor recovery. Arch Phys Med Rehabil 2002; 83:683–691.
45. Macko RF, DeSouza CA, Tretter LD, Silver KH, Smith GV, Anderson PA, Tomoyasu N, Gorman P, Dengel DR. Treadmill aerobic exercise training reduces the energy expenditure and cardiovascular demands of hemiparetic gait in chronic stroke patients. A preliminary report. Stroke 1997; 28:326–330.
46. Macko RF, Smith GV, Dobrovolny CL, Sorkin JD, Goldberg AP, Silver KH. Treadmill training improves fitness reserve in chronic stroke patients. Arch Phys Med Rehabil 2001; 82:879–884.
47. Hesse S, Bertelt C, Jahnke MT, Schaffrin A, Baake P, Malezic M, Mauritz KH. Treadmill training with partial body weight support compared with physiotherapy in nonambulatory hemiparetic patients. Stroke 1995; 26:976–981.
48. Visintin M, Barbeau H, Korner-Bitensky N, Mayo NE. A new approach to retrain gait in stroke patients through body weight support and treadmill stimulation. Stroke 1998; 29:1122–1128.
49. da Cunha IT Jr, Lim PA, Qureshy H, Henson H, Monga T, Protas EJ. Gait outcomes after acute stroke rehabilitation with supported treadmill ambulation training: a randomized controlled pilot study. Arch Phys Med Rehabil 2002; 83:1258–1265.
50. Waagfjord J, Levangie PK, Certo CM. Effects of treadmill training on gait in a hemiparetic patient. Phys Ther 1990; 70:549–558; discussion 558–560.
51. Smith GV, Silver KH, Goldberg AP, Macko RF. "Task-oriented" exercise improves hamstring strength and spastic reflexes in chronic stroke patients. Stroke 1999; 30:2112–2118.
52. Laufer Y, Dickstein R, Chefez Y, Marcovitz E. The effect of treadmill training on the ambulation of stroke survivors in the early stages of rehabilitation: a randomized study. J Rehabil Res Dev 2001; 38:69–78.
53. Spilg EG, Martin BJ, Mitchell SL, Aitchison TC. A comparison of mobility assessments in a geriatric day hospital. Clin Rehabil 2001; 15:296–300.

54. Norman KE, Pepin A, Ladouceur M, Barbeau H. A treadmill apparatus and harness support for evaluation and rehabilitation of gait. Arch Phys Med Rehabil 1995; 76:772–778.

55. Wernig A, Muller S. Laufband locomotion with body weight support improved walking in persons with severe spinal cord injuries. Paraplegia 1992; 30:229–238.

56. Visintin M, Barbeau H. The effects of body weight support on the locomotor pattern of spastic paretic patients. Can J Neurol Sci 1989; 16:315–325.

57. Hesse S, Konrad M, Uhlenbrock D. Treadmill walking with partial body weight support versus floor walking in hemiparetic subjects. Arch Phys Med Rehabil 1999; 80:421–427.

58. Hesse S, Bertelt C, Schaffrin A, Malezic M, Mauritz KH. Restoration of gait in nonambulatory hemiparetic patients by treadmill training with partial body-weight support. Arch Phys Med Rehabil 1994; 75:1087–1093.

59. Hassid E, Rose D, Commisarow J, Guttry M, Dobkin BH. Improved gait symmetry in hemiparetic stroke patients induced during body weight-supported treadmill stepping. NeuroRehabilitation 1997; 11:21–26.

60. Dietz V, Colombo G. Influence of body load on the gait pattern in Parkinson's disease. Mov Disord 1998; 13:255–261.

61. Dietz V, Leenders KL, Colombo G. Leg muscle activation during gait in Parkinson's disease: influence of body unloading. Electroencephalogr Clin Neurophysiol 1997; 105:400–405.

62. Winter DA. Biomechanics of normal and pathological gait: implications for understanding human locomotor control. J Mot Behav 1989; 21:337–356.

63. Taub E, Goldberg IA. Use of sensory recombination and somatosensory deafferentation techniques in the investigation of sensory-motor integration. Perception 1974; 3:393–405.

64. Taub E, Miller NE, Novack TA, Cook EW, Fleming WC, Nepomuceno CS, Connell JS, Crago JE. Technique to improve chronic motor deficit after stroke. Arch Phys Med Rehabil 1993; 74:347–354.

65. Cavagna GA, Willems PA, Heglund NC. The role of gravity in human walking: pendular energy exchange, external work and optimal speed. J Physiol 2000; 528:657–668.

66. Griffin TM, Tolani NA, Kram R. Walking in simulated reduced gravity: mechanical energy fluctuations and exchange. J Appl Physiol 1999; 86: 383–390.

67. Farley CT, McMahon TA. Energetics of walking and running: insights from simulated reduced-gravity experiments. J Appl Physiol 1992; 73:2709–2712.

68. Colby SM, Kirkendall DT, Bruzga RF. Electromyographic analysis and energy expenditure of harness supported treadmill walking: implications for knee rehabilitation. Gait Posture 1999; 10:200–205.

69. Danielsson A, Sunnerhagen KS. Oxygen consumption during treadmill walking with and without body weight support in patients with hemiparesis after stroke and in healthy subjects. Arch Phys Med Rehabil 2000; 81:953–957.

70. Ivanenko YP, Grasso R, Macellari V, Lacquaniti F. Control of foot trajectory in human locomotion: role of ground contact forces in simulated reduced gravity. J Neurophysiol 2002; 87:3070–3089.

71. Harkema SJ, Hurley SL, Patel UK, Requejo PS, Dobkin BH, Edgerton VR. Human lumbosacral spinal cord interprets loading during stepping. J Neurophysiol 1997; 77:797–811.
72. Finch L, Barbeau H, Arsenault B. Influence of body weight support on normal human gait: development of a gait retraining strategy. Phys Ther 1991; 71:842–855; discussion 855–856.
73. Flynn TW, Canavan PK, Cavanagh PR, Chiang JH. Plantar pressure reduction in an incremental weight-bearing system. Phys Ther 1997; 77:410–416.
74. Threlkeld AJ, Cooper LD, Monger BP, Craven AN, Haupt HG. Temporospatial and kinematic gait alterations during treadmill walking with body weight suspension. Gait Posture 2003; 17:235–245.
75. Lamontagne A, Fung J. Faster is better: Implications for speed-intensive gait training after stroke. Stroke 2004; 35:2543–2548.
76. Hesse S, Helm B, Krajnik J, Gregoric M, Mauritz KH. Treadmill training with partial body weight support: influence of body weight release on the gait of hemiparetic patients. J Neurol Rehabil 1997; 11:15–20.
77. Murray MP, Mollinger LA, Gardner GM, Sepic SB. Kinematic and EMG patterns during slow, free, and fast walking. J Orthop Res 1984; 2:272–280.
78. Murray MP, Kory RC, Clarkson BH, Sepic SB. Comparison of free and fast speed walking patterns of normal men. Am J Phys Med 1966; 45:8–24.
79. Fung J, Barbeau H, Roopchand S. Partial weight support improves force generation and postural alignment during overground locomotion following stroke. Abstr Soc Neurosci 1999; 25:907.
80. Nadeau S, Gravel D, Arsenault AB, Bourbonnais D. Plantarflexor weakness as a limiting factor of gait speed in stroke subjects and the compensating role of hip flexors. Clin Biomech (Bristol, Avon) 1999; 14:125–135.
81. Visintin M, Barbeau H. The effects of parallel bars, body weight support and speed on the modulation of the locomotor pattern of spastic paretic gait. A preliminary communication. Paraplegia 1994; 32:540–553.
82. Pitkanen K, Tarkka IM, Sivenius J. Walking training with partial body weight support vs. conventional walking training of chronic stroke patients: preliminary findings. Third World Congress in Neurological Rehabilitation, Venice, Italy, 2002.
83. Nilsson L, Carlsson J, Danielsson A, Fugl-Meyer A, Hellstrom K, Kristensen L, Sjolund B, Sunnerhagen KS, Grimby G. Walking training of patients with hemiparesis at an early stage after stroke: a comparison of walking training on a treadmill with body weight support and walking training on the ground. Clin Rehabil 2001; 15:515–527.
84. Werner C, Bardeleben A, Mauritz KH, Kirker S, Hesse S. Treadmill training with partial body weight support and physiotherapy in stroke patients: a preliminary comparison. Eur J Neurol 2002; 9:639–644.
85. Werner C, Von Frankenberg S, Treig T, Konrad M, Hesse S. Treadmill training with partial body weight support and an electromechanical gait trainer for restoration of gait in subacute stroke patients: a randomized crossover study. Stroke 2002; 33:2895–2901.
86. Trueblood PR. Partial body weight treadmill training in persons with chronic stroke. NeuroRehabilitation 2001; 16:141–153.

87. Winchen Miller E, Quinn ME, Gawlik P. Body weight support treadmill over ambulation training for two patients with disability secondary to stroke. Phys Ther 2002; 82:53–61.
88. Moseley AM, Stark A, Cameron ID, Pollock A. Treadmill training and body weight support for walking after stroke. Cochrane Database Syst Rev 2003; CD002840.
89. Tinson DJ. How stroke patients spend their days. An observational study of the treatment regime offered to patients in hospital with movement disorders following stroke. Int Disabil Stud 1989; 11:45–49.
90. Mackey F, Ada L, Heard R, Adams R. Stroke rehabilitation: are highly structured units more conducive to physical activity than less structured units? Arch Phys Med Rehabil 1996; 77:1066–1070.
91. MacKay-Lyons MJ, Makrides L. Cardiovascular stress during a contemporary stroke rehabilitation program: is the intensity adequate to induce a training effect? Arch Phys Med Rehabil 2002; 83:1378–1383.
92. Potempa K, Lopez M, Braun LT, Szidon JP, Fogg L, Tincknell T. Physiological outcomes of aerobic exercise training in hemiparetic stroke patients. Stroke 1995; 26:101–105.
93. Yang JF, Winter DA. Surface EMG profiles during different walking cadences in humans. Electroencephalogr Clin Neurophysiol 1985; 60:485–491.
94. Winter DA. The Biomechanics and Motor Control of Human Gait: Normal, Elderly and Pathological. 2nd ed. Waterloo: University of Waterloo Press, 1991.
95. Hirasaki E, Moore ST, Raphan T, Cohen B. Effects of walking velocity on vertical head and body movements during locomotion. Exp Brain Res 1999; 127:117–130.
96. van Emmerik RE, Wagenaar RC. Effects of walking velocity on relative phase dynamics in the trunk in human walking. J Biomech 1996; 29:1175–1184.
97. Lamoth CJ, Beek PJ, Meijer OG. Pelvis–thorax coordination in the transverse plane during gait. Gait Posture 2002; 16:101–114.
98. Hesse S, Werner C, Paul T, Bardeleben A, Chaler J. Influence of walking speed on lower limb muscle activity and energy consumption during treadmill walking of hemiparetic patients. Arch Phys Med Rehabil 2001; 82:1547–1550.
99. Ingles JL, Eskes GA, Phillips SJ. Fatigue after stroke. Arch Phys Med Rehabil 1999; 80:173–178.
100. Drew T. Motor cortical cell discharge during voluntary gait modification. Brain Res 1988; 457:181–187.
101. Armstrong DM. The supraspinal control of mammalian locomotion. J Physiol 1988; 405:1–37.
102. Bohannon RW, Larkin PA. Lower extremity weight bearing under various standing conditions in independently ambulatory patients with hemiparesis. Phys Ther 1985; 65:1323–1325.
103. Dickstein R, Nissan M, Pillar T, Scheer D. Foot-ground pressure pattern of standing hemiplegic patients. Major characteristics and patterns of improvement. Phys Ther 1984; 64:19–23.
104. Shumway-Cook A, Anson D, Haller S. Postural sway biofeedback: its effect on reestablishing stance stability in hemiplegic patients. Arch Phys Med Rehabil 1988; 69:395–400.

105. Diller L, Weinberg J. Evidence for accident-prone behavior in hemiplegic patients. Arch Phys Med Rehabil 1970; 51:358–363.

106. Fung J, Boonsinsukh R, Rapagna M. Postural responses triggered by surface perturbations are task-specific and goal directed. In: Levin M, ed. Progress in Motor Control. Effects of Age, Disorders, and Rehabilitation. Vol. 3. Champaign: Human Kinetics, 2003:237–251.

107. Boonsinsukh R, Rapagna M, De Serres S, Fung J. Postural responses triggered by multi-axial surface perturbations during standing and walking in stroke patients. Abstr Soc Neurosci 2002; 28:169.11.

108. Cozean CD, Pease WS, Hubbell SL. Biofeedback and functional electrical stimulation in stroke rehabilitation. Arch Phys Med Rehabil 1988; 69:401–405.

109. Wannstedt GT, Herman RM. Use of augmented sensory feedback to achieve symmetrical standing. Phys Ther 1978; 58:533–539.

110. Winstein CJ, Gardner ER, McNeal DR, Barto PS, Nicholson DE. Standing balance training: effect on balance and locomotion in hemiparetic adults. Arch Phys Med Rehabil 1989; 70:755–762.

111. Karnath HO, Sievering D, Fetter M. The interactive contribution of neck muscle proprioception and vestibular stimulation to subjective "straight ahead" orientation in man. Exp Brain Res 1994; 101:140–146.

112. Jeka JJ, Lackner JR. Fingertip contact influences human postural control. Exp Brain Res 1994; 100:495–502.

113. Jeka JJ, Lackner JR. The role of haptic cues from rough and slippery surfaces, a human postural control. Brain Res 1995; 103:267–276.

114. Slijper H, Latash M. The effects of instability and additional hand support on anticipatory postural adjustments in leg, trunk, and arm muscles during standing. Exp Brain Res 2000; 135:81–93.

115. Rogers MW, Wardman DL, Lord SR, Fitzpatrick RC. Passive tactile sensory input improves stability during standing. Exp Brain Res 2001; 136:514–522.

116. Jeka JJ, Schoner G, Dijkstra T, Ribeiro P, Lackner JR. Coupling of fingertip somatosensory information to head and body sway. Brain Res 1997; 113: 475–483.

117. Jeka JJ, Oie K, Schoner G, Dijkstra T, Henson E. Position and velocity coupling of postural sway to somatosensory drive. J Neurophysiol 1998; 79:1661–1674.

17

Optimizing Gait in Peripheral Neuropathy

James K. Richardson

Department of Physical Medicine and Rehabilitation, University of Michigan, Ann Arbor, Michigan, U.S.A.

I. CHALLENGE OF WALKING AND IMPORTANCE OF SOMATOSENSORY INFORMATION

Walking is deceptively difficult. Even a cursory inspection allows some insight into the challenges of upright gait. It is not by accident that humans, when compared with other species, take much longer time to achieve proficiency with regard to mobility. Most other mammalian species have a low center of mass, and four limbs are used as a base of support; therefore, the ability to maintain the center of mass within this broad base of support, a definition of balance, is relatively easy. In contrast, human bipedal ambulation requires the ability to control and propel an elevated center of mass over just two limbs, which provides a narrow and variable base of support. In order to reliably accomplish this covertly athletic feat, the central nervous system requires timely and accurate information so as to make the motor adjustments necessary to maintain balance (1). This information arrives via the somatosensory, visual, and vestibular systems. Given the difficulty of the bipedal walking task, any distortion in this afferent flow of information may lead to impairments in balance and difficulty with mobility.

In this chapter we will review the epidemiology of PN, how PN-related impairment affects balance, gait and fall risk, and the evaluation of, and interventions to improve gait, balance, and reduce falls in PN.

Of the three sources of afferent information, there is a variety of evidence that the somatosensory source is of greatest importance. Among the most compelling and elegant of this evidence, Fitzpatrick and McCloskey (2) demonstrated that healthy persons could perform an equivalent standing task, which eliminated both visual and vestibular input, with solely somatosensory information. Furthermore, this task was still adequately performed after ischemically induced cutaneous anesthesia of the feet, suggesting that the subjects required just a portion of somatosensory input to maintain balance (3).

II. EPIDEMIOLOGY AND CLINICAL IDENTIFICATION OF PERIPHERAL NEUROPATHY

A diffuse peripheral neuropathy (PN), which reduces distal somatosensory function and strength, is a common neurologic finding among older persons. Diabetes mellitus is the most common underlying etiology among more socioeconomically developed societies. Epidemiologic studies suggest that the prevalence of diabetes mellitus and impaired glucose tolerance are increasing and affect over 40% of U.S. citizens in the 60 to 74 years of age group (4). Further research suggests that the prevalence of PN in this age group is between 32% and 50% for persons with diabetes mellitus, 11% for persons with impaired glucose tolerance, and 7.1% for normoglycemic persons (5). Collectively, these data suggest that the prevalence of PN in the 60–74 years of age group is ~22%.

The detection of PN is an important contribution to the health care of the older person. Apart from its effect on mobility, PN contributes to or causes foot deformity and pain, skin ulceration (6), and lower extremity amputation (7) and is often associated with treatable systemic disorders (8). However, clinical history is unreliable (9) and physical examination is confounded by the "normal" decrement in peripheral nerve function that occurs with aging, making the clinical recognition of PN in older persons challenging. Age-related changes in peripheral nerve have been detected clinically (10), anatomically (11), and electrophysiologically (12), rendering indistinctly the boundary between normal peripheral nerve function for age and PN.

There are drawbacks to many recommended techniques for the clinical detection of PN among older patients. Some recommended examinations are lengthy and require expertise, time, and/or equipment not readily available (13,14), whereas others are simpler but have been used only in the evaluation of diabetic neuropathy among relatively young persons (15–19). Given that other causes of PN are common among older persons (20,21), the application of the techniques described in these studies to older persons, with and without diabetes, is uncertain.

One-hundred subjects between the ages of 50 and 80 years were studied so as to compare clinical findings among older patients with and

Table 1 Absence/Presence of PN for Discrete and Continuous Clinical Variables, Using Optimal Cut-Off Values for the Latter (22)

	PN absent	PN present	p value[a]	Sensitivity (%)	Specificity (%)
Achilles			< 0.001	72.1	90.6
Absent	3	49			
Present	29	19			
Vibration toe			< 0.001	95.6	75
Decreased (< 8 sec)	8	65			
Normal (> 8 sec)	24	3			
Position toe			< 0.001	88.2	68.8
Decreased (< 8 out of 10)	10	60			
Normal (≥ 8 out of 10)	22	8			
Of these 3 signs			< 0.0001	94.1	84.4[b]
0 or 1 present	27	4			
2 or 3 present	5	64			

[a]Chi-square test.
[b]Positive and negative predictive values are 92.8% and 87.1%, respectively.

without PN (22). Sixty-eight of the subjects had electrodiagnostic evidence of PN and 32 who did not, and approximately one-half of the subjects had diabetes mellitus. Three signs, Achilles reflex (absent, despite facilitation via gentle plantar flexion, performed using both tendon-strike and plantar-strike techniques), vibration (128 hz tuning fork perceived for < 8 sec at the great toe), and position sense (< 8 out of 10 1-cm trials at the great toe), were the best predictors of PN on both univariate and logistic regression analyses, the latter using age and body mass index (BMI) as covariates (pseudo $R^2 = 0.744$). The presence of 2 or 3 signs vs. 0 or 1 sign identified PN with reasonable sensitivity and specificity (Table 1). Values were similar among sub-groups with and without diabetes mellitus. It is anticipated that the sensitivity and specificity of these signs would decrease in the office setting, given differences in prior probabilities of finding PN. Patients with equivocal findings, or those with abnormal findings but no obvious reason for PN, should be considered for electrodiagnostic testing so as to confirm the presence of PN in the former and characterize the PN in the latter.

III. STATIC BALANCE AND PN

Quantified parameters of standing sway have been found to be greater (indicating worse balance) among subjects with PN, when compared with similarly aged diabetic subjects without PN and subjects with neither. These

Table 2   Effect of PN on Measures of Balance

Balance task	PN subjects	Control	Signifi-cance, p
Bipedal stance			
Force platform measured	Eyes open: 550 ± 50^a	350 ± 20^a	< 0.05
center of pressure excursion	Eyes closed 1100 ± 100^a	600 ± 50^a	< 0.01
(sway trace in cm) (23)			
Center of pressure excursion	Eye open: 35 ± 12^a	20 ± 8^a	< 0.01
(in cm) (24)	Eye closed: 55 ± 18^a	30 ± 10^a	< 0.01
Unipedal stance			
Balancing 3 sec on command	0.12	0.58	0.021
(success rate) (26)			
Subject controlled (sec) (26)	3.8 ± 3.5	32.2 ± 17.7	≤ 0.001
Lateral leans			
Subjects recovering successfully	5% lean, 0/6	5% lean,	0.068
for a given %foot width (48)	10% lean, 0/6	3/6	
		10% lean,	
		1/6	

^{a}Approximations from graphs from Refs. 36 and 38.

findings have been identified among both younger (23) and older (24) populations (Table 2). In addition to alterations in standing sway, our laboratory
has identified decrements in clinical and high-technology measures of one-
legged balance among older PN patients when compared with age-matched
controls (25,26). Although it is reasonable to suspect that PN is simply a
marker for other disease processes that are the true cause of these balance
impairments, such as diabetes mellitus or central nervous system pathology,
this does not appear to be the case. A variety of posturographic parameters
showed strong correlations with peripheral, but not central, nerve conduction parameters (27) indicating that peripheral nerve dysfunction underlies
the impairment in balance. Moreover, subjects with diabetic PN, but not
subjects with diabetes and healthy peripheral nerves, demonstrated abnormalities of static and dynamic balance as compared to controls (28).

IV.   EFFECT OF PN ON MOBILITY

There is also evidence that PN affects function. Studies have demonstrated
that among older subjects, PN is associated with difficulty rising from a
chair (29), decreased gait speed and stride length (30–33), and swing limb
propulsion strategies based more on hip flexion than ankle plantar flexion
(33). The decreased gait speed often falls well below 1.22 m/sec though
necessary for safe crossing of streets (34). Subjects with PN demonstrated

increased verbal reaction times to auditory stimuli during gait when compared with controls, suggesting that walking requires increased attention for PN patients (35). Despite these high-technology measures of gait aberrancies among PN patients, truncal stability appears to remain normal when patients walk on a flat surface with good lighting at a self-selected speed (31), suggesting that PN patients can compensate for their neurologic impairments under ideal conditions. This finding resonates with clinical experience suggesting that patients with all but the most severe PN do well on a firm, flat, familiar surface with good lighting when not distracted and walking at a self-selected pace.

To investigate neuropathic gait under more challenging conditions, we observed 12 older women PN patients and 12 similarly aged healthy older women ambulating under two conditions: (1) with normal lighting on a flat surface and (2) with low lighting (50 lux) on an irregular surface produced by placing wooden prisms under dark industrial carpeting (Fig. 1). Although both PN and control women demonstrated decreased speed and step length and increased step time and step width variabilities (as measured by standard deviations) on the irregular surface when compared with the flat, the PN subjects made significantly greater changes in their gait on the irregular surface (36). Furthermore, the magnitude of the changes in gait parameters among the PN subjects correlated well with the severity of clinical neuropathy as determined by the Michigan Diabetic Neuropathy Score (15). These findings suggest that gait differences between older persons with and without PN are minimal under ideal conditions but magnified by challenging, as well as realistic, conditions. The findings assume greater clinical relevance when it is understood that among older persons most falls occur during ambulation, particularly on non-flat surfaces (37).

V. PERIPHERAL NEUROPATHY AND FALL RISK

Given abnormalities in bipedal balance, unipedal balance, and gait, it is expected that PN patients would demonstrate an increased rate of falls. Relatively young patients with diabetic PN are 15 times more likely to have an injurious fall than age-matched controls with and without diabetes who do not have PN (38). Similarly, older subjects with PN are 15 to 20 times more likely to fall and six times more likely to be injured from a fall than age-matched controls without PN (39,40). Analysis of skeletal remains from a medieval leprosy hospital, as compared to a control medieval skeletal sample, suggests that even ancient populations with PN from leprosy fell and fractured more frequently (41). As with all persons at increased risk for falls, there is concern regarding the potential for injury and loss of function due to injury or fear. Perhaps, of even greater concern to the patient with diabetic PN, there is also the potential loss of a ubiquitous form of

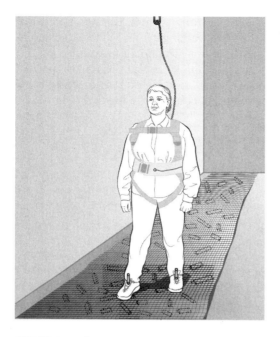

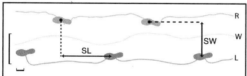

Figure 1   The irregular walkway PN patients traversed under low light conditions. Note the optoelectronic markers over the midline of the trunk and the ankles. Schematic diagram demonstrates the manner in which step width and step length were determined.

exercise, walking, which can help control the diabetic metabolic derangements that influence overall health and survival.

VI.   AFFERENT AND EFFERENT IMPAIRMENTS ASSOCIATED WITH PN

Efforts have been made to quantify the afferent deficit behind the decrement in function described earlier. Cavanagh and colleagues (42) found that ankle dorsiflexion/plantar flexion proprioceptive thresholds were increased (worse) among older subjects with diabetic PN when compared with control groups of similarly aged subjects with non-neuropathic diabetes and without diabetes or PN. PN subjects' perception thresholds were in the range of 3 to 5 degrees when compared with a threshold of 1 to 5 degrees for the subjects without PN (Table 3). It was noted that quantitative sensory testing of

Optimizing Gait in Peripheral Neuropathy   *345*

Table 3 Functionally Significant Sensory and Motor Impairments Associated with PN

Impairment	PN subjects	Control subjects	Significance, p
Sensory			
Ankle proprioceptive thresholds (degrees) (42,43)	Dorsi/plantar flexion, 4.6 ± 4.5	1.4 ± 0.7	< 0.01
	Inversion, 1.30 ± 1.06	0.21 ± 0.19	0.048
	Eversion, 2.57 ± 2.90	0.39 ± 0.10	0.036
Motor			
Maximal isokinetic strength [open chain (Nm)] (45)	Dorsiflexion, 24.3 ± 6.8	30.7 ± 7.5	< 0.0001
	Plantar flexion, 87.8 ± 23.2	111.0 ± 28.7	< 0.01
	Knee extension, 150.8 ± 38.5	178.6 ± 52.8	< 0.0001
	Knee flexion, 82.4 ± 20.2	99.6 ± 31.0	< 0.01
	Wrist extension, 8.5 ± 2.4	9.5 ± 3.2	NS
Peak acceleration [open chain (m/sec^2)] (46)	Dorsiflexion, 4765 ± 1681	6343 ± 1524	< 0.001
	Plantar flexion, 5737 ± 1977	7601 ± 1825	< 0.001
	Knee extension, 4737 ± 1820	5899 ± 2013	< 0.05
Rate of torque development [closed chain inversion (Nm/sec)] (48)	78.2 ± 50.8	152.7 ± 54.6	0.016

Abbreviation: NS, Non-significant.

vibration and touch explained only about 20–45% of the variance in ankle proprioception. Our laboratory quantified ankle inversion/eversion proprioceptive thresholds in older subjects with PN and age-matched controls. Overall, the PN group demonstrated thresholds that were 4.6 times greater (worse) than controls subjects (Table 3) (43). Moreover, the PN subjects were found to have significantly decreased clinical toe position sense (number correct of 10 1-cm trials at great toe) but normal clinical ankle position sense, suggesting that decreased clinical position sense at the toe is associated with impaired sub-clinical ankle proprioception.

Motor abnormalities have been identified electrophysiologically in patients with solely sensory signs and by means of quantified strength testing in PN patients with normal clinical muscle testing (Table 3) (44,45). Furthermore, these motor deficits occurred not only in plantar flexion and dorsiflexion, but also in knee extension/flexion (45,46). These abnormalities correlated with clinical measures of PN severity, but not with retinopathy or nephropathy, and were not found among diabetic patients without PN. The findings contrasted markedly from the usual clinical perspective that reduced dorsiflexion strength is the first sign of strength loss at the ankle, and that the knee extensors and flexors are usually unaffected.

Because of the shape of the foot and the frequency with which lateral falls lead to injury (47), ankle inversion strength is of particular importance in terms of arresting a lateral perturbation. Therefore, our laboratory quantified closed chain ankle inversion strength in six pairs of diabetic age-matched older women (one of each pair with and without PN), with clinically normal ankle strength under two different conditions (48). In the first test, the subjects were required to recover from a lateral lean, induced by the release of a horizontal lean control cable attached to a pelvic belt, and in the second test, the subjects voluntarily moved the center of reaction as quickly as possible to the lateral edge of their foot, by performing an ankle inversion maneuver during a 10-sec trial. The women with PN were never able to recover from the lateral leans test, whereas some of the older women without PN were able to do so (Table 2). Somewhat surprisingly, the two groups did not differ in terms of closed chain ankle inversion strength (Nm). However, the rate of strength development (determined by the slope of the tangent of the force/time curve, in Nm/sec) was markedly decreased for the PN group (Table 3). Furthermore, this measure of ankle rate of strength development, but not ankle strength, strongly correlated with clinical unipedal stance time (Fig. 2). Taken together, the data suggest that strength that is rapidly available is of greater assistance in the maintenance of balance than ankle strength that is only slowly available, and that PN patients with clinically normal ankle strength have impairments in rapidly available ankle strength. Similarly, recent research among older persons without PN has demonstrated that power, a measure of speed of force

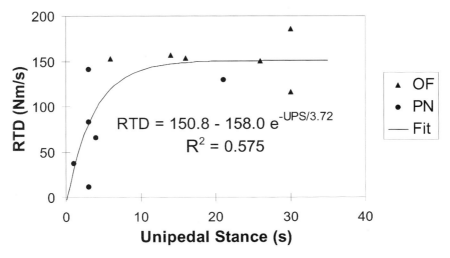

Figure 2 The relationship between rate of torque development and unipedal stance time among 12 diabetic women, six with PN and six without (17). Rate of strength development at the ankle explained more of the variance in unipedal stance time than did ankle strength (17).

production, is an entity distinct from strength that may have a greater influence on mobility function (49).

It is likely that the impairments in ankle proprioceptive thresholds and strength interact to cause impairments in balance. A useful analogy with which to visualize this interaction is to imagine the center of mass (anterior to L5) as a randomly moving but tightly bunched flock of sheep on top of a small plateau, which in turn represents the base of support. The center of ground reaction force is imagined to be a sheepdog whose job is to keep the sheep on the plateau. When the sheep wander too near the edge of the plateau, the sheepdog must position itself between the sheep and the edge and compel the sheep to move back to the middle of the plateau. Similarly, when the center of mass moves, for example, too anteriorly, the plantar flexors must quickly contract so that the ground reaction force moves ahead of the center of mass and forces it posteriorly. To be successful, the sheepdog must be vigilant and fast. Unfortunately, for PN patients, the sheepdog/ground reaction force is not vigilant and does not perceive the position of the sheep/center of mass until they are near the edge because of the afferent impairment discussed earlier. When the location of the sheep/center of mass is finally apparent, the sheepdog/ground reaction force moves slowly, due to the efferent impairment discussed earlier, and the sheep fall off before the sheepdog/ground reaction force can position itself between the sheep and the abyss. This interaction between afferent and efferent impairments likely underlies the marked difficulty that PN patients have with one-legged stance (25,26). Furthermore, there is evidence that when ankle muscles fatigue, as likely happens more rapidly among those with PN than those without, position sense worsens still further (50).

VII. WHICH PATIENTS WITH PN ARE MORE LIKELY TO FALL?

Because not all patients with PN fall, it would be convenient if it were possible to identify those at greatest risk. To address this question, 83 patients with PN were studied, none of whom had evidence of central neurologic or significant musculoskeletal abnormalities (51). Forty (48.8%), 28 (34.1%), and 18 (22.0%) subjects reported a history of at least one, multiple, and injurious falls, respectively, over the previous 2 years. Factors associated with single and multiple falls were similar and so, only results for multiple and injurious falls are reported. Using logistic regression controlling for age, sex, comorbidities, and use of medications associated with falls, an increased BMI and more severe PN (as determined clinically by the Michigan Diabetes Neuropathy Score) (15) were associated with both fall categories (pseudo $R^2 = 0.458$ and 0.484, respectively, for multiple and injurious falls). Medications associated with fall risk demonstrated a trend toward association with falls among the PN subjects, but age, gender, nerve conduction study parameters, Romberg testing, and comorbidities were not consistently associated with either fall category during bivariate or multivariate analysis. When the genders were analyzed separately, BMI appeared to be the stronger risk among women and PN severity the stronger risk among men. In addition, men with a history of falls demonstrated shorter unipedal stance times (3.7 vs. 7.8 sec, fallers vs. non-fallers; $p = 0.025$).

VIII. CLINICAL EVALUATION OF BALANCE

If PN is suspected due to history or positive findings on examination, then a functional evaluation is indicated. Chair rise should be evaluated and, in one study of older women, has been related more strongly to PN than knee extensor strength (29). Romberg testing is insensitive to mild to moderate PN and so, if positive, the test indicates severe PN or the presence of more proximal disease such as myelopathy. Unipedal stance testing (three attempts on the foot of choice) is most helpful when normal. Clinical experience suggests that if the older patient can achieve unipedal balance for > 10 sec, it is likely that the PN is of minimal functional significance, but if the PN patient cannot achieve ≥5 sec on any attempt, they should be considered at increased fall risk (51,52). It is important that the patient re-sets and equally distributes weight on both feet prior to each attempt. Unipedal stance testing may assess fall risk better in men than in women (51,52). Unipedal stance should also be used to evaluate hip abductor strength. A drop in the non-weight-bearing side of the pelvis, or an excessive lateral trunk shift toward the weight-bearing side, indicates hip abductor weakness on the stance side, a treatable finding that will lessen contralateral limb clearance during the swing phase of gait.

IX. EVALUATION OF GAIT

A. Foot Clearance

Watching the patient ambulates several lengths of a hallway is the most important part of the evaluation. When considering the PN patient, special attention should be paid to forefoot clearance initially and at the end of the walk, because it is common for clearance to lessen over time as the anterior tibialis and/or hip abductors fatigue. If forefoot clearance is decreased unilaterally, then the strength of the dorsiflexors ipsilateral to the side of reduced clearance should be evaluated. Strength may be normal with one repetition and is therefore more effectively evaluated with 10 consecutive resistance maneuvers. Asymmetric strength may represent an L5 radiculopathy or, more likely a peroneal mononeuropathy at the fibular head, superimposed on the PN. If the latter is identified, then causes of pressure over the lateral aspect of the knee, due to activities such as leg crossing, or episodes of prolonged knee flexion should be sought and corrected. A lightweight ankle foot orthosis, custom fabricated so as to prevent skin injury and ongoing pressure over the fibular head, will be helpful and has been demonstrated to increase speed and step length and to decrease energy expenditure during gait among patients with lower motor neuron disorders (53,54). Acceptance of orthoses may improve if the patient understands that the device need only be worn during times of anticipated fatigue. If forefoot clearance is decreased bilaterally due to dorsiflexor weakness, it is likely that the patient has severe PN. Such patients will likely benefit from bilateral ankle–foot orthoses and will likely also need a cane or touch of some other surface for balance. The strength of the hip abductors contralateral to the side(s) of reduced clearance should also be evaluated. A drop in the non-weight-bearing side of the pelvis, or an excessive lateral trunk shift toward the weight-bearing side, indicates hip abductor weakness on the stance side, a treatable finding that will lessen contralateral limb clearance during the swing phase of gait. Hip abductor weakness may be due to underlying hip arthritis, a gluteus medius tear or tendonitis, which often presents as a refractory greater trochanteric "bursitis" (55), L5/S1 radiculopathy, myopathy or simple deconditioning. Regardless of the etiology, if hip abductor strengthening is not successful, a cane in the contralateral upper extremity will effectively lessen demands on the affected hip abductors (56). Leg length discrepancy may also be responsible for asymmetric foot clearance, with the longer side demonstrating less clearance. A heel wedge

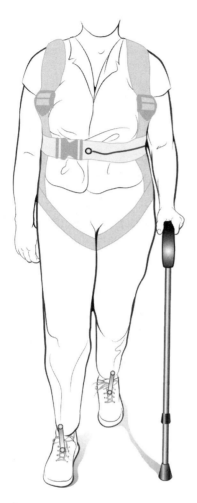

Figure 3   The cane height is adjusted to the level of the wrist and the patient places the cane forward in synchrony with the contralateral lower extremity.

on the shorter side, which corrects about one-half of the discrepancy, is often helpful and may reduce energy expenditure (57).

B.   Step Variability

The examiner should also focus on step-width variability. Patients with functionally significant PN will typically demonstrate variable foot place- ment in the frontal plane, with steps varying excessively in width. The rele- vance of this finding is underscored by biomechanical studies that indicate medial–lateral alteration of foot placement to be the most effective and efficient way to control lateral motion during ambulation (58), and frontal plane balance to be primarily determined by medial–lateral foot placement relative to the center of mass (59). Of particular concern is a step so medially directed that it crosses into the path of the stance limb when it transits into swing phase. Such a step brings about the possibility of a collision, a common and destabilizing event among older persons presented with lateral perturbations (60), between the stance and swing limb with the next step.

Therefore, correcting step-width and step-time variabilities, the latter being less clinically detectable than the former but strongly and prospectively associated with falls (61), in older patients with PN is of interest. We recently studied the effect of a cane (Fig. 3), touch of a vertical surface (Fig. 4), and ankle orthoses (Fig. 5) that supported the medial and lateral aspect of the distal lower leg (62) on step-width and step time variabilities in 42 PN subjects as they traversed a walkway with an irregular surface under low light conditions (as described in Fig. 1) (63). The subjects demonstrated significantly decreased step-width variability and step-width range with each of the interventions on the irregular surface, when compared with the control condition without the interventions. Step-time variability also decreased with use of all three interventions; however, the decrease was significant only for the orthoses and vertical surface, whereas the decrease in step-time variability with cane use was only a trend. The cane significantly slowed gait speed when compared with the control condition, whereas the orthosis and vertical surface did not change gait speed. Overall, the results suggest that with just brief (5 min) practice, each of the interventions improved medial–lateral stability and reduced temporal variability of PN patients during a challenging walking task but at the cost of speed for the cane and availability for the vertical surface. The orthoses had neither of these limitations but carry the concern of skin problems, particularly at the ankle for those patients with both PN and venous insufficiency.

X. GENERAL RECOMMENDATION AND INTERVENTIONS

A. Education

Education of the patient and/or family is universally important. Patients with PN, as well as their physicians, often underestimate their degree of disability due to PN because of its insidious onset and the gradual adaptive response that restricts mobility. The patient and family must be made to understand that the PN patient has lost a special sense, as well as likely rapidly available strength, in the lower extremities and will need to compensate for that loss if the patient is to regain or retain previous levels of function. If the use of adaptive aids to compensate for PN is described as being analogous to the use of spectacles for decreased vision or a hearing aid for

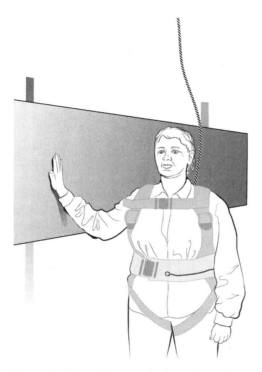

Figure 4 The subject touched a wall at about shoulder height as they walked on the irregular surface. Subjects used the dorsal or palmar surface of their hands, on the basis of their preference.

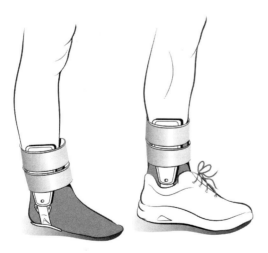

Figure 5 The ankle orthoses in place, with foam-lined shells on the medial and lateral aspects of the lower leg.

loss of hearing acuity, compliance may be better. It is also important to communicate that PN patients generally do well when undistracted, walking at a self-selected speed on a surface that is firm, flat, familiar, and well lit. Interventions are used for all other times.

B. Environmental Modification

Convenient and reliable surfaces for upper extremity touch or support should be arranged, particularly adjacent to stairs and any other irregular surfaces. The support need not always be obvious, such as grab bars in the bathroom, but can be solid furniture such as sofa arms. A home visit by an occupational or physical therapist is often fruitful. The patient's intrinsic environment should be modified as well, and medications associated with falls (hypnotics, anxiolytics, anti-hypertensives, anti-depressants, anti-convulsants) should be discontinued whenever possible (51).

C. Maximizing Visual Input

Because somatosensory information is impaired, vision must be maximized intrinsically through proper refraction and ophthalmologic consultation and extrinsically through lighting. In particular, the path for nocturnal trips to the bathroom must be well lit. Recent work has confirmed the clinical suspicion that bifocals or trifocals (including "progressive" lenses) are associated with falls; therefore, reading and "walking" glasses are best used separately (64).

D. Strengthening

Our study of older PN subjects using a cane to recover from a perturbation while performing a transfer from bipedal to unipedal stance demonstrated that patients often put 25% of their body weight onto a cane during recovery (65). Therefore, upper extremity strengthening of grip, elbow extensors, and shoulder depressors will maximize efficacy of canes and walkers. Given the relative lack of healthy axons to distal muscles in the setting of PN, it is unlikely that significant distal muscle hypertrophy can occur in subjects with PN (66). However, strengthening may still occur by means of improved centrally mediated synchronization of motor units (67). Accordingly, knee extensor strength in patients with lower motor neuron disorders has been found to increase with resistance regimen (68). In a single blind study of 20 PN patients, a 3-week program of closed chain ankle strengthening and unipedal balance practice led to improvements in functional reach, tandem stance, and unipedal balance, whereas a control exercise regimen did not (69). Although unstudied, strengthening of the hip abductors and abdominal oblique musculature is also recommended on the basis of the importance of these muscles to, respectively, medial–lateral hip and trunk stability.

E. Balance Training

Little work has been done investigating the effect of balance training on PN populations. Older persons without PN who received balance training have been found to decrease standing sway on a foam surface, a condition that mimics impaired somatosensory input (70). Despite the minimal data in this area, consultation with a physical therapist is often helpful in other ways. Patients may improve their insight into their capabilities and limitations in a safe setting and receive expert assistance in designing strategies for solving unique mobility dilemmas.

F. Enhancing Plantar Surface Sensation

Pilot studies have demonstrated that older persons with decreased plantar sensation demonstrated a more rapid response to mediolateral perturbations when standing on a surface that indented the plantar skin surface (1-mm ball bearings) (71). In addition, recent work evaluated vibratory "noise" applied to the plantar aspects of the feet of older persons during standing. Under these conditions, subjects demonstrated less sway than under the control condition without the noise (72,73). These novel interventions seem promising for patients with mild PN, although their effects on gait had not been investigated at the time of this writing.

G. Foot Pain

Asymmetries in gait may be due to an antalgic pattern. Too often, clinicians assume that foot pain in a patient with PN is due to the PN itself. However, pain that increases with weight-bearing is rarely solely neuropathic and is usually mechanical. Foot intrinsic muscle weakness distorts the normal foot anatomy and weight-bearing forces. These changes render the PN patient susceptible to a variety of disorders, but most commonly meta-tarsal pain, plantar fasciitis, and stress fractures. These sources of pain can usually be identified clinically, despite altered sensation, by palpating the appropriate regions patiently and thoroughly. Patience is required because PN patients are often slow to recognize a pain source. Strong thumb pressure over each of the metatarsal heads and over the origin of the plantar fascia, on the medial aspect of the calcaneus, with the foot maximally dorsiflexed will usually uncover the source of pain. Similarly, thorough palpation of the length of each of the metatarsals from above and below with the thumb and forefinger will identify most stress fractures. Metatarsalgia and plantar fasciitis symptoms improve with in shoe orthoses designed to support the longitudinal arch and off-load the metatarsal heads. Exercise to stretch the Achilles tendon and plantar flexors are recommended but should only be done when wearing the orthoses. When a stress fracture is suspected, the patient should undergo plain films and a bone scan if symptoms have not been prolonged and suspicion remains. The latter is particularly helpful in identifying early Charcot changes. If the scan is positive, off-loading the region with a cast-boot and rocker sole or crutches is recommended, as is referral to an orthopedic specialist.

XI. SUMMARY

PN is a common and readily identifiable finding among older persons that distorts afferent information from the distal lower extremities and blunts rapid motor responses. These changes result in balance impairment and a marked increased risk of falls and fall-related injuries. Patients with PN and their physicians often underestimate the resultant disability because patients have minimal difficulty ambulating in the office setting and other ideal conditions. However, when challenged by an irregular surface and/ or reduced lighting, these patients show marked changes in gait and often fall. Fall risk can be minimized by a program, tailored to the patient's specific vulnerabilities, which may include patient/family education, environmental modification, maximizing visual input, strengthening, and balance training. Patients should be advised that when the walking surface is firm, flat, and familiar, the lighting good and the environment non-distracting, then patients may walk without assistance; however, when these conditions are not present, then older PN patients should use a cane, touch of a stabilizing surface, or use of ankle orthoses that provide medial–lateral support.

ACKNOWLEDGMENT

The author was supported by Public Health Services Grants 1K23 AG00989 and 2P60 AG08808.

REFERENCES

1. Gandevia SG, Burke D. Does the nervous system depend on kinesthetic information to control natural limb movements?. Behav Brain Sci 1992; 15: 615–632.
2. Fitzpatrick R, McCloskey DI. Proprioceptive, visual and vestibular thresholds for the perception of sway during standing in humans. J Physiol 1994; 478(Pt 1): 173–186.
3. Fitzpatrick R, Rogers DK, McCloskey DI. Stable human standing with lower-limb muscle afferents providing the only sensory input. J Physiol 1994; 480(Pt 2):395–403.
4. Harris MI, Flegal KM, Cowie CC, Eberhardt MS, Goldstein DE, Little RR, Wiedmeyer HM, Byrd-Holt DD. Prevalence of diabetes, impaired fasting glucose and impaired glucose tolerance in U.S. adults: The Third National Health and Nutrition Examination Survey, 1988–1994. Diabetes Care 1998; 21(4):518–524.

5. Franklin GM, Kahn LB, Baxter J, Marshall JA, Hamman RF. Sensory neuropathy in non-insulin-dependent diabetes mellitus: The San Luis Valley Diabetes Study. Am J Epidemiol 1990; 131(4):633–643.

6. Boyko EJ, Ahroni JH, Stensel V, Forsberg RC, Davignon DR, Smith DG. A prospective study of risk factors for diabetic foot ulcer. The Seattle Diabetic Foot Study. Diabetes Care 1999; 22(7):1036–1042.

7. Reiber GE, Pecoraro RE, Koepsell TD. Risk factors for amputation in patients with diabetes mellitus. A case control study. Ann Intern Med 1992; 117(2):97–105.

8. Chalk CH. Acquired peripheral neuropathy. Neurol Clin 1997; 15(3):501–528.

9. Franse LV, Valk GD, Dekker JH, Heiner RJ, van Eijik JT. "Numbness of the feet" is a poor indicator for polyneuropathy in type 2 diabetic patients. Diabet Med 2000; 17(2):105–110.

10. Prakash C, Stern G. Neurological signs in the elderly. Age Ageing 1973; 2(1):24–27.

11. Vital A, Vital C, Rigal B, Decamps A, Emeriau JP, Galley P. Morphological study of the aging human peripheral nerve. Clin Neuropathol 1990; 9(1):10–15.

12. Bouch P, Cattelin F, Saint-Jean O, et al. Clinical and electrophysiological study of the peripheral nervous system in the elderly. J Neurol 1993; 240:263–268.

13. American Diabetes Association, American Academy of Neurology. Report and recommendations of the San Antonio Conference on diabetic neuropathy. Diabetes Care 1988; 11:592–597.

14. Dyck PJ, Karnes JL, Daube J, O'Brien P, Service FJ. Clinical and neuropathological criteria for the diagnosis and staging of diabetic polyneuropathy. Brain 1985; 108(4):861–880.

15. Feldman EL, Stevens MJ, Thomas PK, Brown MB, Canal N, Greene DA. A practical two-step quantitative clinical and electrophysiological assessment for the diagnosis and staging of diabetic neuropathy. Diabetes Care 1994; 17(11):1281–1289.

16. Kumar S, Fernando DJ, Veves A, Knowles EA, Young MJ, Boulton AJ. Semmes–Weinstein monofilaments: a simple, effective and inexpensive screening device for identifying diabetic patients at risk of foot ulceration. Diabetes Res Clin Pract 1991; 13(1):63–67.

17. Valk GD, Nauta JJ, Strijers RL, Bertelsmann FW. Clinical examination vs. neurophysiological examination in the diagnosis of diabetic polyneuropathy. Diabet Med 1992; 9(8):716–721.

18. Vinik AI, Suwanwalaikorn S, Stansberry KB, Holland MT, McNitt PM, Colen LE. Quantitative measurement of cutaneous perception in diabetic neuropathy. Muscle Nerve 1995; 18(6):574–584.

19. Valk GD, de Sonnaville JJ, van Houtum WH, Heine RJ, van Eijik JT, Bouter LM, Bertelsmann FW. The assessment of diabetic polyneuropathy in daily clinical practice: reproducibility and validity of Semmes–Weinstein monofilaments examination and clinical neurological examination. Muscle Nerve 1997; 20(1):116–118.

20. George J, Twomey JA. Causes of polyneuropathy in the elderly. Age Ageing 1986; 15(14):247–249.

21. Huang CY. Peripheral neuropathy in the elderly: a clinical and electrophysiologic study. J Am Geriatr Soc 1981; 29(2):49–54.

22. Richardson JK. The clinical identification of peripheral neuropathy among older persons. Arch Phys Med Rehabil 2002; 83(11):1553–1558.

23. Uccioli L, Giacomini PG, Monticone G, Magrini A, Durola L, Bruno E, Parisi L, Di Girolamo S, Menzinger G. Body sway in diabetic neuropathy. Diabetes Care 1995; 18(3):339–344.

24. Simoneau GG, Ulbrecht JS, Derr JA, Becker MB, Cavanagh PR. Postural instability in patients with diabetic sensory neuropathy. Diabetes Care 1994; 17(12):1411–1421.

25. Hurvitz EA, Richardson JK, Werner RA. Unipedal stance testing in the assessment of peripheral neuropathy. Arch Phys Med Rehabil 2001; 82(2):198–204.

26. Richardson JK, Ashton-Miller JA, Lee SG, Jacobs K. Moderate peripheral neuropathy impairs weight transfer and unipedal balance in the elderly. Arch Phys Med Rehabil 1996; 77(11):1152–1156.

27. Uccioli L, Gicomini PG, Pasqualetti P, Di Girolamo S, Ferrigno P, Monticone G, Bruno E, Boccasena P, Magrini A, Parisi L, Menzinger G, Rossini PM. Contribution of central neuropathy to postural instability in IDDM patients with peripheral neuropathy. Diabetes Care 1997; 20(6):929–934.

28. Resnick HE, Stansberry KB, Harris TB, Tirivedi M, Smith K, Morgan P, Vinik AI. Diabetes, peripheral neuropathy and old age disability. Muscle Nerve 2002; 25(1):43–50.

29. Resnick HE, Vinik AI, Schwartz AV, Leveille SG, Brancati FL, Balfour J, Guralnik JM. Independent effects of peripheral nerve dysfunction on lower-extremity physical function in old age: the Women's Health and Aging Study. Diabetes Care 2000; 23(11):1642–1647.

30. Dingwell JB, Cavanagh PR. Increased variability of continuous overground walking in neuropathic patients is only indirectly related to sensory loss. Gait Posture 2001; 14(1):1–10.

31. Dingwell JB, Cusumano JP, Sternad D, Cavanagh PR. Slower speeds in patients with diabetic neuropathy lead to improved local dynamic stability of continuous overground walking. J Biomech 2000; 33(10):1269–1277.

32. Katoulis EC, Ebdon-Parry M, Lanshammar H, Vileikyte L, Kulkarni J, Boulton AJ. Gait abnormalities in diabetic neuropathy. Diabetes Care 1997; 20(12):1904–1907.

33. Mueller MJ, Minor SD, Sahrmann SA, Schaaf JA, Strube MJ. Differences in the gait characteristic of patients with diabetes and peripheral neuropathy compared with age-matched controls. Phys Ther 1994; 74(4):299–308; discussion 309–313.

34. Langlois JA, Keyl PM, Guralnik JM, Foley DJ, Marottoli RA, Wallace RB. Characteristics of older pedestrians who have difficulty crossing the street. Am J Public Health 1997; 87(3):393–397.

35. Courtemanche R, Teasdale N, Boucher P, Fleury M, Lajoie Y, Bard C. Gait problems in diabetic neuropathic patients. Arch Phys Med Rehab 1996; 77(9):849–855.

36. Richardson JK, Thies SB, DeMott T, Ashton-Miller JA. A comparison of gait characteristic between older women with and without peripheral neuropathy in standard and challenging environments. J Am Geriatr Soc 2004; 52(92): 1532–1537.

37. Berg WP, Alessio HM, Mills EM, Tong C. Circumstances and consequences of falls in independent community-dwelling older adults. Age Aging 1997; 26(4):261–268.

38. Cavanagh PR, Derr JA, Ulbrecht JS, Maser RE, Orchard TJ. Problems with gait and posture in neuropathic patients with insulin-dependent diabetes mellitus. Diabet Med 1992; 9(5):469–474.

39. Richardson JK, Ching C, Hurvitz EA. The relationship between electromyographically documented peripheral neuropathy and falls. J Am Geriatr Soc 1992; 40(10):1008–1012.

40. Richardson JK, Hurvitz EA. Peripheral neuropathy: a true risk factor for falls. J Gerontol A Biol Sci Med Sci 1995; 50A(4):M211–M215.

41. Judd MA, Roberts CA. Fracture patterns at the Medieval Leper Hospital in Chichester. Am J Phys Anthropol 1998; 105(1):43–55.

42. Simoneau GG, Derr JA, Ulbrecht JS, Becker MB, Cavanagh PR. Diabetic sensory neuropathy effect on ankle joint movement perception. Arch Phys Med Rehabil 1996; 77(5):453–460.

43. Van den Bosch CG, Gilsing MG, Lee SG, Richardson JK, Ashton-Miller JA. Peripheral neuropathy effect on ankle inversion and eversion detection thresholds. Arch Phys Med Rehabil 1995; 76(9):850–856.

44. Wolfe GI, Baker NS, Amato AA, Jackson CE, Nations SP, Saperstein DS, Cha CH, Katz JS, Bryan WW, Barohn RJ. Chronic cryptogenic sensory polyneuropathy: clinical and laboratory characteristics. Arch Neurol 1999; 56(5):540–547.

45. Andersen H, Poulsen PL, Mogensen CE, Jakobsen J. Isokinetic muscle strength in long-term IDDM patients in relation to diabetic complications. Diabetes 1996; 45(4):440–445.

46. Andersen H, Mogensen PH. Disordered mobility of large joints in association with neuropathy in patients with long-standing insulin-dependent diabetes. Diabet Med 1997; 14(3):221–227.

47. Greenspan SL, Myers ER, Maitland LA, Resnick NM, Hayes WC. Fall severity and bone mineral density as risk factors for hip fracture in ambulatory elderly. JAMA 1994; 271(2):128–133.

48. Gutierrez EM, Helber MD, Dealva D, Ashton-Miller JA, Richardson JK. Mild diabetic neuropathy affects ankle motor function. Clin Biomech 2001; 16(6): 522–528.

49. Bean JF, Leveille SG, Kiely DK, Bandinelli S, Guralnik J, Ferrucci L. A comparison of leg power and leg strength within the InCHIANTI study: which influences mobility more? J Gerontol: Bio Med Sci 2003; 58(8):728–733.

50. Forestier N, Teasdale N, Nougier V. Alteration of the position sense at the ankle induced by muscular fatigue in humans. Med Sci Sports Exerc 2002; 34(1):117–122.

51. Richardson JK. Factors associated with falls in older patients with diffuse polyneuropathy. J Am Geriatr Soc 2002; 50(11):1767–1773.

52. Vellas BJ, Wayne SJ, Romero L, Baumgartner RN, Rubenstein LZ, Garry PJ. One-leg balance is an important predictor of injurious falls in older persons. J Am Geriatr Soc 1997; 45(6):735–738.

53. Duffy CM, Graham HK, Cosgrove AP. The influence of ankle–foot orthoses on gait and energy expenditure in spina fibida. J Pediatr Orthop 2000; 20(3):356–361.

54. Bean J, Walsh A, Frontera W. Brace modification improves aerobic performance in Charcot–Marie-Tooth disease: a single-subject design. Am J Phys Med Rehabil 2001; 80(8):578–582.

55. Kingzett-Taylor A, Tirman PF, Feller J, McGann W, Prieto V, Wischer T, Cameron JA, Cvitanic O, Genant HK. Tendinosis and tears of gluteus medius and minimus muscles as a cause of hip pain: MR imaging findings. Am J Roentgenol 1999; 173(4):1123–1126.

56. Joyce BM, Kirby RL. Canes, crutches and walkers. Am Fam Physician 1991; 43(2):535–542.

57. Abdulhadi HM, Kerrigan DC, LaRaia PJ. Contralateral shoe-lift: effect on oxygen cost of walking with an immobilized knee. Arch Phys Med Rehabil 1996; 77(7):670–672.

58. Kuo AD. Stabilization of lateral motion in passive dynamic walking. Int J Robot Res 1999; 18(9):917–930.

59. MacKinnon CD, Winter DA. Control of whole body balance in the frontal plane during human walking. J Biomech 1993; 26(6):633–644.

60. Maki BE, Edmonstone MA, McIlroy WE. Age-related differences in laterally directed compensatory stepping behavior. J Gerontol: Med Sci 2000; 55A(5):M270–M277.

61. Hausdorff JM, Rios DA, Edelberg HK. Gait variability and fall risk in community-living older adults: a 1-year prospective study. Arch Phys Med Rehabil 2001; 82(8):1050–1056.

62. Active Ankle Systems Inc., 509 Barrett Ave., Louisville, KY 40204.

63. Richardson JK, Thies S, DeMott T, Ashton-Miller JA. Interventions improve gait regularity in patients with peripheral neuropathy while walking on an irregular surface under low light. J Am Geriatr Soc 2004; 52(4):510–515.

64. Lord SR, Dayhew J, Howland A. Multifocal glasses impair edge-contrast sensitivity and depth perception and increase the risk of falls in older people. J Am Geriatr Soc 2002; 50(11):1760–1766.

65. Ashton-Miller JA, Yeh MW, Richardson JK, Galloway T. A cane reduces loss of balance in patients with peripheral neuropathy: results from a challenging unipedal balance test. Arch Phys Med Rehabil 1996; 77(5):446–452.

66. Carlson BM, Faulkner JA. Muscle regeneration in young and old rats: effects of motor nerve transection with and without marcaine treatment. J Gerontol A Biol Sci Med Sci 1998; 53(1):B52–B57.

67. Rutherford OM, Jones DA. The role of learning and coordination in strength training. Eur J Appl Occup Physiol 1986; 55(1):100–105.

68. Lindeman E, Leffers P, Spaans F, Drukker J, Reulen J, Kerckhoffs M, Koke A. Strength training in patients with myotonic dystrophy and hereditary motor and sensory neuropathy: a randomized clinical trial. Arch Phys Med Rehabil 1995; 76(7):612–620.

69. Richardson JK, Sandman D, Vela S. A focused exercise regimen improves clinical measures of balance in patients with peripheral neuropathy. Arch Phys Med Rehabil 2001; 82(2):205–209.

70. Hu MH, Woollacott MH. Multisensory training of standing balance in older adults: I. Postural stability and one-leg stance. J Gerontol: Med Sci 1994; 49(2):M52–M61.
71. Maki BE, McIlroy WE. Postural control in the older adult. Clin Geriatr Med Studenski S, ed. 1996; 12(4):635–658.
72. Dhruv NT, Niemi JB, Harry JD, Lipsitz LA, Collins JJ. Enhancing tactile sensation in older adults with electrical noise stimulation. Neuroreport 2002; 13(5):597–600.
73. Priplata AA, Niemi JB, Harry JD, Lipsitz LA, Collins JJ. Vibrating insoles and balance control in elderly people. Lancet 2003; 362(9390):2003–2004.

18

Posthip Fracture and Hip Replacements

Jeremy A. Idjadi and Joseph D. Zuckerman

*NYU—The Hospital for Joint Diseases Orthopedic Institute, New York,
New York, U.S.A.*

Kenneth Koval

*Dartmouth-Hitchcock Medical Center, Orthopedic Surgery, Lebanon,
New Hampshire, U.S.A.*

I. INTRODUCTION

Disease of the hip, whether from osteoarthritis, hip fracture, or another etiology, is a significant source of morbidity and mortality. The burden on both patients and the health care system is immense. Some authors estimate that by the year 2040, over 500,000 hip fractures will occur in the United States, incurring $16 billion in health care expenses (1). Furthermore, over 250,000 total hip arthroplasties are performed in the United States each year for osteoarthritis and a variety of other diseases.

In light of the obvious impact that these diseases and their treatment have on patients as well as society, attempts at decreasing morbidity by implementing safe, efficient, and effective rehabilitation programs is paramount. Loss of mobility is a factor that contributes to the prolonged recovery following hip fractures, as well as to the increased one-year mortality rate (2). Additionally, pre and postoperative ambulatory ability has been shown to correlate with survival time (3). Gait, along with balance, is one of the major components of mobility (4). The effective and efficient evaluation and management of gait disorders, in patients who have undergone total hip replacement and the operative treatment of hip fractures, is essential to improve outcomes and to lessen the burden on the patient and on society.

II. GOALS

As is often the case in medicine, the goal of the orthopedic surgeon, the physiatrist, and other healthcare workers, is to help return the patient to their premorbid level of function.

Due to the nature of the diseases contributing to the need for hip arthroplasty, many candidates for the procedure have some element of gait dysfunction prior to surgery. Thus, the goal should be to regain the level of gait function that preceded any manifestation of the underlying disease process. There are many factors that may affect return to premorbid function. Bilateral disease is one such factor that can have a dramatic effect on return of function. In these patients, optimal gait function is not achieved until both hips have been treated and have recovered. As expected, patients with unilateral disease show better gait analysis results postarthroplasty, than patients with bilateral disease after either side has been treated (5). Furthermore, though gait efficiency has been shown to improve after total hip arthroplasty, the level of recovery generally does not quite attain premorbid gait status (6,7). It has also been shown that, as compared to healthy women, patients who underwent total hip arthroplasty show a significantly decreased hip extensor force as well as a significantly decreased gait speed (8).

The goal of rehabilitation after hip fracture should be a return to prefracture ambulatory status, whether this represents independent community ambulation or household ambulation with a walker (9). As has been shown in many different studies, one of the most important predictors of ambulation progress after hip fractures, is the level of premorbid ambulation. Age, ASA rating, fracture type, and nursing home residence prior to hip fracture have also been shown to be predictors of postoperative ambulation (10–13). In one study, 41% of patients regained prefracture level of ambulation while 59% lost some degree of ambulatory ability (12). Though general conditioning and fitness may be promoted for at risk groups, practically speaking, it is difficult to alter these preinjury factors in the population of patients who sustain hip fractures. The importance of maximizing postoperative recovery of ambulation is emphasized by the fact that gait function has been shown to be predictive of long-term hospital care vs. discharge to home (4,14).

III. PREOPERATIVE

As in all of medicine, evaluation of the entire patient is of the utmost importance. While the majority of patients undergoing hip replacement will have a diagnosis of unilateral osteoarthritis, it is important to consider other diagnoses which may affect the surgical plan, rehabilitation plan, and expected outcome. Bilateral disease is one situation in which gait analysis has shown that patients reach optimal function only after bilateral total hip arthroplasty has been performed. Patients with unilateral disease have superior postoperative gait patterns as compared to those with bilateral disease who have undergone unilateral surgery (5). The primary diagnosis may also help predict the expected outcome for specific groups. For example, it has been shown that patients with rheumatoid arthritis, who often have multiple involved joints, walk slower, are weaker preoperatively, and have less increase in strength postoperatively (15). Other concurrent pathology such as that of the ipsilateral or contralateral knee, or lumbar spine, must also be considered.

Careful consideration of comorbidities is also important, as some have been found to be associated with compromised gait function. For example, Parkinsonism, age, American Society of Anesthesiology rating of operative risk, and delirium have been found to be associated with poor functional outcome, including decline in ambulation, following operative management of hip fractures (10,12,16–18).

Because the occurrence of hip fractures is not predictable, little can be done preoperatively to optimize the patient's condition before surgery. Though the operative treatment of hip fractures may be considered urgent, an attempt to medically optimize patients prior to surgery is imperative (19–23).

In contrast to the need for urgent treatment of hip fractures, the conditions leading to total hip arthroplasty are usually much more chronic in nature. It has been demonstrated on a number of occasions, that ambulatory function prior to total hip replacement is predictive of function afterwards. More specifically, patients with greater walking disability prior to surgery were found to function at lower levels postoperatively (12,15). Thus, though some studies have shown that preoperative muscle output is not predictive of postoperative strength (15), it may be prudent to maximize gait function with attention to strength, range of motion, and endurance, prior to elective surgery. One such study compared three gait parameters (cadence, stride length, and gait velocity) as well as walk distance between exercise protocol groups and control groups, both preoperatively and postoperatively. Though there were no significant differences between the groups preoperatively, the exercise group had significantly higher postoperative scores on every parameter, at nearly every time point examined. Furthermore, a preoperative exercise program was shown to result in an approximately three month earlier return of gait function, as compared to routine preoperative and postoperative care (24).

With regards to total hip arthroplasty, an obvious caveat is that one of the major indications is to relieve pain and restore function so that a patient may mobilize and optimize independence (24–26). It can be expected that preoperative musculoskeletal optimization may be limited by pain and decreased fitness (24). Therefore, any preoperative exercise regimen must be individualized and carefully consider the patient's discomfort and functional status.

IV. INTRAOPERATIVE

Intraoperatively, there are many variables that may affect outcome. In total hip arthroplasty (Figs. 1 and 2), both the procedure performed, and the implant used, have been shown to affect gait (27–30). Although the indications of staged vs. simultaneous bilateral hip replacement for patients with bilateral disease is beyond the scope of this discussion, as mentioned above, it has been shown that patients do not gain optimal gait function until both hips are replaced (5).

With regards to intertrochanteric hip fractures (Figs. 3 and 4), it has been suggested that the quality of fracture reduction is more predictive of better walking performance than the type of device used (31). In general, for both intertrochanteric and femoral neck fractures (Figs. 3 through 6),

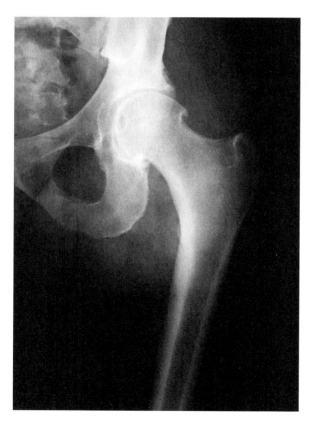

Figure 1 Radiograph of a hip with osteoatrthritis.

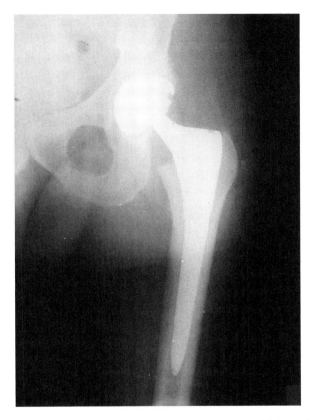

Figure 2 Radiograph of an uncemented total hip replacement used to treat an osteoarthritic hip.

no significant difference has been noted between internal fixation and prosthetic replacement with regards to ambulatory ability outside of the early postoperative period (1,9,32–35).

V. POSTOPERATIVE

A. Early Mobilization

Postoperatively, there are many ways to improve function and decrease morbidity. Early mobilization out of bed after hip surgery, whether for fracture fixation or arthroplasty, is imperative for the welfare of the patient. This reduces the risk of deep-vein thrombosis, pulmonary complications, skin breakdown, and decline in mental status (36,37). Furthermore, mobilizing a patient encourages one to begin the recovery process.

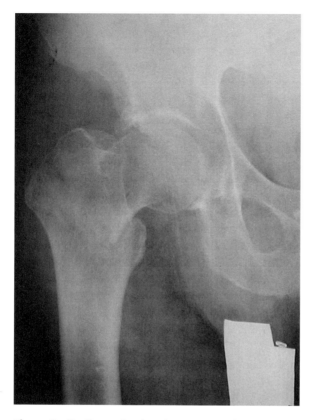

Figure 3 Radiograph of an intertrocanteric hip fracture.

B.   Early Physiatry Evaluation

Rehabilitation after hip surgery should be started on postoperative day 1. After an appropriate referral, the physiatrist and physical therapist should conduct a complete evaluation. This acute care evaluation should include a review of the patient's diagnosis, the surgical procedure done, and the patient's weight bearing status. The therapist should assess the patient's medical status so that they may be aware of any conditions that could adversely affect the rehabilitation process. Furthermore, it is imperative that the therapist take note of the patient's premorbid level of function, as well as their social and living situation, both of which will determine their ambulatory needs and goals.

A careful physical assessment should also be performed and documented. It should include: joint range of motion, muscle strength, and flexibility. Particular attention should be directed toward the operative lower extremity, as well as to the upper extremities, which will be invaluable during

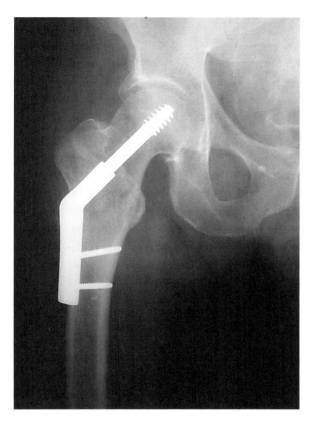

Figure 4 Radiograph of an intertrochanteric hip fracture after internal fixation with a sliding hip screw device.

transfers as well as with the use of assistive devices. Further, neurologic, balance, and functional assessments may also be made. The therapist should take note of the surgical wound or dressing and any deformities that may be present. The above evaluation, in conjunction with the orthopaedist's or physiatrist's physical therapy order, is then used in formulating a physical therapy treatment plan customized for each patient.

Though gait training may be one of the ultimate goals, mobilization and transfer training, strength training, balance training, and maintenance of joint range of motion must be an essential part of a comprehensive rehabilitation program. The patient should be assisted out of bed to a chair on postoperative day 1. If unable to tolerate this transfer, the patient may be helped to the edge of the bed into a dangling position. The therapist should also provide instruction in bed mobility. As recovery progresses, the amount of assistance given to the patient by the therapist gradually decreases until he or she can transfer independently.

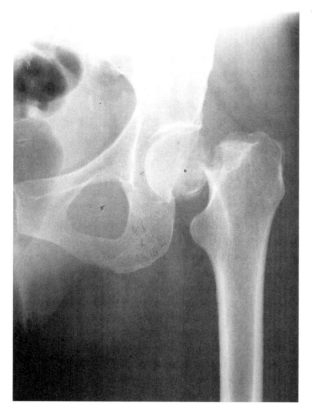

Figure 5   Radiograph of a femoral neck fracture.

Exercise and strength training is started on the acute care service for both hip fracture and total hip replacement patients. Instruction is provided for an exercise program in three positions: supine, sitting, and standing. The exercises are administered on a daily basis. Supine exercises include quadriceps sets, heel slides, active assisted hip flexion, active assisted straight leg raising, active hip extension and abduction, and ankle pumps. Quadriceps strengthening is important to facilitate independent transfer ability. A significant relationship between hip abductor strength and ambulation without supervision has been found by some investigators (9). In a sitting position, exercises start with active knee extension. Self-assisted hip flexion with a towel (in patients who had internal fixation) is an effective way to increase the patient's hip flexion strength.

Standing exercises include straight leg raises while the patient holds onto parallel bars, hip abduction, hip flexion, and quarter-knee bends. Stand-

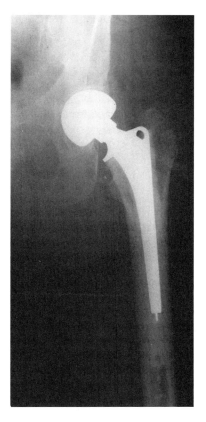

Figure 6 Radiograph of a cemented hemi-arthroplasty used to treat a femoral neck fracture.

ing exercises are performed concentrically with a 3 or 5 seconds isometric hold and then continued eccentrically as the lower extremity is lowered. Exercises progress from active assisted, to active, and then resistive. Repetitions are increased to enhance the patient's endurance. Patients whose balance is impaired may require contact guarding when performing standing exercises.

Activity precautions must be considered, depending on the injury or procedure performed. Patients with hip fractures treated with internal fixation generally have no restriction regarding hip range of motion. Patients who have had a prosthetic replacement using the posterior approach, whether a total hip arthroplasty or a hemiarthroplasty, are limited to 90° of hip flexion for six weeks. In addition, hip adduction and internal rotation are contraindicated. These patients are instructed to keep their legs apart and to place a pillow between their legs when lying on the uninjured side to prevent hip adduction, which could lead to prosthetic dislocation. Conversely, external rotation and extension are contraindicated if the procedure was performed using an anterior approach.

C. Weight Bearing as Appropriate

Gait training is initiated on the first or second postoperative day. The majority of patients who have been surgically treated with either internal fixation or prosthetic replacement, should be allowed to bear weight as tolerated. Although in the past, partial weight bearing was frequently utilized, we now understand that a weight bearing as tolerated protocol is appropriate. It has been shown that even partial weight bearing involves the generation of considerable force across the hip by the lower extremity musculature. The forces exerted across the hip when a patient uses his upper extremities to transfer onto a bedpan approach four times body weight (38). Studies have also demonstrated that unrestricted weight bearing does not increase complication rates following internal fixation or prosthetic replacement after femoral neck or intertrochanteric fracture (39–44). It has also been suggested that early full weight bearing helps rehabilitation and discharge of patients (45–47). Furthermore, with gait analysis, it has been shown that patients that are allowed to bear weight as tolerated after femoral neck or intertrochanteric fractures, will self limit the loading of the injured limb. Specifically, patients who underwent internal fixation of an unstable intertrochanteric fracture or a displaced femoral neck fracture, initially placed significantly less weight on the injured extremity than patients who sustained a femoral neck fracture which was treated with prosthetic replacement (48). Over time, the patients progressed their weight bearing to full status.

With regards to total hip arthroplasty, weight-bearing status is again dependent on many variables. In general, cemented or hybrid total hip arthroplasty patients are allowed weight bearing as tolerated in the early postoperative period (49). In uncemented total hip arthroplasty, the weight-bearing recommendations are a bit more complex. In light of the fact that early weight bearing may lead to movement at the bone–prosthesis interface and thereby inhibit bone ingrowth (50), limiting the weight bearing in these patients has been suggested. However, there is no general agreement on this. Many surgeons will allow full weight bearing following noncemented arthroplasty. However, later weight bearing has been shown to have detrimental effects on gait, hip extension, and strength (51–53). Although by 24 weeks after surgery, no significant functional consequences persist (54).

The goal of weight bearing as tolerated (WBAT) ambulation, following internal fixation or arthroplasty, might be modified if fixation stability is compromised or if an intraoperative fracture occurred, requiring additional fixation. Although older patients are allowed to weight bear as tolerated, regardless of fracture pattern or implant selection, weight bearing may be limited in younger patients who sustain a displaced femoral neck or unstable intertrochanteric fracture. Limited weight bearing is much better performed and tolerated in younger patients than older patients, although there is no data as yet to confirm a beneficial effect in outcome. Younger patients are restricted to foot-flat weight bearing until there is radiographic evidence of healing—unless the fracture was stabilized with an interlocked nail and bone-to-bone contact was achieved at surgery.

If there is no contraindication to unrestricted weight bearing, patient's goals are set to ambulate weight bearing as tolerated 15 ft with moderate assistance on postoperative day 1, progressing to 20 ft with minimal assistance on day 2 and 40 ft on day 3. On postoperative day 3 or 4, the patient is instructed in stair climbing with maximal supervision. Subsequent patient goals include progression of ambulation to crutches as tolerated and progression of stair climbing with decreased supervision. These goals are to be taken as general guidelines. Every patient's rehabilitation program must be tailored to the individual's physical, psychological, and social situation.

D. Adaptive Equipment

Adaptive equipment and assistive devices are routinely prescribed for patients to aid in gait performance. These devices are used to increase stability and lower the weight bearing forces across the operative extremity. Standard walkers provide the greatest base of support, however, they tend to be more cumbersome and may be difficult to advance. Though rolling walkers may be moved forward more easily, they should only be prescribed for individuals with sufficient coordination to stop the motion when needed. Axillary and forearm crutches are less cumbersome than walkers and can be used to provide either unilateral or bilateral support. Canes, four-pronged or straight, offer the least degree of stability. However, they are the least cumbersome and therefore the easiest to manipulate. The cane is held in the hand opposite the impaired side.

Ambulatory status, as it pertains to the use of assistive devices and functional domain (community vs. household), has been studied in patients with hip fractures. In general, it has been found that the majority of patients lose at least one level of ambulatory function after sustaining a hip fracture. For example, if a patient was a community ambulatory without an assistive device preinjury, they may require a walking aid postoperatively. Likewise, if a patient was a community ambulator with an assistive device preinjury, they may become a household ambulator postoperatively (12). Similarly, other studies have found that increased dependence (>50%), in lower extremity physical activities of daily living such as walking 10 ft, walking one block, and climbing five stairs, persists at two year follow up. Perhaps the most striking finding was a new dependency (>89%) in climbing five stairs at one year, for patients who required no prefracture assistance (55).

Assistive devices benefit patients with regards to stability and safety. However, it has been shown that their use may be detrimental to gait and muscular training in some patients following total hip arthroplasty. In one study, though patients with crutches walked more symmetrically and with a longer stride length, they reduced the activity of pelvi-trochanteric muscles and abductor muscles on the operative side, thus adversely affecting rehabilitation of these groups (56). Others have also found that the prolonged use of crutches may inhibit function (54).

E. Disposition

Postoperatively, a social worker should meet with the patient and family to assess the patient's needs and resources following hospital discharge. The goal of treatment is to return the patient to his or her premorbid level of independence. Depending on the patient's ambulatory ability, social support network, and financial resources, discharge disposition may be to a variety of settings. Inpatient rehabilitation is a setting where patients may receive intense daily physical and occupational therapy for at least three hours per day. Subacute rehabilitation units provide at least one hour of daily therapy. Skilled nursing facilities offer various degrees of rehabilitation, ranging from little or no therapy to daily sessions. These facilities may function to fine-tune skills learned in an acute rehabilitation program before discharge home. Day hospitals allow individuals with good social support systems to receive a full day of therapeutic activity in a hospital setting while being able to return home at night. Outpatient facilities may offer less comprehensive interdisciplinary therapeutic programs than may be provided on an inpatient basis, yet are ideal for individuals requiring limited rehabilitative intervention. Finally, physical and occupational therapy can be provided in the home environment where individuals have the opportunity to make functional gains in familiar surroundings until they are sufficiently mobile and independent to progress to an outpatient program.

The effect of inpatient rehabilitation on patient outcome and gait function following hip fracture has been examined. In one such study, patients who received two hours of inpatient physical therapy seven days a week for gait training, stair climbing, transfers, joint range of motion, and upper and lower extremity strengthening, were compared to those discharged to an outside rehabilitation facility. No differences were found in the patients' ambulatory ability at 6- and 12-months follow up (48). Other authors believe that aggressive and intense physical therapy is responsible for the high percentage of independent ambulation that permeated all types of hip fractures as well as surgical treatments (9). Furthermore, other studies have suggested that patients who attended more physical therapy visits had a greater likelihood of returning to prefracture ambulatory status (32).

Though intuition may suggest that more intense physical therapy would accelerate rehabilitation and subsequent hospital discharge, studies have not confirmed this. In one study, 88 patients with operatively treated hip fractures were randomized to 3.6 hr per week of physical therapy vs. 1.9 hr per week. When using the criteria of: (1) walking 50 m without resting in two minutes, with assistive device if necessary and (2) climbing one flight of stairs, with assistive device if necessary, as well as other nongait functional measures, no difference was noted between the groups with regard to duration of physical rehabilitation. In this case, the findings were thought to be due to the considerable dropout rate in the intervention group. These findings suggested that a focus on out-patient rehabilitation may be in order (57).

The results for hip fracture have been mixed with regards to patients that are discharged home and receive standard physical therapy vs. specialized home rehabilitation programs. Some have shown increased walking velocity and mobility (58), while others have shown no significant difference in gait performance (59). One study of patients undergoing total hip arthroplasty showed that a home based perioperative exercise intervention program both before and up to 24 weeks postoperatively yielded patients with greater stride length and gait velocity at three weeks post surgery and greater gait velocity and walking distance at 12 and 24 weeks. Subjects in the intervention program also benefited from a 3 month earlier return of gait function as compared to controls (24).

With regard to disposition and postoperative rehabilitation, it is clear that there are a significant number of variables, most of which have not been studied in randomized controlled clinical trials. Thus, the individual, as well as their financial resources and social support systems, should be considered when determining the appropriate disposition and rehabilitation in any given case.

VI. SUMMARY

Though gait evaluation and treatment for patients who have undergone total hip replacement and the operative treatment of hip fracture is a complex matter, it can be approached in a straightforward manner so that safe, efficient, and effective rehabilitation can be implemented. The goal is to return all patients to their premorbid level of function. Weight-bearing status and precautions should be determined on an individual basis. With the approach discussed above, realistic outcomes may be expected, gait function may be improved, and associated morbidity may be lessened.

REFERENCES

1. Cummings SR, Rubin SM, Black D. The future of hip fractures in the United States. Numbers, costs, and potential effects of postmenopausal estrogen. Clin Orthop 1990; 252:163–166.

2. Wallace WA. The increasing incidence of fractures of the proximal femur: an orthopaedic epidemic. Lancet 1983; 1(8339):1413–1414.
3. Crane JG, Kernek CB. Mortality associated with hip fractures in a single geriatric hospital and residential health facility: a ten-year review. J Am Geriatr Soc 1983; 31(8):472–475.
4. Fox KM, Hawkes WG, Hebel JR, Felsenthal G, Clark M, Zimmerman SI, Kenzora JE, Magaziner J. Mobility after hip fracture predicts health outcomes. J Am Geriatr Soc 1998; 46(2):169–173.
5. Wykman A, Olsson E. Walking ability after total hip replacement. A comparison of gait analysis in unilateral and bilateral cases. J Bone Joint Surg Br 1992; 74(1):53–56.
6. Stauffer RN, Smidt GL, Wadsworth JB. Clinical and biomechanical analysis of gait following Charnley total hip replacement. Clin Orthop 1974; 99:70–77.
7. Brown M, Hislop HJ, Waters RL, Porell D. Walking efficiency before and after total hip replacement. Phys Ther 1980; 60(10):1259–1263.
8. Perron M, Malouin F, Moffet H, McFadyen BJ. Three-dimensional gait analysis in women with a total hip arthroplasty. Clin Biomech (Bristol, Avon) 2000; 15(7):504–515.
9. Barnes B, Dunovan K. Functional outcomes after hip fracture. Phys Ther 1987; 67(11):1675–1679.
10. Cheng CL, Lau S, Hui PW, Chow SP, Pun WK, Ng J, Leong JC. Prognostic factors and progress for ambulation in elderly patients after hip fracture. Am J Phys Med Rehabil 1989; 68(5):230–233.
11. Mossey JM, Mutran E, Knott K, Craik R. Determinants of recovery 12 months after hip fracture: the importance of psychosocial factors. Am J Public Health 1989; 79(3):279–286.
12. Koval KJ, Skovron ML, Aharonoff GB, Meadows SE, Zuckerman JD. Ambulatory ability after hip fracture. A prospective study in geriatric patients. Clin Orthop 1995; 310:150–159.
13. Hannan EL, Magaziner J, Wang JJ, Eastwood EA, Silberzweig SB, Gilbert M, Morrison RS, McLaughlin MA, Orosz GM, Siu AL. Mortality and locomotion 6 months after hospitalization for hip fracture: risk factors and risk-adjusted hospital outcomes. JAMA 2001; 285(21):2736–2742.
14. Friedman PJ, Richmond DE, Baskett JJ. A prospective trial of serial gait speed as a measure of rehabilitation in the elderly. Age Ageing 1988; 17(4):227–235.
15. Murray MP, Brewer BJ, Gore DR, Zuege RC. Kinesiology after McKee-Farrar total hip replacement. A two-year follow-up of one hundred cases. J Bone Joint Surg Am 1975; 57(3):337–342.
16. Hammer AJ. Intertrochanteric and femoral neck fractures in patients with parkinsonism. S Afr Med J 1991; 79(4):200–202.
17. Marcantonio ER, Flacker JM, Michaels M, Resnick NM. Delirium is independently associated with poor functional recovery after hip fracture. J Am Geriatr Soc 2000; 48(6):618–624.
18. Shah MR, Aharonoff GB, Wolinsky P, Zuckerman JD, Koval KJ. Outcome after hip fracture in individuals ninety years of age and older. J Orthop Trauma 2001; 15(1):34–39.

19. Fox HJ, Pooler J, Prothero D, Bannister GC. Factors affecting the outcome after proximal femoral fractures. Injury 1994; 25(5):297–300.
20. Bray TJ. Femoral neck fracture fixation. Clinical decision making. Clin Orthop 1997; 339:20–31.
21. Hamlet WP, Lieberman JR, Freedman EL, Dorey FJ, Fletcher A, Johnson EE. Influence of health status and the timing of surgery on mortality in hip fracture patients. Am J Orthop 1997; 26(9):621–627.
22. Hoenig H, Rubenstein LV, Sloane R, Horner R, Kahn K. What is the role of timing in the surgical and rehabilitative care of community-dwelling older persons with acute hip fracture? Arch Intern Med 1997; 157(5):513–20. Erratum in: Arch Intern Med 1997; 157(13):1444.
23. Morrison RS, Chassin MR, Siu AL. The medical consultant's role in caring for patients with hip fracture. Ann Intern Med 1998; 128(12 Pt 1):1010–1020. Review. Erratum in: Ann Intern Med 1998; 129(9):755.
24. Wang AW, Gilbey HJ, Ackland TR. Perioperative exercise programs improve early return of ambulatory function after total hip arthroplasty: a randomized, controlled trial. Am J Phys Med Rehabil 2002; 81(11):801–806.
25. Vaz MD, Kramer JF, Rorabeck CH, Bourne RB. Isometric hip abductor strength following total hip replacement and its relationship to functional assessments. J Orthop Sports Phys Ther 1993; 18(4):526–531.
26. Loizeau J, Allard P, Duhaime M, Landjerit B. Bilateral gait patterns in subjects fitted with a total hip prosthesis. Arch Phys Med Rehabil 1995; 76(6):552–557.
27. Murray MP, Gore DR, Brewer BJ, Gardner GM, Sepic SB. A comparison of the functional performance of patients with Charnley and Muller total hip replacement. A two-year follow-up of eighty-nine cases. Acta Orthop Scand 1979; 50(5):563–569.
28. Olsson E, Goldie I, Wykman A. Total hip replacement. A comparison between cemented (Charnley) and non-cemented (HP Garches) fixation by clinical assessment and objective gait analysis. Scand J Rehabil Med 1986; 18(3):107–116.
29. Wykman A, Olsson E, Axdorph G, Goldie I. Total hip arthroplasty. A comparison between cemented and press-fit noncemented fixation. J Arthroplasty 1991; 6(1):19–29.
30. Menon PC, Griffiths WE, Hook WE, Higgins B. Trochanteric osteotomy in total hip arthroplasty: comparison of 2 techniques. J Arthroplasty 1998; 13(1):92–96.
31. Barrios C, Walheim G, Brostrom LA, Olsson E, Stark A. Walking ability after internal fixation of trochanteric hip fractures with Ender nails or sliding screw plate. A comparative study of gait. Clin Orthop 1993; 294:187–192.
32. Barnes B. Ambulation outcomes after hip fracture. Phys Ther 1984; 64(3):317–323.
33. Jette AM, Harris BA, Cleary PD, Campion EW. Functional recovery after hip fracture. Arch Phys Med Rehabil 1987; 68(10):735–740.
34. Clayer MT, Bauze RJ. Morbidity and mortality following fractures of the femoral neck and trochanteric region: analysis of risk factors. J Trauma 1989; 29(12):1673–1678.

35. Walheim G, Barrios C, Stark A, Brostrom LA, Olsson E. Postoperative improvement of walking capacity in patients with trochanteric hip fracture: a prospective analysis 3 and 6 months after surgery. J Orthop Trauma 1990; 4(2):137–143.

36. Allman RM, Laprade CA, Noel LB, Walker JM, Moorer CA, Dear MR, Smith CR. Pressure sores among hospitalized patients. Ann Intern Med 1986; 105(3):337–342.

37. Parker MJ, Pryor GA. Hip Fracture Management. Oxford, London: Blackwell Scientific Publication, 1993:212–261.

38. Nordin M, Frankel VH. Biomechanics of the hip. In: Nordin M, Frankel VH, eds. Basic Biomechanics of the Musculoskeletal System. Malvern, PA: Lea and Febiger, 1989:135–151.

39. Abrami G, Stevens J. Early weight bearing after internal fixation of transcervical fracture of the femur: preliminary report of a clinical trial. J Bone Joint Surg Br 1964; 46:204–205.

40. Ainsworth TH Jr. Immediate full weight-bearing in the treatment of hip fractures. J Trauma 1971; 11(12):1031–1040.

41. Ecker ML, Joyce JJ III, Kohl EJ. The treatment of trochanteric hip fractures using a compression screw. J Bone Joint Surg Am 1975; 57(1):23–27.

42. Neiman S. Early weightbearing after classical internal fixation of medial fractures of the femoral neck. Acta Ortha Scand 1975; 46:782–794.

43. Moller BN, Lucht U, Grymer F, Bartholdy NJ. Instability of trochanteric hip fractures following internal fixation. A radiographic comparison of the Richards sliding screw-plate and the McLaughlin nail-plate. Acta Orthop Scand 1984; 55(5):517–520.

44. Koval KJ, Friend KD, Aharonoff GB, Zukerman JD. Weight bearing after hip fracture: a prospective series of 596 geriatric hip fracture patients. J Orthop Trauma 1996; 10(8):526–530.

45. Ceder L, Thorngren KG, Wallden B. Prognostic indicators and early home rehabilitation in elderly patients with hip fractures. Clin Orthop 1980; 152:173–184.

46. Ceder L, Thorngren KG. Rehabilitation after hip repair. Lancet 1982; 2(8307):1097–1098.

47. Johnell O, Nilsson B, Obrant K, Sernbo I. Age and sex patterns of hip fracture—changes in 30 years. Acta Orthop Scand 1984; 55(3):290–292.

48. Koval KJ, Sala DA, Kummer FJ, Zuckerman JD. Postoperative weight-bearing after a fracture of the femoral neck or an intertrochanteric fracture. J Bone Joint Surg Am 1998; 80(3):352–356.

49. Demopoulos JT, Selman L. Rehabilitation following total hip replacement. Arch Phys Med Rehabil 1972; 53(2):51–59.

50. Pilliar RM, Lee JM, Maniatopoulos C. Observations on the effect of movement on bone ingrowth into porous-surfaced implants. Clin Orthop 1986; 208:108–113.

51. Johnsson R, Melander A, Onnerfalt R. Physiotherapy after total hip replacement for primary arthrosis. Scand J Rehabil Med 1988; 20(1):43–45.

52. Long WT, Dorr LD, Healy B, Perry J. Functional recovery of noncemented total hip arthroplasty. Clin Orthop 1993; 288:73–77.

53. Shih CH, Du YK, Lin YH, Wu CC. Muscular recovery around the hip joint after total hip arthroplasty. Clin Orthop 1994; 302:115–120.

54. Andersson L, Wesslau A, Boden H, Dalen N. Immediate or late weight bearing after uncemented total hip arthroplasty: a study of functional recovery. J Arthroplasty 2001; 16(8):1063–1065.

55. Magaziner J, Hawkes W, Hebel JR, Zimmerman SI, Fox KM, Dolan M, Felsenthal G, Kenzora J. Recovery from hip fracture in eight areas of function. J Gerontol Ser A Biol Sci Med Sci 2000; 55:M498–M507.

56. Sonntag D, Uhlenbrock D, Bardeleben A, Kading M, Hesse S. Gait with and without forearm crutches in patients with total hip arthroplasty. Int J Rehabil Res 2000; 23(3):233–243.

57. Lauridsen UB, de la Cour BB, Gottschalck L, Svensson BH. Intensive physical therapy after hip fracture. Dan Med Bull 2002; 49:70–72.

58. Sherrington C, Lord SR. Home exercise to improve strength and walking velocity after hip fracture: a randomized controlled trial. Arch Phys Med Rehabil 1997; 78(2):208–212.

59. Tinetti ME, Baker DI, Gottschalk M, Williams CS, Pollack D, Garrett P, Gill TM, Marottoli RA, Acampora D. Home-based multicomponent rehabilitation program for older persons after hip fracture: a randomized trial. Arch Phys Med Rehabil 1999; 80(8):916–922.

19

Optimizing Gait in Older People with Foot and Ankle Disorders

Hylton B. Menz

Musculoskeletal Research Centre, School of Physiotherapy, La Trobe University, Bundoora, Victoria, Australia

Stephen R. Lord

Prince of Wales Medical Research Institute, Randwick, North South Wales, Sydney, Australia

I. INTRODUCTION

The human foot plays an important role in all weight-bearing tasks, as it provides the only direct source of contact between the body and the supporting surface. When walking, the foot contributes to shock absorption, adapts to irregular surfaces, and provides a rigid lever for forward propulsion (1). Any disruption to the precise timing of foot and ankle motion has the potential to decrease both the stability and efficiency of gait patterns.

The aging process is associated with significant alterations to the cutaneous, vascular, neurological, and musculoskeletal characteristics of the foot and ankle. These changes include a decreased number and output of sweat and sebaceous glands, leading to dryness and an increased likelihood of fissuring (2), degradation of sensory receptors in the skin, leading to impaired tactile and vibration sensitivity (3,4), reduction in penetration of capillary loops leading to reduced epidermal blood supply (2,5–7), reduced joint range of motion (8–10), which may impair the ability of the lower limb to absorb shock (1) and reduced strength of lower limb muscles (11–15). As a consequence of these age-related changes, foot pain and deformity are a common accompaniment of advancing age, and many of these problems are compounded by underlying systematic disease and ill-fitting footwear. The aim of this chapter is to briefly outline the prevalence and consequences of foot problems in older people, and to discuss the management of some of the more common musculoskeletal conditions observed in the elderly foot.

II. PREVALENCE AND CONSEQUENCES OF FOOT PROBLEMS IN OLDER PEOPLE

Foot problems have long been recognized as being very common in older people. Studies conducted in hospitals or clinical settings have reported very high rates of foot problems—up to 80% of older people (16–18)—whereas larger community studies (often involving telephone interviews) report lower rates of foot problems, generally in the range of 30–40% (19). Women are more likely to suffer from foot problems than men, possibly due to the detrimental influence of wearing ladies' fashion footwear with elevated heels and a constrictive toebox (20–22). The prevalence of foot problems has been shown to increase with age, however in the very old, foot problems become less prevalent as a consequence of reduced mobility and the increased number of older people who are confined to bed (23). The most commonly observed and reported problems are hyperkeratotic lesions (corns and calluses), followed closely by nail disorders and structural deformities such as hallux valgus ("bunions") and lesser toe deformities (hammertoes and clawtoes) (23). However, a number of other conditions commonly diagnosed in the clinical setting (such as plantar heel pain) are rarely included in epidemiological surveys, and as a consequence, the prevalence of some of the more complex foot disorders in older people is largely unknown.

Numerous investigations conducted in a range of different countries have shown that foot problems contribute to impaired physical functioning and ability to perform basic activities of daily living. In an epidemiological study of 459 elderly residents in a small Italian town, Benvenuti et al. (24) reported significant associations between the presence of clinically assessed foot problems and self-reported difficulty in performing housework, shopping and walking 400 m. An evaluation of gait patterns also revealed that those with foot pain required a greater number of steps to walk three meters than those free of foot problems. A similar study of 1002 elderly women in the United States reported that women with chronic and severe foot pain walked more slowly and took longer to rise from a chair. After controlling for age, body mass index, co-morbidities and pain in other sites, severe foot pain was independently associated with increased risk for walking difficulty and disability in activities of daily living (25). More recently, a population-based cross-sectional survey conducted in the Netherlands of 7200 people aged 65 years and older reported that the 20% of subjects with foot problems were more likely to suffer from limited mobility and poor perceived well-being than those without foot problems (26).

Foot problems may also contribute to impaired balance and increase the risk of suffering a fall. A recent cross-sectional study of 135 older people reported that people with foot problems performed poorly in functional tasks and balance tests, the most detrimental foot conditions being the presence of pain and hallux valgus (27,28). Three retrospective studies have shown that older people who suffer from foot problems are more likely to have a history of recurrent falls (29–31), and prospective studies have confirmed this association. Gabell et al.(32) reported that "foot trouble" was associated with a threefold increased risk of falling in a sample of 100 older people, Tinetti et al. (33) found that the presence of a "serious foot problem" (defined as a bunion, toe deformity, ulcer or deformed nail) doubled the risk of falling, and Koski et al. (34) found that older people with bunions were twice as likely to fall than those without. More recently, a study of musculoskeletal pain in 1002 elderly women found that foot pain was the only site of pain that was significantly associated with an increased risk of falling (35). These results indicate that foot problems are a falls risk factor, presumably mediated by impaired balance and ability to perform daily functional tasks.

III. EVALUATION OF FOOT AND ANKLE PROBLEMS IN OLDER PEOPLE

Physical examination is the basis for diagnosing foot and ankle disorders. Simple observation and palpation techniques, in conjunction with detailed history taking and observation of gait patterns, are generally sufficient to diagnose most common conditions (36). The standard physical examination of the older patient with foot problems involves assessment of skin and appendages, vascular status (including pulse palpation and ankle-brachial index measurement), neurological status (including sensory testing with graded monofilaments and reflex testing), orthopedic examination (including foot posture, range of motion measurement of the ankle, subtalar, midtarsal and metatarsophalangeal joints), manual muscle testing, footwear assessment, and gait analysis (37). The reliability of simple clinical tests of foot and ankle characteristics in older people is generally good (38,39), although foot posture assessment remains a difficult issue (40). Footwear assessment is useful in order to identify the contribution of ill-fitting footwear to foot problems (22) and inappropriate footwear to balance difficulties (41), however, the diagnostic value of assessing wear patterns of footwear is questionable (42).

Gait analysis of older people with foot and ankle disorders in clinical practice is generally observational, however the use of video analysis of treadmill walking has been widely adopted by podiatrists and physical therapists (43,44). The relatively recent development of instrumentation for measuring pressure distribution under the foot has provided some useful insights into gait dysfunction associated with diabetic neuropathy, rheumatoid arthritis, foot posture variations and first ray deformity, and in-shoe systems have been used to assess the effects of various footwear and orthotic interventions (45). Generally speaking, however, the cost of these systems prevents their widespread, routine clinical use.

Conventional plain radiography remains the routine imaging technique for diagnosing common skeletal problems, although other techniques may offer additional benefits for certain conditions. Bone scanning has good sensitivity but poor specificity for detecting inflammatory conditions, infection, and osseus tumors, ultrasonography may be beneficial in diagnosing tendon trauma, plantar fasciitis, and interdigital neuritis, computed tomography offers enhanced imaging of trabeculae of bone and is particularly useful in diagnosing tarsal coalitions, and magnetic resonance imaging offers very clear images of bony and soft tissue disorders (36).

IV.   COMMON MUSCULOSKELETAL FOOT AND ANKLE PROBLEMS THAT CAN AFFECT BALANCE AND GAIT

A wide range of cutaneous, vascular, neurological, and musculoskeletal conditions are often manifest in the foot, and indeed, observation of lower limb problems can assist in the initial diagnosis of underlying systemic conditions in elderly patients (46). While it is beyond the scope of this chapter to discuss the management of the myriad of foot and ankle problems that may impair gait in older people, the following section provides a brief overview of some of the more common musculoskeletal conditions, divided into the regions of the foot they affect. A more comprehensive list of these conditions is provided in Figure 1.

A.   Forefoot

1.   Hallux Valgus

More commonly referred to as "bunions" (from the Greek *bunios*, meaning "turnip"), hallux valgus is the most common deformity of the first ray segment of the foot and refers to the lateral deviation of the hallux and subsequent abnormal medial prominence of the first metatarsal head. Although the most visible consequence of the deformity is the bulbous, often inflamed great toe joint, the condition frequently involves the progressive structural deformation of the entire forefoot. Hallux valgus is a multifactorial condition, which can be caused by trauma, muscle imbalance, structural deformity of the metatarsals, arthritic conditions (such as rheumatoid arthritis and gout), faulty foot mechanics, and, the detrimental effects of ill-fitting footwear (47,48).

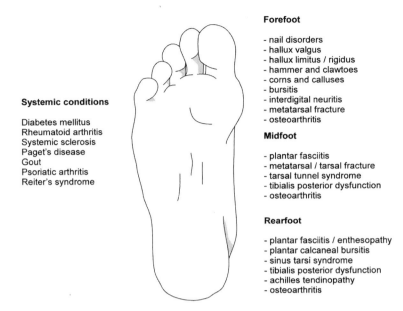

Systemic conditions

Diabetes mellitus
Rheumatoid arthritis
Systemic sclerosis
Paget's disease
Gout
Psoriatic arthritis
Reiter's syndrome

Forefoot

- nail disorders
- hallux valgus
- hallux limitus / rigidus
- hammer and clawtoes
- corns and calluses
- bursitis
- interdigital neuritis
- metatarsal fracture
- osteoarthritis

Midfoot

- plantar fasciitis
- metatarsal / tarsal fracture
- tarsal tunnel syndrome
- tibialis posterior dysfunction
- osteoarthritis

Rearfoot

- plantar fasciitis / enthesopathy
- plantar calcaneal bursitis
- sinus tarsi syndrome
- tibialis posterior dysfunction
- achilles tendinopathy
- osteoarthritis

Figure 1 Common foot and ankle problems that may affect gait in older people.

We have previously shown that older people with severe hallux valgus
are more likely to have lesser toe deformities and plantar calluses, and
demonstrate worse balance when performing a coordinated leaning task
compared to those without the condition (28). Few investigations have been
performed to assess the impact of hallux valgus on gait patterns. A number
of plantar pressure analyses have been performed on subjects with and without hallux valgus, however, the results have been inconsistent. While some
studies have reported an overall medial shift in pressure distribution
(49,50), others have found a greater tendency to increased lateral loading
in subjects with hallux valgus (51,52). These inconsistencies are likely to
be due to inadequate adjustment for confounding variables and/or differences in the severity of hallux valgus in the study samples. While increased
medial loading may contribute to the initial development of the deformity
(48), with further progression the first ray segment of the foot often becomes
hypermobile, thereby resulting in greater lateral loading.

More recently, significant differences in temporo-spatial gait parameters and upper body movement patterns have been reported between
older people with and without hallux valgus. After adjusting for potential
confounders, subjects with moderate to severe hallux valgus were found
to exhibit reduced velocity and step length and less rhythmic acceleration
patterns in the vertical plane. These differences were particularly

pronounced when subjects walked on an irregular surface, suggesting that older people with hallux valgus may have an increased risk of falling when traversing uneven terrain (53).

In addition to potential gait and balance problems, the enlarged first metatarsal head associated with hallux valgus creates difficulties with finding suitable footwear, and the friction created by the shoe often leads to the formation of a bursa over the site that may become inflamed or ulcerated. Treatment of hallux valgus involves changing footwear to that with a broader forefoot, the application of foam or silicon pads over the joint, foot orthoses and surgery. Surgery has been shown to provide better long-term results than foot orthoses (54); however, pressure distribution is not always normalized following surgery (51,52), and subsequently the development of transfer lesions to the lesser metatarsophalangeal joints is common. Unfortunately, the evidence pertaining to the efficacy of hallux valgus surgery is generally of low quality, and the most recent Cochrane review concluded that inadequate evidence exists to indicate significant benefits of any one surgical technique vs. another (55).

2. Hallux Limitus/Rigidus

Hallux limitus is an arthritic condition in which there is limited range of motion at the first metatarsophalangeal joint of the hallux. If this progresses to complete fusion of the joint, it is termed hallux rigidus (56). The pathogenesis of the condition is unknown, however, postulated risk factors include flat foot, metatarsus elevatus, and excessively long first metatarsal (56). Pressure distribution studies indicate that feet with hallux limitus generate much larger forces under the hallux but lower forces under the first metatarsophalangeal joint, which is likely to represent compensatory dorsiflexion of the interphalangeal joint to enable forward propulsion (50). Proximal compensation for inadequate metatarsophalangeal dorsiflexion during propulsion has been postulated as a contributing factor to the development of upper body postural symptoms (57). In a recent study, restriction of first metatarsophalangeal joint motion using a specially designed insole resulted in increased ankle dorsiflexion and knee extension and less hip extension during the midstance phase of gait, indicating that hallux limitus/rigidus does have the potential to alter movement patterns of proximal segments (58).

For hallux limitus, treatment involves foot orthoses to facilitate more normal propulsion through the first metatarsophalangeal joint, or manipulation and injection with corticosteroid (59). For hallux rigidus, footwear modifications or surgery may be necessary. However, in a recent 14-year follow-up study of patients who had chosen not to have surgery, few reported that their condition had worsened, and 75% would still choose not to have surgery if they had to make the decision again. A large proportion of these patients had changed their footwear to that with a more ample toebox, suggesting that selection of appropriate footwear may be a sufficient treatment in many people (60). Indeed, a recent retrospective analysis of 772 patients with hallux limitus reported that 55% were successfully treated with conservative measures, including change of footwear, foot orthoses, and corticosteroid injection (61).

3. Lesser Toe Deformity

Long-term wearing of ill-fitting footwear, in association with faulty foot mechanics and intrinsic muscle atrophy, can lead to the development of clawing, hammering, and retraction of the lesser toes (62). Hammertoes and clawtoes are one of the most common foot complaints in older people, and can lead to the development of corns on the dorsum of the interphalangeal joints and calluses under the metatarsal heads. There is also evidence to suggest that toe deformity may impair balance and mobility in older people. We recently found that older people with lesser toe deformity demonstrated poorer balance and took longer to ascend and descend stairs than those without toe deformity (28). Gait studies have shown that the toes accept a large proportion of bodyweight during the propulsive phase of gait (63), so in the presence of toe deformity, the ability to generate sufficient power for normal forward motion may be impaired (23). Treatment of lesser toe deformity involves footwear modification, various splinting devices, stretching and strengthening exercises, and management of secondary lesions. The efficacy of these approaches has not been fully evaluated, however, there is preliminary evidence that silicon devices placed under the toe sulcus significantly reduce pressure loading of the toes during gait (64), and that a toe strengthening program may improve standing balance in older people (65). Severe cases often require surgery to realign and stabilize the affected metatarsophalangeal or interphalangeal joints and/or lengthen the long flexor or extensor tendons. Outcomes of lesser toe surgery vary considerably, depending on the nature of the deformity (i.e., flexible or rigid), the choice of surgical procedure, and the presence of associated conditions, however, complications such as transfer lesions, floating digits, and residual clawing are relatively common (66).

4. Interdigital Neuritis

Interdigital neuritis (also referred to as *Morton's neuroma*) is the term given to plantar digital neuritis affecting the 3rd/4th interdigital space (67). The pain associated with this condition frequently has a "pins and needles" quality and radiates towards the toes. While the etiology is uncertain, this condition is thought to result from the pinching of a plantar digital nerve caused by excessively narrow footwear or abnormal foot mechanics. Treatment involves footwear advice and/or modification, padding to redistribute weight-bearing pressure away from the affected area, or surgical excision (68).

5.   Stress/Insufficiency Fracture

Stress fractures are most commonly caused by healthy bones being exposed to intense and/or repetitive loads for which the bone is not prepared, such as a rapid increase in training intensity in a competitive athlete. Insufficiency stress fractures, however, result from normal loads to bones weakened by genetic, metabolic, nutritional, or endocrine processes. As bone mineral density decreases with age, older people develop an increased risk of insufficiency fracture, particularly older women with osteoporosis. Insufficiency fractures can occur in the bones of the foot, most commonly the metatarsals (69–71), but occasionally the talus (72) or calcaneus (73). Treatment involves a period of non-weightbearing, foot orthoses and appropriate management of osteoporosis (71).

B.   Midfoot

Pain in the midfoot is less common than forefoot or rearfoot pain. The most commonly diagnosed condition responsible for pain in this area is plantar fasciitis (see section on "Rearfoot"). Less common causes include stress fractures of the tarsal bones, tarsal tunnel syndrome, and tibialis posterior dysfunction. Tarsal tunnel syndrome is a well known but rare entrapment neuropathy involving the posterior tibial nerve in the tarsal tunnel, a fibro-osseous channel extending from the medial aspect of the ankle to the midfoot. Tarsal tunnel syndrome can result from a range of conditions such as ganglia, sarcoma, talocalcaneal coalition, and the presence of an accessory flexor digitorum longus muscle (74). Treatment involves surgical decompression of the neurovascular bundle and/or resection of the osseous coalition or accessory muscle.

Tibialis posterior dysfunction is a condition in which the tibialis posterior muscle, which plays a major role in maintaining the medial arch of the foot, weakens and may partially rupture, leading to a progressive and disabling flatfoot deformity (75). While the exact cause is unknown, tendon degeneration due to reduced blood supply has been implicated (76), and the condition is more common in people with obesity, hypertension, diabetes, or previous trauma (77). Treatment options include foot orthoses, physical therapy, tendon reconstruction, or surgical fixation of joints in the rearfoot (75).

C.   Rearfoot

Pain in the region of the heel is one of the most common presentations to foot specialist clinics, and it has been estimated that the prevalence of heel pain in older people lies between 12% and 15% (78). There are a range of causes of heel pain, including proximal plantar fasciitis (also referred to as heel spur syndrome or enthesopathy), nerve entrapment, calcaneal stress fracture, and plantar calcaneal bursitis. A number of systemic conditions can also lead to heel pain, including Paget's disease, rheumatoid arthritis, psoriatic arthritis, gout, and Reiter's syndrome (79). Heel pain can be quite disabling and impair normal gait patterns. In the presence of heel pain, patients compensate by reducing the single limb support duration of the affected side and by reducing the unaffected side's swing phase and single limb support as a percentage of the gait cycle, possibly in an attempt to minimize loading on the affected area (80).

Older people may be more likely to develop heel pain due to the effects of aging on the structure and function of the plantar heel pad, a specialized soft tissue structure under the calcaneus consisting of closely packed fat cells that is responsible for shock attenuation when walking. Older people have thicker, but more compressible heel pads that dissipate more energy than younger people (81), which may result in greater impact being applied to the musculoskeletal and neural structures in the heel region. The other likely contributor to heel pain in older people is excess bodyweight, as many patients with heel pain have a higher body mass index than controls (82).

A wide range of treatments have been reported for plantar heel pain, including stretching the calf muscles, foot orthoses/insoles, heel cups, tension night splints, corticosteroid injection, therapeutic ultrasound, nonsteroidal anti-inflammatory drugs, galvanic currents, shoe modifications, acupuncture, laser therapy, extracorporeal shock-wave therapy, and surgery (83). However, the quality of evidence for each of these interventions is generally poor, and the most recent Cochrane review on the topic concluded that although there is some evidence for the effectiveness of cortisone administered via iontophoresis, the efficacy of other frequently employed treatments has not been fully established in comparative studies (84).

V. FOOT PROBLEMS ASSOCIATED WITH SYSTEMIC DISEASE

A. Rheumatoid Arthritis

Foot involvement affects 53–92% of people with rheumatoid arthritis (85–87) and the associated pain leads to significant impairment in ambulation (88). The first metatarsophalangeal joint is commonly affected, leading to synovitis, hallux valgus, or hallux rigidus (89). As the condition progresses, the entire forefoot may be affected, leading to lesser toe deformity and displacement of the fibrofatty tissue under the metatarsal heads. Rearfoot involvement is common and often results in valgus heel deformity (90). As a consequence of these changes, people with rheumatoid arthritis often exhibit a slow and shuffling gait pattern, with reduced velocity, shortened stride length, and delayed heel lift (88). Kinematic analyses of the foot have also revealed significantly increased eversion of the foot and internal rotation of the tibia (91), and plantar pressure studies have revealed significantly elevated medial forefoot pressures in people with valgus heel deformity (92). Management of foot problems in rheumatoid arthritis involves regular debridement of calluses, which provides effective, if short-term relief (93), and the prescription of foot orthoses, which have been found to be effective in decreasing pain and improving gait and general mobility (94,95).

B.   Diabetes Mellitus

The common and serious consequences of diabetes on the foot are well known. Between 15% and 20% of people with diabetes are admitted to hospital at some stage in their life as a consequence of a foot-related complication such as neuropathic ulceration, infection, and ischemia (96). These complications result from a combination of factors, including sensory, motor and autonomic neuropathy, foot deformity, and limited joint mobility. Many of these changes, particularly sensory neuropathy, are also associated with characteristic changes in gait, including reduced velocity, step length and cadence, decreased power generation at the ankle, decreased knee joint flexion, and decreased ground reaction forces (97–99). In a recent study, we also found that people with diabetic peripheral neuropathy demonstrate less rhythmic accelerations of the upper body, a factor that may predispose to falls (100).

Management of the diabetic foot requires a multi-disciplinary approach involving satisfactory control of blood sugar levels, patient education regarding foot hygiene, appropriate footwear and exercise, and ulcer management involving debridement, wound care and pressure redistribution techniques such as foot orthoses and modified footwear (101–103). Plantar pressure measurement systems may be useful in determining the optimum design of offloading devices (45). Gait instability associated with diabetic peripheral neuropathy may also be managed by the use of walking sticks or ankle braces (104).

C.   Other Systemic Conditions

As shown in Figure 1, a wide range of other systemic conditions may lead to foot problems, including skin lesions, joint pain, and vascular changes associated with systemic sclerosis (105,106), heel pain associated with Paget's disease (107), tophus formation associated with gout (108), nail and joint involvement in psoriatic arthritis (109), and, although uncommon in older people, inflammatory heel pain associated with Retier's syndrome (110). Successful treatment of these conditions requires a combination of medical management of the underlying disease process and conservative management of foot complications.

VI. THE ROLE OF FOOTWEAR AND FOOT ORTHOSES

A. Footwear

Footwear advice and modification play an important role in optimizing gait in elderly people. Between 50% and 80% of elderly people wear ill-fitting shoes (21,22,111), and there is a strong association between inappropriate footwear and foot problems (21,22). Certain footwear characteristics, such as high heels, soles with poor grip and inadequate fixation, may also be associated with impaired gait, balance, falls, and hip fracture (112–116). We have previously shown that balance is maximized in shoes with low heels (112) and high heel collars (i.e., boot) (113), and that the addition of a bevel to the rear section of a shoe can improve slip resistance (115). More recently, we also reported an association between wearing shoes with inadequate fixation and suffering a trip-related hip fracture (116). Older people should therefore generally be advised to wear appropriately fitting shoes with low heels, textured soles, laces, and if feasible, a high heel collar for additional ankle support (114).

Footwear modification (*pedorthics*) is also a useful conservative management strategy for older people with foot problems. The aim of footwear modification is to reduce shock and shear, to relieve excessive pressure from sensitive or painful areas, to accommodate, correct, and support deformities, and to control or limit painful motion of joints (117). This may be achieved by the prescription of shoes with extra depth in the forefoot, the addition of balloon patches to the upper part of the shoe to accommodate prominent toe deformities, adding a lateral flare to the midsole to enhance stability, inserting a wedge of soft material into the heel region to improve shock absorption, and adding an external "rockerbar" to the sole of the shoe to enhance propulsion (Fig. 2). These approaches are particularly useful in the management of diabetic foot ulcers (118,119), chronic arthritic conditions such as rheumatoid arthritis (120,121), and following surgical fusion of the tarsal joints (122). Plantar pressure measurement systems have proven to be very useful in optimizing the design of rockerbars (123–125).

B. Foot Orthoses

Foot orthoses are devices placed within the shoe that aim to decrease pain and improve function by altering the biomechanical function of the lower limb (126). Although a wide range of styles of foot orthoses are currently in use, broadly speaking, they can be divided into two functional categories; those that aim to improve function by redistributing pressure beneath the foot (*pressure redistributing orthoses*), and those that improve function by limiting excessive motion of tarsal joints (*motion controlling orthoses*). Pressure redistributing orthoses are generally made from compressible materials and are commonly used to offload sites of high pressure in the diabetic

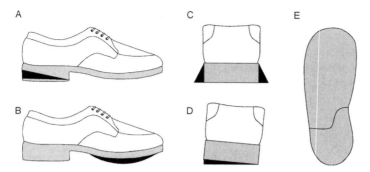

Figure 2 Footwear modifications for optimizing gait. A: Shock absorbing cushioned heel to improve shock absorption, B: Rockersole to improve propulsion, C: Lateral sole flaring to increase stability, D: External wedging to correct varus or valgus heel deformity, E: Thomas heel to control pes planus ("flat foot").

foot, while motion controlling orthoses are made from firmer materials and are commonly used to manage conditions related to pes planus ("flat foot").

Numerous studies have shown that pressure redistributing orthoses are very effective in moving pressure away from high-pressure sites such as prominent metatarsal heads (127–131), and as such can be very useful in the management of forefoot pain in rheumatoid arthritis (131) and plantar forefoot lesions associated with diabetes (132,133). Figure 3 shows some of the more common designs of pressure redistributing orthoses. Motion-controlling orthoses have been found to be effective in limiting excessive motion of the lower limb (134), and appear to be effective in decreasing pain associated with conditions such as plantar fasciitis (135–137). Although

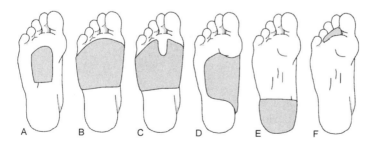

Figure 3 Common designs of plantar pressure redistributing orthoses. A: plantar metatarsal pad to elevate central metatarsal heads, B: plantar cover for additional cushioning, C: U-shaped plantar cover for redirecting pressure away from 2nd metatarsal head, D: valgus pad to support medial arch, E: plantar heel pad for heel elevation and increased cushioning of heel, F: toe prop to straighten 2nd–4th toes and redirect pressure from apices of toes.

most studies of these devices have been performed in healthy young people, recent randomized controlled trials have reported that motion-controlling orthoses are effective in limiting deformity, decreasing pain and improving function in patients with rheumatoid arthritis (94,95,138), and there is some preliminary evidence that foot orthoses may also be useful in managing osteoarthritis of the tarsal joints (139).

VII. CONCLUSIONS

Foot problems are very common in older people and are associated with impaired gait and mobility. However, many foot problems can be adequately managed with conservative interventions such as physical therapy modalities, footwear advice and modification, and prescription of foot orthoses. The recent development of plantar pressure analysis systems has provided a useful tool for assessing the biomechanical changes associated with these interventions.

REFERENCES

1. Saltzman CL, Nawoczenski DA. Complexities of foot architecture as a base of support. J Orthop Sports Phys Ther 1995; 21:354–360.
2. Muehlman C, Rahimi F. Aging integumentary system. Podiatric review. J Am Podiatr Med Assoc 1990; 80:577–582.
3. Rosenberg G. Effect of age on peripheral vibratory perception. J Am Geriatr Assoc 1958; 6:471–481.
4. Stevens JC, Choo KK. Spatial acuity of the body surface over the life span. Somatosens Motor Res 1996; 13:153–166.
5. Gilchrest BA. A review of skin ageing and its medical therapy. Br J Dermatol 1996; 135:867–875.
6. Glogau RG. Physiologic and structural changes associated with aging skin. Dermatol Clin 1997; 15:555–559.
7. Jenkins G. Molecular mechanisms of skin ageing. Mech Ageing Dev 2002; 123:801–810.
8. Nigg BM, Fisher V, Allinger TL, Ronsky JR, Engsberg JR. Range of motion of the foot as a function of age. Foot Ankle 1992; 13:336–343.
9. James B, Parker AW. Active and passive mobility of lower limb joints in elderly men and women. Am J Phys Med Rehabil 1989; 68:162–167.
10. Vandervoort AA, Chesworth BM, Cunningham DA, Paterson DH, Rechnitzer PA, Koval JJ. Age and sex effects on mobility of the human ankle. J Gerontol 1992; 47:M17–M21.
11. Jennekens FGI, Tomlinson BE, Walton JN. Histochemical aspects of five limb muscles in old age. J Neurol Sci 1971; 14:259–276.
12. McDonagh MJN, White MJ, Davies CTM. Different effects of ageing on the mechanical properties of human arm and leg muscles. Gerontology 1984; 30:49–54.

13. Davies CTM, White MJ. Contractile properties of elderly human triceps surae. Gerontology 1983; 29:19–25.

14. Vandervoort AA, McComas AJ. Contractile changes in opposing muscles of the human ankle joint with aging. J Appl Physiol 1986; 61:361–367.

15. Endo M, Ashton-Miller J, Alexander N. Effects of age and gender on toe flexor muscle strength. J Gerontol 2002; 57A:M392–M397.

16. Ebrahim SBJ, Sainsbury R, Watson S. Foot problems of the elderly: a hospital survey. Br Med J 1981; 283:949–950.

17. Hung L, Ho Y, Leung P. Survey of foot deformities among 166 geriatric inpatients. Foot Ankle 1985; 5:156–164.

18. Crawford VLS, Ashford RL, McPeake B, Stout RW. Conservative podiatric medicine and disability in elderly people. J Am Podiatr Med Assoc 1995; 85:255–259.

19. Greenberg L. Foot care data from two recent nationwide surveys—a comparative analysis. J Am Podiatr Med Assoc 1994; 84:365–370.

20. Gorecki GA. Shoe related foot problems and public health. J Am Podiatry Assoc 1978; 4:245–247.

21. Frey CC, Thompson F, Smith J, Sanders M, Horstman H. American Orthopedic Foot and Ankle Society women's shoe survey. Foot Ankle 1993; 14:78–81.

22. Burns SL, Leese GP, McMurdo MET. Older people and ill-fitting shoes. Postgrad Med J 2002; 78:344–346.

23. Menz HB, Lord SR. Foot problems, functional impairment and falls in older people. J Am Podiatr Med Assoc 1999; 89:458–461.

24. Benvenuti F, Ferrucci L, Guralnik J, Gangemi S, Baroni A. Foot pain and disability in older persons: an epidemiologic survey. J Am Geriatr Soc 1995; 43:479–484.

25. Leveille SG, Guralnik JM, Ferrucci L, Hirsch R, Simonsick E, Hochberg MC. Foot pain and disability in older women. Am J Epidemiol 1998; 148:657–665.

26. Gorter KJ, Kuyvenhoven MM, deMelker RA. Nontraumatic foot complaints in older people. A population-based survey of risk factors, mobility, and well-being.. J Am Podiatr Med Assoc 2000; 90:397–402.

27. Menz HB, Lord SR. The contribution of foot problems to mobility impairment and falls in older people. J Am Geriatr Soc 2001; 49:1651–1656.

28. Menz HB, Lord SR. Foot pain impairs balance and functional ability in community-dwelling older people. J Am Podiatr Med Assoc 2001; 91:222–229.

29. Wild D, Nayak US, Isaacs B. Characteristics of old people who fell at home. J Clin Exp Gerontol 1980; 2:271–287.

30. Blake A, Morgan K, Bendall M, Dalloso H, Ebrahim S, Arie T, Fentem F, Bassey E. Falls by elderly people at home—prevalence and associated factors. Age Ageing 1988; 17:365–372.

31. Dolinis J, Harrison JE. Factors associated with falling in older Adelaide residents. Aust N Z J Public Health 1997; 21:462–468.

32. Gabell A, Simons MA, Nayak USL. Falls in the healthy elderly: predisposing causes. Ergonomics 1985; 28:965–975.

33. Tinetti ME, Speechley M, Ginter SF. Risk factors for falls among elderly persons living in the community. N Engl J Med 1988; 319:1701–1707.

34. Koski K, Luukinen H, Laippala P, Kivela S-L. Physiological factors and medications as predictors of injurious falls by elderly people: a prospective population-based study. Age Ageing 1996; 25:29–38.

35. Leveille SG, Bean J, Bandeen-Roche K, Jones R, Hochberg M, Guralnik JM. Musculoskeletal pain and risk of falls in older disabled women living in the community. J Am Geriatr Soc 2002; 50:671–678.

36. Balint GP, Korda J, Hangody L, Balint PV. Foot and ankle disorders. Best Pract Res Clin Rheumatol 2003; 17:87–111.

37. Merriman LM, Turner W. Assessment of the Lower Limb. New York: Churchill Livingstone, 2002.

38. VanGisbergen MJ, Dekker J, Zuijderduin W. Reliability of the diagnosis of impairments in survey research in the field of chiropody. Disabil Rehabil 1993; 15:76–82.

39. Menz HB, Tiedemann A, Kwan MMS, Latt MD, Sherrington C, Lord SR. Reliability of clinical tests of foot and ankle characteristics in older people. J Am Podiatr Med Assoc 2003; 93:380–387.

40. Razeghi M, Batt ME. Foot type classification: a critical review of current methods. Gait Posture 2002; 15:282–291.

41. Menz HB, Sherrington C. The Footwear Assessment Form: a reliable clinical tool to assess footwear characteristics of relevance to postural stability in older adults. Clin Rehabil 2000; 14:657–664.

42. Vernon W, Parry A, Potter M. A theory of shoe wear pattern influence incorporating a new paradigm for the podiatric medical profession. J Am Podiatr Med Assoc 2004; 94:261–268.

43. Payne C. Methods of analysing gait. In: Merriman LM, Turner W, eds. Assessment of the Lower Limb. New York: Churchill Livingstone, 2002.

44. Toro B, Nester CJ, Farren PC. The status of gait assessment among physiotherapists in the United Kingdom. Arch Phys Med and Rehabil 2003; 84:1878–1884.

45. Orlin MN, McPoil TG. Plantar pressure assessment. Phys Ther 2000; 80: 399–409.

46. Tarara EL, Spittel JA. Clues to systemic diseases from examination of the foot in geriatric patients. J Am Podiatry Assoc 1978; 68:424–430.

47. Inman VT. Hallux valgus: a review of etiologic factors. Orthop Clin N Am 1974; 5:59–66.

48. Kilmartin TE, Wallace WA. The aetiology of hallux valgus: a critical review of the literature. Foot 1993; 3:157–167.

49. Plank MJ. The pattern of forefoot pressure distribution in hallux valgus. Foot 1995; 5:8–14.

50. Bryant A, Tinley P, Singer K. Plantar pressure distribution in normal, hallux valgus and hallux limitus feet. Foot 1999; 9:115–119.

51. Stokes IAF, Hutton WC, Stott JRR, Lowe LW. Forces under the hallux valgus foot before and after surgery. Clin Orthop Relat Res 1979; 142:64–72.

52. Resch S, Stenstrom A. Evaluation of hallux valgus surgery with dynamic foot pressure registration with the F-Scan system. Foot 1995; 5:115–121.

53. Menz HB, Lord SR. Gait instability in older people with hallux valgus. Foot Ankle Int 2005. In press.

54. Torkki M, Malmivaara A, Seitsalo S, Hoikka V, Laippala P, Paavolainen P. Surgery vs orthosis vs watchful waiting for hallux valgus: a randomized controlled trial. J Am Med Assoc 2001; 285:2474–2480.
55. Ferrari J, Higgins JPT, Prior TD. Interventions for treating hallux valgus (abductovalgus) and bunions. Cochrane Database Syst Rev 2004; 1:CD000964.
56. Weinfeld SB, Schon LC. Hallux metatarsophalangeal arthritis. Clin Orthop Relat Res 1998; 349:9–19.
57. Dananberg HJ. Gait style as an etiology to chronic postural pain: part II. Postural compensatory process. J Am Podiatr Med Assoc 1993; 83:615–624.
58. Hall C, Nester CJ. Sagittal plane compensations for artificially induced limitation of the first metatarsophalangeal joint—a preliminary study. J Am Podiatr Med Assoc 2004; 94:269–274.
59. Solan M, Calder J, Bendall S. Manipulation and injection for hallux rigidus. Is it worthwhile? J Bone Joint Surg 2001; 83B:706–708.
60. Smith R, Katchis S, Ayson L. Outcomes in hallux rigidus patients treated nonoperatively: a long-term follow-up study. Foot Ankle Int 2000; 21:906–913.
61. Grady JF, Axe TM, Zager EJ, Sheldon LA. A retrospective analysis of 772 patients with hallux limitus. J Am Podiatr Med Assoc 2002; 92:102–108.
62. Coughlin MJ. Mallet toes, hammer toes, claw toes and corns. Postgrad Med 1984; 75:191–198.
63. Hughes J, Clark P, Klenerman L. The importance of the toes in walking. J Bone Joint Surg 1990; 72B:245–251.
64. Claisse PJ, Binning J, Potter J. Effect of orthotic therapy on claw toe loading. Results of significance testing at pressure sensor units.. J Am Podiatr Med Assoc 2004; 94:246–254.
65. Kobayashi R, Hosoda M, Minematsu A, Sasaki H, Maejima H, Tanaka S, Kanemura N, Matsuo A, Shirahama K, Ueda T, Kamoda C, Yoshimura O. Effects of toe grasp training for the aged on spontaneous postural sway. J Phys Ther Sci 1999; 11:31–34.
66. Femino JE, Mueller K. Complications of lesser toe surgery. Clin Orthop Relat Res 2001; 391:72–78.
67. Youngswick FD. Intermetatarsal neuroma. Clin Podiatr Med Surg 1994; 11:579–592.
68. Wu KK. Morton's interdigital neuroma: a clinical review of its etiology, treatment, and results. J Foot Ankle Surg 1996; 35:112–119.
69. Varenna M, Binelli L, Zucchi F, Beltrametti P, Gallazzi M, Sinigaglia L. Is the metatarsal fracture in postmenopausal women an osteoporotic fracture? A cross-sectional study on 113 cases. Osteoporos Int 1997; 7:558–563.
70. Kaye RA. Insufficiency stress fractures of the foot and ankle in postmenopausal women. Foot Ankle Int 1988; 19:221–224.
71. Freeman D, Randall DB. Stress fracture of the foot secondary to osteoporosis: an atypical presentation. J Am Podiatr Med Assoc 2001; 91:99–101.
72. Umans H, Pavlov H. Insufficiency fracture of the talus: diagnosis with MR imaging. Radiology 1995; 197:439–442.
73. Ito K, Hori K, Terashima Y, Sekine M, Kura H. Insufficiency fracture of the body of the calcaneus in elderly patients with osteoporosis. Clin Orthop Relat Res 2004; 422:190–194.

74. Lau JT, Daniels TR. Tarsal tunnel syndrome: a review of the literature. Foot Ankle Int 1999; 20:201–209.
75. Mendicino SS. Posterior tibial tendon dysfunction. Diagnosis, evaluation, and treatment. Clin Podiatr Med Surg 2000; 17:33–54.
76. Frey CC. Vascularity of the posterior tibial tendon. J Bone Joint Surg 1990; 72A:884–888.
77. Holmes GB, Mann RA. Possible epidemiological factors associated with rupture of the posterior tibial tendon. Foot Ankle 1992; 13:70–79.
78. Black JR, Bernard JM, Williams LA. Heel pain in the older patient. Clin Podiatr Med Surg 1993; 10:113–119.
79. Barrett SL, O'Malley R. Plantar fasciitis and other causes of heel pain. Am Fam Physician 1999; 59:2200–2206.
80. Levins AD, Skinner HB, Caiozzo VJ. Adaptive gait responses to plantar heel pain. J Rehabil Res Dev 1998; 35:289–293.
81. Hsu TC, Wang CL, Tsai WC, Kuo JK, Tang FT. Comparison of the mechanical properties of the heel pad between young and elderly adults. Arch Phys Med Rehabil 1998; 79:1101–1104.
82. Rano JA, Fallat LM, Savoy-Moore RT. Correlation of heel pain with body mass index and other characteristics of heel pain. J Foot Ankle Surg 2001; 40:351–356.
83. Young CC, Rutherford DS, Niedfeldt MW. Treatment of plantar fasciitis. Am Fam Physician 2001; 63:467–474,477–478.
84. Crawford F, Thomson C. Interventions for treating plantar heel pain. Cochrane Database Syst Rev 2003; 3:CD000416.
85. Fleming A, Benn RT, Corbett M, Wood PH. Early rheumatoid disease. II. Patterns of joint involvement. Ann Rheum Dis 1976; 35:361–364.
86. Jahss MH. Foot and ankle pain resulting from rheumatic conditions. Curr Opin Rheumatol 1992; 4:233–240.
87. Michelson J, Easley M, Wigley FM, Hellmann D. Foot and ankle problems in rheumatoid arthritis. Foot Ankle Int 1994; 15:608–613.
88. Platto MJ, O'Connell PG, Hicks JE, Gerber LH. The relationship of pain and deformity of the rheumatoid foot to gait and an index of functional ambulation. J Rheumatol 1991; 18:38–43.
89. Woodburn J, Helliwell PS. Foot problems in rheumatology. Br J Rheumatol 1997; 36:932–934.
90. Keenan MAE, Peabody TD, Gronley JK, Perry J. Valgus deformities of the feet and characteristics of gait in patients who have rheumatoid arthritis. J Bone Joint Surg 1991; 73A:237–247.
91. Woodburn J, Helliwell PS, Barker S. Three-dimensional kinematics at the ankle joint complex in rheumatoid arthritis patients with painful valgus deformity of the rearfoot. Rheumatology 2002; 41:1406–1412.
92. Woodburn J, Helliwell PS. Relation between heel position and the distribution of forefoot plantar pressures and skin callosities in rheumatoid arthritis. Ann Rheum Dis 1996; 55:806–810.
93. Woodburn J, Stableford Z, Helliwell PS. Preliminary investigation of debridement of plantar callosities in rheumatoid arthritis. Rheumatology 2000; 39:652–654.

94. Chalmers AC, Busby C, Goyert J, Porter B, Schulzer M. Metatarsalgia and rheumatoid arthritis—a randomized, single blind, sequential trial comparing 2 types of foot orthoses and supportive shoes. J Rheumatol 2000; 27: 1643–1647.
95. Woodburn J, Barker S, Helliwell PS. A randomized controlled trial of foot orthoses in rheumatoid arthritis. J Rheumatol 2002; 29:1377–1383.
96. Reiber GE. The epidemiology of diabetic foot problems. Diab Med 1996; 13:S6–S11.
97. Mueller MJ, Minor SS, Sahrmann SA, Schaaf JA, Strube MJ. Differences in the gait characteristics of patients with diabetes and peripheral neuropathy compared with age-matched controls. Physical Ther 1994; 74:299–313.
98. Courtemanche R, Teasdale N, Boucher P, Fleury M, Lajoie Y, Bard C. Gait problems in diabetic neuropathic patients. Arch Phys Med Rehabil 1996; 77:849–855.
99. Katoulis EC, Ebdon-Parry M, Lanshammar H, Vileikyte L, Kulkarni J, Boulton AJ. Gait abnormalities in diabetic neuropathy. Diab Care 1997; 20: 1904–1907.
100. Menz HB, Lord SR, St George R, Fitzpatrick RC. Walking stability and sensorimotor function in older people with diabetic peripheral neuropathy. Arch Phys Med Rehabil 2004; 85:245–252.
101. Spencer S. Pressure relieving interventions for preventing and treating diabetic foot ulcers. Cochrane Database Syst Rev 2000; 3:CD002302.
102. Valk GD, Kriegsman DM, Assendelft WJ. Patient education for preventing diabetic foot ulceration. Cochrane Database Syst Rev 2001; 4:CD001488.
103. Smith J. Debridement of diabetic foot ulcers. Cochrane Database Syst Rev 2002; 4:CD003556.
104. Richardson JK, Thies SB, DeMott TK, Ashton-Miller JA. Interventions improve gait regularity in patients with peripheral neuropathy while walking on an irregular surface under low light. J Am Geriatr Soc 2004; 52:510–515.
105. Sari-Kouzel H, Hutchinson CE, Middleton AL, Webb F, Moore T, Griffin K, Herrick A. Foot problems in patients with systemic sclerosis. Rheumatology 2001; 40:410–413.
106. LaMontagna G, Baruffo A, Tirri R, Buono G, Valentini G. Foot involvement in systemic sclerosis: a longitudinal study of 100 patients. Semin Arthritis Rheum 2002; 31:248–255.
107. Lichniak JE. The heel in systemic disease. Clin Podiatr Med Surg 1990; 7: 225–241.
108. Thomas E, Olive P, Canovas F, Medioni D, Leroux JL, Baldet P, Bonnel F, Blotman F. Tophaceous gout of the navicular bone as a cause of medial inflammatory tumor of the foot. Foot Ankle Int 1998; 19:48–51.
109. Hammerschlag WA, Rice JR, Caldwell DS, Goldner JL. Psoriatic arthritis of the foot and ankle: analysis of joint involvement and diagnostic errors. Foot Ankle 1991; 12:35–39.
110. Zatourian J, Finelli LF, Blumethal D. Reiter's syndrome. A review and case report. J Am Podiatr Med Assoc 1987; 77:653–657.
111. Chung S. Foot care—a health care maintenance program. J Gerontol Nurs 1983; 9:213–227.

112. Lord SR, Bashford GM. Shoe characteristics and balance in older women. J Am Geriatr Soc 1996; 44:429–433.
113. Lord SR, Bashford GM, Howland A, Munro B. Effects of shoe collar height and sole hardness on balance in older women. J Am Geriatr Soc 1999; 47: 681–684.
114. Menz HB, Lord SR. Footwear and postural stability in older people. J Am Podiatr Med Assoc 1999; 89:346–357.
115. Menz HB, Lord SR. Slip resistance of casual footwear: implications for falls in older adults. Gerontology 2001; 47:145–149.
116. Sherrington C, Menz HB. An evaluation of footwear worn at the time of fall-related hip fracture. Age Ageing 2003; 32:310–314.
117. Janisse D. Prescription footwear for arthritis of the foot and ankle. Clin Orthop Relat Res 1998; 349:100–107.
118. Mueller MJ. Therapeutic footwear helps protect the diabetic foot. J Am Podiatr Med Assoc 1997; 87:360–364.
119. Pinzur MS, Dart HC. Pedorthic management of the diabetic foot. Foot Ankle Clin 2001; 6:205–214.
120. Shrader J, Siegel K. Postsurgical hindfoot deformity of a patient with rheumatoid arthritis treated with custom-made foot orthoses and shoe modifications. Phys Ther 1997; 77:296–305.
121. Shrader JA. Nonsurgical management of the foot and ankle affected by rheumatoid arthritis. J Orthop Sports Physical Ther 1999; 29:703–717.
122. Marzano R. Orthotic considerations and footwear modifications following ankle fusions. Tech Foot Ankle Surg 2002; 1:46–49.
123. van Schie C, Ulbrecht JS, Becker MB, Cavanagh PR. Design criteria for rigid rocker shoes. Foot Ankle Int 2000; 21:833–844.
124. Brown D, Wertsch JJ, Harris GF, Klein J, Janisse D. Effect of rocker soles on plantar pressures. Arch Physical Med Rehabil 2004; 85:81–86.
125. Hsi WL, Chai HM, Lai JS. Evaluation of rocker sole by pressure–time curves in insensate forefoot during gait. Am J Physical Med Rehabil 2004; 83: 500–506.
126. Root ML. Development of the functional foot orthosis. Clin Podiatr Med Surg 1994; 11:183–210.
127. Holmes GB, Timmerman L. A quantitative assessment of the effect of metatarsal pads on plantar pressures. Foot Ankle Int 1990; 11:141–145.
128. Hayda R, Tremaine MD, Tremaine K, Banco S, Teed K. Effect of metatarsal pads and their positioning: a quantitative assessment. Foot Ankle Int 1994; 15:561–566.
129. Chang AH, Abu-Faraj ZU, Harris GF, Nery J, Shereff MJ. Multistep measurement of plantar pressure alterations using metatarsal pads. Foot Ankle Int 1994; 15:654–660.
130. Abu-Faraj ZO, Harris GF, Chang AH, Shereff MJ. Evaluation of a rehabilitative pedorthic: plantar pressure alterations with scaphoid pad application. IEEE Trans Rehabil Eng 1996; 4:328–336.
131. Hodge MC, Bach TM, Carter GM. Orthotic management of plantar pressure and pain in rheumatoid arthritis. Clin Biomech 1999; 14:567–575.

132. Kato H, Takada T, Kawamura T, Hotta N, Torri S. The reduction and redistribution of plantar pressures using foot orthoses in diabetic patients. Diab Res Clin Pract 1996; 31:115–118.

133. Raspovic A, Newcombe L, Lloyd J, Dalton E. Effect of customized insoles on vertical plantar pressures in sites of previous neuropathic ulceration in the diabetic foot. Foot 2000; 10:133–138.

134. Landorf KB, Keenan A-M. Efficacy of foot orthoses—what does the literature tell us? J Am Podiatr Med Assoc 2000; 90:149–158.

135. Pfeffer G, Bacchetti P, Deland J, Lewis A, Anderson R, Davis W, Alvarez R, Brodsky J, Cooper P, Frey C, R RH, Myerson M, Sammarco J, Janecki C, Ross S, Bowman M, Smith R. Comparison of custom and prefabricated orthoses in the initial treatment of proximal plantar fasciitis. Foot Ankle Int 1999; 20:214–221.

136. Lynch DM, Goforth WP, Martin JE, Odom RD, Preece CK, Kotter MW. Conservative treatment of plantar fasciitis. A prospective study. J Am Podiatr Med Assoc 1998; 88:375–380.

137. Martin JE, Hosch JC, Goforth WP, Murff RT, Lynch DM, Odom RD. Mechanical treatment of plantar fasciitis. A prospective study. J Am Podiatr Med Assoc 2001; 91:55–62.

138. Conrad KJ, Budiman-Mak E, Roach KE, Hedeker D. Impacts of foot orthoses on pain and disability in rheumatoid arthritis. J Clin Epidemiol 1996; 49:1–7.

139. Thompson JA, Jennings MB, Hodge W. Orthotic therapy in the management of osteoarthritis. J Am Podiatr Med Assoc 1992; 82:136–139.

Index

About the Editors

JEFFREY M. HAUSDORFF is the Director of the Laboratory for the Analysis of Gait and Neurodynamics, Movement Disorders Unit, Tel Aviv Sourasky Medical Center, Israel; Senior Lecturer in the Department of Physical Therapy at the Sackler School of Medicine, Tel Aviv University, Israel; and Lecturer in Medicine at Harvard Medical School, Boston, Massachusetts. He received the M.S.M.E. degree from the Massachusetts Institute of Technology, Cambridge, and the Ph.D. degree from Boston University, Massachusetts. For more than twenty years, Dr. Hausdorff has studied gait and its changes with aging and disease. His work has focused on neurodynamics and the application of time series analysis and statistical physics to the study of gait and brain function, with a special emphasis on gait variability and falls in older adults. His investigations have been funded by the NIH and private agencies and have prompted awards from the American Physiological Society, the Biomedical Engineering Society, and the American Geriatrics Society.

NEIL B. ALEXANDER is a Professor in the Division of Geriatric Medicine and the Department of Internal Medicine, as well as Senior Research Professor at the Institute of Gerontology, University of Michigan, Ann Arbor; Director of the Mobility Research Center at the University of Michigan Geriatrics Center; and Associate Director of Research at the Ann Arbor VA Health Care System, GRECC, Michigan. He has extensive experience in assessment and enhancement of mobility in older adults, including the ability to rise from a chair, a bed, and from the floor; maintain upright stance and avoid falls; walk safely; and improve postural control, strength, physical activity, and aerobic capacity. Funded by multiple NIA and VA Merit grants, he has received two NIA research career awards (K08 and K24), chairs the NIA Clinical Review Committee, and serves on the editorial board of the *Journal of the American Geriatrics Society* and as an associate editor for the *Journal of Gerontology Medical Sciences*. He received his M.D. degree (1983) from the University of Minnesota, an M.S. degree (1989) in biostatistics and research design from the University of Michigan, Ann Arbor, and is board certified in internal medicine and geriatric medicine.

About the Book

With chapters by many of the foremost international authorities on aging, neurology, physical therapy, rehabilitation, and mobility research, this reference provides an up-to-date review of approaches to gait disorders and falls. This volume presents the fundamental concepts of gait and describes the changes in mobility with aging and disease. A focus is placed on recent assessment and intervention practices for common gait disorders, especially those seen in older adults, including sections on neuro-psychological influences, fear of falling and exercise, and strategies for specific disease groups, such as patients with neurological disorders or those recovering from stroke or hip surgery.

Describing a wide range of assessment tools, diagnostic evaluation strategies, and clinical approaches to gait, this reference introduces a new classification scheme to encompass the full range of mobility capacity in all older adults . . . reviews the physiology of gait, the factors that contribute to gait disorders, and the epidemiology of gait disorders . . . covers cognitive and behavioral influences on gait and falling . . . describes methods for analyzing gait in the clinic and the laboratory . . . details clinical and evidence-based methods for gait disorder and fall analysis, as well as techniques for gait optimization in patients with neurological disorders and foot and ankle, post-hip, and surgical injuries . . . considers a state-of-the-art strategy for multidimensional fall risk assessment . . . and includes a set of recommended fall reduction strategies.